POSTPARTUM DEPRESSION
AND CHILD DEVELOPMENT

Postpartum Depression and Child Development

Edited by

LYNNE MURRAY
PETER J. COOPER

Foreword by Eugene Paykel
Afterword by Sir Michael Rutter

THE GUILFORD PRESS
New York   London

©1997 The Guilford Press
A Division of Guilford Publications, Inc.
72 Spring Street, New York, NY 10012

Printed in the United States of America

This book is printed on acid-free paper.

Last digit is print number: 9 8 7 6 5 4 3 2 1

Library of Congress Cataloging-in-Publication Data

Postpartum depression and child development
  / edited by Lynne Murray, Peter J. Cooper
    p.   cm.
    Includes bibliographical references and index.
    ISBN 1-57230-197-X
    1. Postpartum depression. 2. Infant psychology. 3. Mother
and infant   4. Children of depressed parents. I. Murray, Lynne.
II. Cooper, Peter J.
RG852.P684   1997   96-39987
618.7'6—dc21   CIP

Contributors

Susan B. Campbell, PhD, Department of Psychology, University of Pittsburgh, Pittsburgh, Pennsylvania, United States

Jeffrey F. Cohn, PhD, Department of Psychology, University of Pittsburgh, Pittsburgh, Pennsylvania, United States

Peter J. Cooper, PhD, Winnicott Research Unit, Department of Psychology, University of Reading, Reading, United Kingdom

Bertrand Cramer, MD, Department of Psychiatry, University of Geneva, Geneva, Switzerland

Tiffany Field, PhD, Touch Research Institute, School of Medicine, University of Miami, Miami, Florida, United States

Donna M. Gelfand, PhD, Department of Psychology, University of Utah, Salt Lake City, Utah, United States

Dale F. Hay, PhD, Faculty of Social and Political Science, University of Cambridge, Cambridge, United Kingdom

Alison E. Hipwell, PhD, Winnicott Research Unit, Department of Psychiatry, University of Cambridge, Cambridge, United Kingdom

R. Channi Kumar, PhD, MD, Institute of Psychiatry, University of London, London, United Kingdom

Lynne Murray, PhD, Winnicott Research Unit, Department of Psychology, University of Reading, Reading, United Kingdom

Michael W. O'Hara, PhD, Department of Psychology, University of Iowa, Iowa City, Iowa, United States

Hanuš Papoušek, ScD, MD, Developmental Psychobiology Unit, University of Munich, Munich, Germany

Mechthild Papoušek, PhD, Developmental Psychobiology Unit, University of Munich, Munich, Germany

E. S. Paykel, MD, Department of Psychiatry, University of Cambridge, Cambridge, United Kingdom

Michael Rutter, MD, Institute of Psychiatry, University of London, London, United Kingdom

Douglas M. Teti, PhD, Department of Psychology, University of Maryland, Baltimore, Maryland, United States

E. Z. Tronick, PhD, Child Development Unit, Harvard Medical School, Cambridge, Massachusetts, United States

M. Katherine Weinberg, PhD, Child Development Unit, Harvard Medical School, Cambridge, Massachusetts, United States

Foreword

The period following the birth of a child is the hardest time to be depressed. The expected joys of motherhood (and of fatherhood) and the hopes which have accompanied pregnancy may be replaced by feelings of desperation, of failure, inability to function, and perhaps inability to provide love to one's partner or to the baby.

For many years, research on postpartum depression has focused on its frequency, its causes, and whether it is different in nature from other forms of depression. Thus, the impact of postpartum depression has been viewed as falling primarily on the mother. Only comparatively recently has there been the realization that another important feature of postpartum depression is that there is a new child. What is the potential impact of a parent's postpartum depression on the infant? There is evidence of major effects, and the study of them has become the most active and important research in the field of postpartum disorders.

The editors of this volume, Lynne Murray and Peter J. Cooper, have worked at the forefront of this field since its inception. They jointly founded the influential Winnicott Research Unit in the Department of Psychiatry at Cambridge, and recently established its successor at Reading. They have assembled an authoritative group of contributors, who are doing the best and most influential work in this rapidly advancing field. In their preface, Murray and Cooper point out that the question is no longer whether depression has an effect on the child, but of understanding the effects in detail. In the penultimate section of the book they and their colleagues take the field further forward into an exploration of different treatment modalities.

Postpartum problems concern adults, children, and families. This is a book for psychologists, psychiatrists, and others working both in child and adult fields. It has a great deal to offer researchers in child development, and for astute clinicians in many other fields who want to stay in touch with the latest developments in this area of transgenerational impact.

E. S. PAYKEL, M.D.
UNIVERSITY OF CAMBRIDGE
CAMBRIDGE, UNITED KINGDOM

Preface

There was an explosion of infancy research in the 1970s. One of the most striking findings to emerge concerned the degree of infant sensitivity to the quality of interpersonal communication. This finding raised the clinical issue of the impact on the infant of prolonged disturbances in caregiving. This issue has been addressed in a number of contexts. Clinicians and researchers have paid particular attention to the impact of postpartum depression on parenting and child developmental progress. Postpartum depression is relatively common and easily identified, and although it is associated with significant disturbances in functioning, these disturbances are generally not so severe as to necessitate removal of the infant and the consequent difficulties of disentangling the effects of the maternal disorder from those of separation experiences.

In the 1980s, a number of seminal studies concerned with postpartum depression and infant caregiving were undertaken. The work of Tiffany Field, E. Z. Tronick, and Jeffrey F. Cohn, for example, established profiles of impairments in maternal communication occurring in the context of depressed mood and identified associated infant disturbance. The recent work reflected in this volume has readdressed these phenomena, applying more rigorous and sophisticated research methods. Depression is now defined according to well-established criteria; the samples studied include low-risk as well as high-risk groups; sample sizes are larger than was the case in the early studies, allowing us to look at how depression interacts with other important variables, such as social adversity; and longitudinal designs allow investigation of the consequences of early environmental disturbance. The conceptual developments in recent years have principally concerned the elucidation of the mechanisms mediating infant outcome. The question is no longer whether depression has an effect on the child, but one of understanding how the proximal mother–infant interactions affect infant functioning, of what the importance of the course of the maternal mood disorder might be, of the extent to which the effects of such disorder are mediated by particular cognitions, and, finally, of what the role of infant variables is in determining the course of maternal mood and of child developmental progress.

The introductory chapter in this volume, by Michael W. O'Hara, provides a comprehensive review of research on the epidemiology of postpartum depression, its etiology, and its course. Research in this field has seen radical shifts from the time of Pitt's seminal paper in 1968, in which he argued for a distinct category of "postnatal depressions," to a skeptical position advanced in the 1980s, to the current view that, for a subgroup of women, childbirth does appear to be of specific etiological significance.

The introduction is followed by two chapters that provide the intellectual and empirical background for thinking about how maternal depression might influence the mother–infant dyad and the potential consequences for the infant. First, Hanuš Papoušek and Mechthild Papoušek (Chapter 2), pioneers in this field of work, review the research, including their own spanning 30 years, on the fine-grained regulation of early parent–infant contacts. They elaborate the basis for a system of "intuitive parenting" and specify various conditions, some in the infant and some parental, including maternal depression, that may challenge the balance of the system and lead to vicious cycles of impaired patterns of relating. E. Z. Tronick and M. Katherine Weinberg (Chapter 3) then provide a review of how early parent–infant interactions have been conceived by developmental psychologists. Like the Papoušeks, they point to a system that is mutually regulated and finely tuned and emphasize that minor misattunements are common and quite normal; they note that these misattunements offer opportunities for repair that may be particularly important in the development of the infant's sense of self-efficacy. They present a new theoretical formulation, informed by systems theory, of why *mutual* experience may be of particular importance in infant psychological development. They also offer an explanation, embedded in their model of mutual regulation, of the different development trajectories of male and female offspring of depressed mothers.

The next four chapters concern research into the development of children of women with postpartum depression. Dale F. Hay (Chapter 4) sets out the findings of three British longitudinal community studies concerned with the cognitive development of the children of mothers with postpartum depression; she considers possible mechanisms that may mediate the association between the maternal depression and compromised cognitive outcome. In particular, she emphasizes the way in which infant attention and emotion may be regulated during early interactions with the mother, and makes the case for a sensitive period in infant cognitive development. Lynne Murray and Peter J. Cooper (Chapter 5) draw on their prospective longitudinal studies tracking development from early infancy to 5 years in the context of postpartum depression. Using neonatal assessments and measures of infant interactive behavior independent of the mother, the role of infant and maternal factors is examined. Their findings suggest that although infant factors are important in the onset of maternal depression, these factors contribute little to face-to-face interactions and child outcome.

The third chapter in this section, by Douglas M. Teti and Donna M. Gelfand (Chapter 6), provides a comprehensive review of the literature on the cognitions associated with depression. From their research with a clinically referred sample, they show that the mother's feelings of self-efficacy are central in mediating the impact of depression, marital quality, and support on maternal caretaking competence. They highlight maternal perceptions of the infant as an important component of the process and consider both the research and treatment implications that follow from this formulation. In the final chapter in this section, Susan B. Campbell and Jeffrey F. Cohn (Chapter 7) emphasize the importance of taking into account the course of maternal mood disorder in understanding mother–infant interactions and infant outcome. Thus, in their low-risk community sample, only those mothers whose depression persisted for at least 6 months showed impairments in parenting. This finding, arising from a sample selected to eliminate the impact of social and economic adversity, contrasts with those from other studies and underlines the importance of studying demographically arid clinically diverse samples in which the impact of the maternal disorder may be variously mediated.

The next section of this volume comprises three chapters concerned with the treatment of postpartum depression. In the first of these, Peter J. Cooper and Lynne Murray (Chapter 8) describe a randomized controlled trial in which three different types of brief psychotherapy were compared in the treatment of a community sample of women with postpartum depression. Although it is clear that the forms of treatment studied were highly effective in alleviating the maternal depressive symptoms, mother–infant interactions and certain infant outcomes were found to be more resistant to the interventions. The next chapter, by Tiffany Field (Chapter 9), reviews a considerable body of treatment research and points to the importance of taking infant factors into account and matching particular forms of mother–infant intervention to particular profiles of interactional disturbance.

The final chapter in this section, by Bertrand Cramer (Chapter 10), provides a psychodynamic formulation of postpartum depression (in language comprehensible to the general audience) and outlines a psychodynamic approach to disturbances in the mother–infant relationship, including those that occur in the context of maternal depression. It is evident that this form of treatment is associated with significant shifts in maternal functioning.

The final chapter, by Alison E. Hipwell and R. Channi Kumar (Chapter 11), provides a review of the limited research concerning the impact on parenting and child development of psychotic disorders arising after childbirth. Because the occurrence of psychotic disorder is significantly associated with childbirth and difficult decisions concerning child management have to be made, this is an important area of investigation and the authors' review of this complex subject highlights the way forward for future research.

Contents

IV. THE TREATMENT OF POSTPARTUM DEPRESSION AND ASSOCIATED MOTHER–INFANT DISTURBANCES

V. POSTPARTUM PSYCHOSIS

I

*

INTRODUCTION TO POSTPARTUM DEPRESSIVE DISORDER

1

~

The Nature of Postpartum
Depressive Disorders

Michael W. O'Hara
University of Iowa

Postpartum depression is an important social and health problem for women and their families (Boyce & Stubbs, 1994; Cox, 1986; O'Hara, 1994, 1995). Depression tears at the fabric of a woman's self-esteem, her marital relationship, and her relationship with her children (Weissman & Paykel, 1974). It can be particularly devastating at a time when a woman and her family expect joy and happiness to be the rule of the day, not sadness and depression. Postpartum depression has many consequences. First among them is the personal suffering of women. In addition, there is growing evidence that the mother–child relationship and the child's social and cognitive development may suffer as a consequence of maternal depression. These issues are explored throughout this volume. The purpose of this chapter is to provide a context for the chapters that follow. To accomplish this task, I characterize the nature of postpartum depression and its consequences, illuminate some of the factors that put women at risk, and briefly discuss its treatment.

Women, and especially women of childbearing age, are at high risk for depression (Kessler et al., 1994; Myers et al., 1984). For example, the 6-month period prevalence of depression among women ages 25–44 is approximately 10% (Myers et al., 1984). Many more women who do not meet criteria for syndromal depression (e.g., criteria according to the fourth edition of the *Diagnostic and Statistical Manual of Mental Disorders* [DSM-IV; American Psychiatric Association, 1994]) experience significant social morbidity associated with high levels of depressive symptoms (Johnson, Weissman, & Klerman, 1992; Wells et al., 1989). Unfortunately, the vast majority of these women receive no care from specialists and, at least in the United States, fewer than half receive any kind of care at all for their depression (Regier et al., 1993).

POSTPARTUM BLUES AND PSYCHOSIS

Because depression is so common among women of childbearing age, it is not surprising that many women are depressed during the puerperium. These depressions range considerably in their severity, duration, and timing (O'Hara, 1994; Watson, Elliott, Rugg, & Brough, 1984). The custom within the literature on postpartum psychiatric disorders has been to distinguish three phenomena: postpartum blues, postpartum psychosis, and postpartum depression. Postpartum blues refers to a relatively mild, transient, and common emotional disturbance that occurs most often in the first week postpartum and is characterized by such symptoms as crying, confusion, mood lability, anxiety, and depressed mood (Kennerley & Gath, 1989; O'Hara, Schlechte, Lewis, & Wright, 1991). These symptoms last from a few hours to a few days and have few negative sequelae (O'Hara, 1994). Postpartum psychosis appears at the other end of the severity continuum; it refers to a severe and relatively rare psychiatric disorder, often affective in nature. Characteristic symptoms of postpartum psychosis include delusions, hallucinations, and gross impairment in functioning (Brockington et al., 1981). Usually, inpatient treatment is necessary for women experiencing a postpartum psychosis.

Although postpartum blues and postpartum psychosis have been the subject of a great many investigations (Hamilton & Harberger, 1992; Kumar & Brockington, 1988; O'Hara, Schlechte, Lewis, & Varner, 1991; O'Hara, 1994), they are not formal diagnostic categories in DSM-IV (American Psychiatric Association, 1994) or the tenth revision of the *International Classification of Diseases* (ICD-10; World Health Organization, 1992). Rather, each term conveys a sense of timing of onset and relative severity. Neither the severity nor the duration of the blues passes the threshold for a psychiatric disorder. Although postpartum psychosis is, by definition, severe and may persist for a considerable period, it is usually diagnosed as, for example, manic episode, depressive episode, or brief psychotic episode. In DSM-IV, each of these disorders may be formally characterized as having a postpartum onset if the episode begins within 4 weeks of childbirth.

DIAGNOSIS

Postpartum depression refers to a nonpsychotic depressive episode that begins in or extends into the postpartum period (Cox, Murray, & Chapman, 1993; O'Hara, 1994; Watson et al., 1984). In past research, these depressions have been defined in a variety of ways (O'Hara & Zekoski, 1988). More recent and rigorous studies have defined postpartum depression based on standardized diagnostic criteria for depression (Cooper & Murray, 1995; Cox et al., 1993; O'Hara, Zekoski, Philipps, & Wright, 1990; Troutman & Cutrona, 1990). A diagnosis of postpartum depression usually requires that a woman be experiencing dysphoric mood along with several other symptoms such as sleep, appetite, or psychomotor disturbance; fatigue; excessive guilt; and suicidal thoughts (American Psychiatric Association, 1994; Spitzer, Endicott, & Robins, 1978). Typically, symptoms must be present for a minimum amount of time (at the very least, 1 week) and must result in some impairment in the woman's functioning (e.g., Cooper & Murray, 1995; O'Hara et al., 1990). A typical case is described in Case History 1.1.

RISK

A number of studies conducted in Great Britain and North America in the 1980s converged to suggest that the prevalence of postpartum depression, defined on the basis of clear diagnostic criteria, was between 8% and 15%. For example, three studies conducted in Great Britain obtained prevalence rates of postpartum depression ranging between 12% and 15% (Cox, Connor, & Kendell, 1982; Kumar & Robson, 1984; Watson et al., 1984). Similar studies carried out in North America yielded somewhat lower prevalence rates (8–12%) (Cutrona, 1983; O'Hara, Neunaber, & Zekoski, 1984). Although there was some question whether these rates

CASE HISTORY 1.1. Mrs. Jones

Mrs. Jones was 26 years old, married, and experiencing her first pregnancy. She had a college degree and was working full time as a pharmacist. Her husband was 36 years old and in school. Mrs. Jones was the oldest of three siblings; her parents were both still living but had separated about 4 years before her pregnancy. She and her husband were actively preparing for childbirth. The pregnancy was planned and Mrs. Jones and her husband were happy about it. She did report some negative feelings, however, about her upcoming experience with childbirth.

The initial interview with Mrs. Jones took place in January and since the previous October, Mrs. Jones reported feeling irritable. She had few other symptoms; however, she did find that some aspects of her work and relationships with her family were mildly impaired. She reported a previous episode of depression about 5 years earlier when she was a college student. It lasted about 5 months and she was seen at the university counseling center for treatment. She reported that she had had many previous similar episodes (six). However, there was no evidence of any other psychiatric difficulty in her history.

Mrs. Jones said that her mother had experienced recurrent unipolar depressions at least once a year over many years beginning at age 33. Her father had a long history of alcoholism, beginning at age 16. Mrs. Jones reported that her father's drinking caused family problems and that he drank every night. There was no evidence of a psychiatric history in her two brothers or her husband.

Mrs. Jones had a full-term male child, who weighed approximately 8 pounds (3,610 grams), through a normal vaginal delivery. She was also on an antibiotic during the latter part of her pregnancy. Her son was hospitalized for 10 days following birth because of an elevated white blood count. She breast-fed the baby and stayed in the hospital with him until day 8 postpartum. Mrs. Jones also noted that the baby experienced colic during at least the first 3 months postpartum.

About day 3 postpartum Mrs. Jones's mood began to sink. She said that her low mood felt almost like physical pain. She also reported feeling anxious and irritable at this time. During the period of her depression, which lasted at least 2 months, she completely lost her appetite. She woke up during the night and could not get back to sleep. She commented that it was almost like not falling asleep. She had no energy and had lost interest in most things. Mrs. Jones reported feeling guilty; in particular, she believed that she was not a good mother and she blamed herself for her son's colic. She also had extreme difficulty concentrating. Finally, she found that her work and family relationships were impaired by her depression. Despite both her mother and husband urging her to seek help for her depression, she did not. At 6 months postpartum she was still reporting a moderate level of depressive symptomatology.

Note: From O'Hara (1994, p. 9). Copyright 1994 by Springer-Verlag. Reprinted by permission.

were higher than what would have been observed in the community (Watson et al., 1984), there did appear to be an increase in rates of depression after delivery relative to pregnancy (Kumar & Robson, 1984; O'Hara et al., 1984). However, none of these early studies could really address the question of the nature of the specific relation between childbearing and depression (O'Hara, 1994).

In contrast to the case for nonpsychotic depression, there is little doubt that for women there is a specific association between childbirth and both psychosis and the blues. Women are between 20 and 30 times more likely to be hospitalized for a psychotic episode in the first 30 days after delivery than at other times before or after childbirth (Kendell, Chalmers, & Platz, 1987). This rise in psychosis admissions is dramatically illustrated in Figure 1.1. The increased risk for "blues-like" symptoms is about fourfold for recently delivered women relative to nonchildbearing controls (O'Hara et al., 1990). Figure 1.2 portrays the distinct pattern of dysphoric mood which characterizes childbearing versus nonchildbearing women over time. To answer the question about the specific association between nonpsychotic depression and childbearing, several controlled studies were undertaken beginning in the mid-1980s.

The first study of postpartum depression to include a comparison group was conducted in Oxford, England (Cooper, Campbell, Day, Kennerley, & Bond, 1988). The estimated point prevalence rate of depression at 3 months postpartum was 8.7%, not significantly different from the 9.9% point prevalence rate obtained from an epidemiologically derived

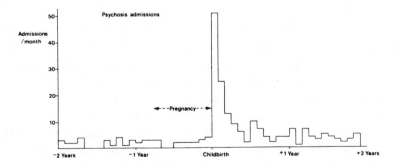

FIGURE 1.1. Risk for hospitalization for psychosis associated with childbirth. Adapted from Kendell, Chalmers, and Platz (1987). Copyright 1987 by the Royal College of Psychiatrists. Adapted by permission.

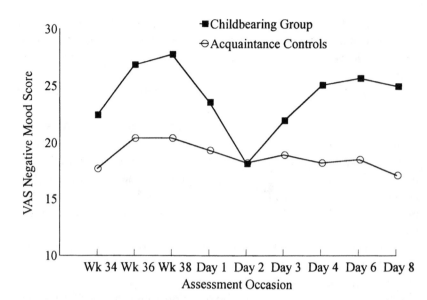

FIGURE 1.2. Visual Analogue Scales (VAS) negative mood scale scores for childbearing and nonchildbearing subjects during pregnancy and after delivery. (Wk 34 = 34th week of pregnancy; Wk 36 = 36th week of pregnancy; Wk 38 = 38th week of pregnancy; Day 1 = day 1 postpartum; Day 2 = day 2 postpartum; Day 3 = day 3 postpartum; Day 4 = day 4 postpartum; Day 6 = day 6 postpartum; Day 8 = day 8 postpartum. Range of VAS negative mood scale is 0–100; higher scores reflect more negative mood.) From O'Hara, Zekoski, Philipps, and Wright (1990). Copyright 1990 by the American Psychological Association. Reprinted by permission.

community sample of childbearing-age women from Edinburgh. Using an acquaintance control group in Iowa in the United States, O'Hara et al. (1990) obtained a 3-month period prevalence of major and minor depression of 10.4% for childbearing women and 7.7% for nonchildbearing controls. These differences were not statistically significant. In a study similar to that of O'Hara et al. (1990), Troutman and Cutrona (1990) compared rates of postpartum depression in a sample of childbearing adolescents (26% major and minor depression at 6 weeks) and an acquaintance control group of nonchildbearing adolescents (15%). Although these differences were striking, they were not statistically significant. Moreover, most of the difference between the two groups was in the form of minor depression. The prevalence rates of major depression (6%

vs. 5%) were similar for the two groups. The most recent controlled study, conducted in the midlands of England, compared the point and 6 month period prevalence of depression in a large sample of childbearing women at 6-months postpartum and an equal-size sample of nonchildbearing women (Cox et al., 1993). The 6-month period prevalences for both groups were similar (13.8% vs. 13.4%).

The results of four major controlled studies of the prevalence of postpartum depression converge to suggest that there is no elevation in the risk for nonpsychotic depression associated with childbearing. Although there are a number of other potential explanations for these findings (e.g., inadequate statistical power to detect true differences), it is unlikely that bigger and better studies would demonstrate the level of increased risk for nonpsychotic depression that has been observed for the blues and psychosis. Nevertheless, these depressions may have characteristics that differ from depressions that emerge at other times with respect to timing of onset, severity, duration, and consequences.

TIMING OF ONSET

If women are not at increased risk for depression during the puerperium, do these depressions tend to occur in close proximity to childbirth rather than being evenly distributed throughout the postpartum period? Several studies have yielded data relevant to the question of timing of onset of postpartum depression. For example, Kumar and Robson (1984) found that more than three times as many new cases were observed at 3 months postpartum as at 6 months and 1 year postpartum. In a similar fashion, Watson et al. (1984) observed that two-thirds of new depressive episodes in the first year postpartum occurred in the first 3 months. For Cooper et al. (1988), 40% of new episodes began in the first 3 months postpartum. In the Cox et al. (1993) study, 50% of episodes for childbearing women began in the first 5 weeks after delivery versus 16% for the control subjects, a significant difference. However, Nott (1987) did not observe any association between childbirth and timing of onset of depression. Moreover, O'Hara et al. (1990) found that although 69% of postpartum depressions began within 3 weeks of delivery, an equal percentage of control subjects had depressions that occurred within the same time frame. These findings suggest that postpartum depression may begin earlier rather than later in the postpartum period. A potential alternative explanation is that depression after childbirth may be particularly salient to a woman (O'Hara, 1994). Some women may be expecting that a depression should occur after delivery or are ready, when asked, to report on symptoms occurring after childbirth. It is also possible that using childbirth as an anchor in an interview to determine the onset of symptoms may cause some women, for example, to identify their symptoms as beginning early in the postpartum period rather than late in pregnancy. Only a phenomenon of this sort would explain the fact that a large number of nonchildbearing controls in O'Hara et al. (1990) reported that their depressions began within the first few weeks of the birth of the baby of the childbearing subject with whom they were yoked in the study. In sum, although several studies have supported the intriguing possibility that depressions that might have otherwise occurred evenly over a several-month period are brought forward in time because of childbirth, the normal insidiousness of depression onset makes exact onsets difficult to determine and increases the probability of judgment biases by both subjects and investigators regarding depression onset.

SYMPTOM PATTERN

Depressions that occur after childbirth may show a symptom pattern different from depressions that occur at other times (O'Hara, 1994). For example, Pitt (1968) argued in his seminal study that depressions occurring after childbirth are "atypical." Atypical depression was meant to characterize those depressions that had prominent neurotic symptoms, such as anxiety, irritability, or phobias, which tended to overshadow the depression. Pitt suggested that many of the women experiencing a postpartum depression in his sample had these atypical characteristics. Similar arguments have been made for the distinctiveness of postpartum psychosis (Dean & Kendell, 1981; Brockington et al., 1981). However, Cooper et al. (1988) found no support for this view in comparing the symptom pictures of depressed childbearing and nonchildbearing women. Moreover, O'Hara et al. (1990) observed little evidence of differences in symptom pictures, with the exception that at 3 weeks postpartum the depressed childbearing subjects had significantly higher levels of depressive symptomatology than did the depressed nonchildbearing subjects. Also, Whiffen and Gotlib (1993) found only a few differences between samples of depressed childbearing and childbearing women. For example, women experiencing postpartum depression tended to have less severe episodes (in contrast to the finding of O'Hara et al., 1990) and better marital relationships than did depressed nonchildbearing subjects. Unfortunately, the other two controlled studies (Cox et al., 1993; Troutman & Cutrona, 1990) did not report on possible symptom differences that may have characterized their depressed childbearing and nonchildbearing subjects. Although there has been little indication of distinct symptoms that characterize depressed childbearing women (Purdy & Frank, 1993), too little research has addressed this question for us to be confident that postpartum depression does not present in some distinctive fashion.

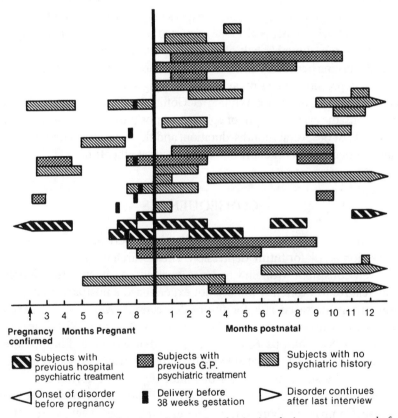

FIGURE 1.3. Onset and duration of depressions beginning during pregnancy and after delivery. Adapted from Watson, Elliott, Rugg, and Brough (1984). Copyright 1984 by the Royal College of Psychiatrists. Adapted by permission.

DURATION OF EPISODE

One index of severity of depression is the length of the episode. In general, postpartum depressions appear to persist over several months (O'Hara, 1994). Figure 1.3 provides a graphical description of the onset and duration of depressions during pregnancy and the puerperium (Watson et al., 1984). Watson et al. reported that one-quarter of their depressed subjects had episodes lasting 3 months or more and another quarter had episodes lasting 6 months or more. Also, Kumar and Robson (1984) found that 50% of their depressed subjects had episodes lasting six months or more. Several other British studies obtained essentially the same results (Cox, Rooney, Thomas, & Wrate, 1984; Pitt, 1968; Wolkind, Coleman, & Ghodsian, 1980). Campbell, Cohn, Flanagan, Popper, and Myers (1992) reported an average duration of 15 weeks with many other women experiencing ongoing symptoms at a subclinical level. Cooper et al. (1988) reported shorter durations of postpartum depression. Roughly half of their postpartum depressed subjects had episodes lasting between 4 and 8 weeks. Two controlled studies found durations of depression to be similar in childbearing and nonchildbearing subjects (O'Hara et al., 1990; Whiffen & Gotlib, 1993). In sum, with a few exceptions, the average length of episodes of postpartum depression seems to be at least of several months' duration, and these durations do not differ much from durations of depressions that occur at other times.

CONSEQUENCES

The major consequence to a woman of having experienced a postpartum depression is risk for future depression. The research in this area has been relatively consistent. Women who have experienced a postpartum depression, relative to women who have not experienced a postpartum depression, are at increased risk for future depressions over a 5-year period (Cooper & Murray, 1995; Ghodsian, Zajicek, & Wolkind, 1984; Kumar & Robson, 1984; Philipps & O'Hara, 1991). For example, Philipps and O'Hara (1991) reported that 80% (8/10) of postpartum depressed women experienced a subsequent major or minor depression during a 4½ year follow-up compared to 42% (25/60) of postpartum nondepressed women. Comparable figures from Cooper and Murray (1995) were a 60% (33/55) recurrence rate for postpartum depressed and 35% (14/40) rate for postpartum nondepressed women. The Cooper and Murray (1995) study is of particular significance because their primiparous postpartum depressed women were distinguished on the basis of whether the postpartum episode was a "first" episode or reflected recurrent depression. Women whose postpartum episode was their first had postpartum depressions of shorter duration, were significantly less likely to experience a subsequent nonpostpartum depression, and were more likely to experience a subsequent postpartum depression than were postpartum depressed women who had experienced previous depressions. The findings of Cooper and Murray (1995) suggest the possibility that some depressions may be specifically caused by some biological or psychosocial element of childbearing and that these depressions may be somewhat less severe but more likely to reoccur during times of childbearing than postpartum depressions that reflect an ongoing vulnerability to depression. This finding is important because it may provide some clues about a distinctive depression that develops in response to childbirth for some women; however, full confidence in the robustness of this finding awaits replication. Whether or not there is a distinctive postpartum depression, women who are depressed during the puerperium are at high risk for future depressions. These episodes of depression have serious implications for the woman's ability to function effectively in all her social roles (e.g., mother, spouse, and worker). In addition, there are many consequences to the child of having a depressed mother. These consequences are discussed throughout the rest of this volume.

CAUSAL FACTORS

Although postpartum depression is increasingly being defined in terms of diagnostic criteria (O'Hara, 1994), studies that have investigated correlates or causal factors in postpartum depression have often used samples defined by indices that measure severity of depression (O'Hara, 1991). Examples of these measures include the Beck Depression Inventory (Beck, Ward, Mendelson, Mock, & Erbaugh, 1961) and the Edinburgh Postnatal Depression Scale (Cox, Holden, & Sagovsky, 1987). These measures, which are used as an index of mood at the time of completion, may be administered at any time during the puerperium and may be taken to reflect severity of postpartum depression. However, the relation between a score on a mood measure and a diagnosis of postpartum depression is usually unclear, making it difficult to generalize from studies defining depression on the basis of a severity measure to the phenomenon of postpartum depression (defined diagnostically). For these reasons, this review of causal factors primarily includes studies that have defined postpartum depression using diagnostic criteria.

Background Factors

Although having few financial resources and caring for a first child are examples of factors that might be expected to increase the stressfulness of the puerperium and thus a woman's risk for blues or depression (Brown & Harris, 1978), there is little evidence that these factors are in fact associated with increased risk for postpartum blues or depression. In two studies, a lower educational level has been found to be significantly associated with postpartum depression (Campbell & Cohn, 1991; Gotlib, Whiffen, Wallace, & Mount, 1991). However, several other sound studies that included measures of background factors found no evidence that any sociodemographic factor was related to risk for postpartum depression (Cox et al., 1982; O'Hara, 1986; O'Hara, Schlechte, Lewis, & Varner, 1991; Watson et al., 1984). What remains to be done with respect to the possible role of demographic factors, particularly given the evidence linking low socioeconomic to depression in young women, is a quantitative analysis (i.e., a meta-analysis) that would provide estimates of the effect sizes of the correlations between the various sociodemographic variables and postpartum depression and the blues (O'Hara & Swain, 1996).

Biological Factors

Many hypotheses accounting for the biological basis of postpartum blues and depression have been tested in a large number of studies, particularly over the past 15 years. Interest in a biological etiology is in part due to the dramatic hormonal changes that occur in women in the first few days after delivery. Levels of progesterone, estradiol, and free estriol drop dramatically, as much as 90–95% (Speroff, Glass, & Kase, 1989). Although these changes occur primarily during a period that many women report symptoms of the postpartum blues rather than at the onset of postpartum depression, hormonal factors have been thought to play an important etiological role in postpartum depression (O'Hara, 1991, 1994). For example, it has been hypothesized that levels of hormones such as the estrogens, progesterone, prolactin, and cortisol are too high—or too low—in the puerperium or that changes in the levels of these hormones occur too quickly—or not quickly enough (Stein, 1982). The hormonal dysfunction hypothesis is similar to that proposed for mood disturbances in the premenstrual period and during menopause (Yalom, Lunde, Moos, & Hamburg, 1968; Carroll & Steiner, 1978; Dalton, 1980). In addition, numerous biological hypotheses derived from the more general depression literature have been tested in childbearing women. Studies testing biological hypotheses are reviewed selectively here, emphasizing progesterone, estrogens, cortisol, prolactin, and thyroid function. (For reviews of this literature, see George & Sandler, 1988, and Hamilton & Harberger, 1992.)

Progesterone

Progesterone withdrawal has been hypothesized as a causal factor in postpartum mood disorders (Dalton, 1980). The evidence for this hypothesis has been decidedly mixed (O'Hara, 1991); only two studies have compared postpartum depressed and nondepressed women with respect to progesterone levels. In a sophisticated study, based on assessments conducted at about 8 weeks postpartum, Harris et al. (1989) reported lower levels of progesterone among depressed breast-feeding women than nondepressed breast-feeding women. Among the bottle-feeding women just the opposite association was observed. However, in another large study ($N > 147$ for all analyses), O'Hara, Schlechte, Lewis, and Varner (1991) observed no differences in progesterone levels between postpartum depressed and nondepressed women. On the whole, findings of other studies of the depressive symptoms or the blues have been similarly inconclusive (Ballinger, Kay, Naylor, & Smith, 1982; Kuevi et al., 1983; Metz et al., 1983; Nott, Franklin, Armitage, & Gelder, 1976).

Estrogens

As noted earlier, estrogen levels, much like progesterone levels, decrease markedly after childbirth. Three studies have investigated the relation between estrogen levels (usually estradiol) and postpartum depression. Two of these studies produced negative findings (Gard, Handley, Parsons, & Waldron, 1986; Harris et al., 1989). However, O'Hara, Schlechte, Lewis and Varner (1991) did observe significantly lower levels of estradiol in postpartum depressed women compared to nondepressed women at week 36 gestation and day 2 postpartum. Despite the relative lack of positive findings for the role of estradiol in postpartum depression, there has been a recent interest in estrogen-based prophylaxis of postpartum depression (Gregoire, Kumar, Fueritt, Henderson, & Studd, 1996).

Cortisol

Abnormalities in the hypothalamic–pituitary–adrenal system have been studied intensively as etiological factors in major depression (Schlesser, 1986). Both free and bound cortisol are elevated during late pregnancy, peak at high levels during labor, drop precipitously after delivery to about late pregnancy levels, and gradually decline over time (Jolivet, Blanchier, & Gautray, 1974). Both overproduction and sudden withdrawal of corticosteroids have been posited as potential causes of postpartum mood disorders (George & Sandler, 1988; Railton, 1961). Studies testing these hypotheses have yielded few positive results with respect to either free or bound cortisol (Harris et al., 1989; O'Hara, Schlechte, Lewis, & Varner, 1991). In a study addressing cortisol and the blues, Handley, Dunn, Waldron, and Baker (1980) did find significantly higher levels of cortisol at 38 weeks gestation in women who later experienced the postpartum blues than in women who did not. However, they did not replicate this finding in a later study (Gard et al., 1986). Finally, disturbances in cortisol dynamics, reflected in dexamethasone nonsuppression, do not appear to distinguish postpartum depressed and nondepressed women in the early puerperium (Greenwood & Parker, 1984; O'Hara, Schlechte, Lewis, & Varner, 1991; Singh et al., 1986).

Prolactin

Levels of prolactin, which are very high by the end of pregnancy, fall more slowly after delivery than do the gonadal hormones. In nonchildbearing women, high levels of prolactin (hyperprolactinemia) are associated with depression, anxiety, and hostility (Campbell & Winokur, 1985). As with the steroid hormones, the findings for prolactin have been mixed. Harris et al. (1989) reported that lower levels of prolactin were associated with higher levels of depression at 8 weeks postpartum. However, O'Hara, Schlechte, Lewis, and Varner (1991) found no association between prolactin levels during pregnancy and after delivery and postpartum depression. Finally, studies of the association between symptom levels and depressive mood have reported mixed results (e.g., George, Copeland, & Wilson, 1980; Nott et al., 1976). It should be noted that prolactin is a difficult hormone to measure well in the puerperium. Breast feeding stimulates prolactin secretion and prolactin levels are significantly higher in breast-feeding than in non-breast-feeding women (Vemer & Rolland, 1981). The literature has also suggested that even slight movement stimulates prolactin secretion (George & Sandler, 1988); however, O'Hara, Schlechte, Lewis, and Varner (1991) found little evidence of this phenomenon.

Thyroid Function

Hamilton (1962) argued that hypothyroidism may be a cause of postpartum depression, particularly when it begins more than 2 weeks after delivery. Harris et al. (1989) reported an association between depression meeting DSM-III (American Psychiatric Association, 1980) criteria and thyroid dysfunction (either hyper- or hypothyroidism) measured at 6 weeks postpartum. Similarly, Pop et al. (1991) found a significant association between depression meeting the research diagnostic criteria and thyroid dysfunction (either hyper- or hypothyroidism) at one of several assessments during the first 34 weeks postpartum. In a second study, Harris et al. (1992) found that the thyroid antibody-positive group of women, compared to the antibody-negative group of women, showed an increased rate of postpartum depression independent of thyroid dysfunction. Several possibilities have been offered for this finding, such as that symptoms of malaise due to the autoimmune disorder (e.g., poor appetite, low energy, and increased irritability) are recorded as symptoms of depression rather than as symptoms of a medical condition (Harris, 1993).

There has been little consistency in the findings of studies of hormonal variables. One major problem with this research has been the inconsistency with which postpartum mood has been measured and the timing of those measurements. This problem is common to all of the research on postpartum depression. A second major problem is that the simple hormonal models are unable to account for much variability in postpartum mood. There may be many reasons for this state of affairs. For example, the wrong hormones may have been studied or the complex interrelationships among hormones, neurotransmitters, and other biological factors may not have been adequately captured. Finally, hormonal factors may only be important for women who are otherwise vulnerable to affective disorder. This vulnerability could be in itself biological/genetic (e.g., reflected in personal or family history of affective disorders) in nature, or it could be psychological (e.g., poor cognitive/social coping with stress) or social/environmental (e.g., poor marital relationship, adverse social circumstances). All three of these possibilities may be true. In the next several sections, I review the potential roles of these other factors.

Gynecological and Obstetric Factors

Several investigators have hypothesized links between menstrual problems and postpartum mood disturbance based on the assumption that similar types of hormonal dysfunction might underlie both premenstrual and postpartum mood disorders (e.g., Yalom et al., 1968; Steiner, 1979). For example, one study (Dennerstein, Morse, & Varnavides, 1988) compared women with prospectively determined premenstrual syndrome and women with no menstrual problems and found only a marginally higher rate of past postpartum depression among the women with premenstrual syndrome. The only other study of the association between premenstrual mood disorder and postpartum depression found no evidence of an association (O'Hara, 1994). Although several other studies reported significant associations between "premenstrual tension" and the postpartum blues or depressive symptoms (Nott et al., 1976; Playfair & Gowers, 1981; Yalom et al., 1968), none provided a description of their criteria for "premenstrual tension."

Obstetric and pregnancy complications, which could be considered stressful life events, have been inconsistently related to postpartum depression, with some studies finding less mood disturbance in women with more stress or delivery complications (Paykel, Emms, Fletcher, & Rassaby, 1980; Pitt, 1968). Other studies found the expected relation between obstetric complications and postpartum mood disturbance (Campbell & Cohn, 1991; Oakley, 1980). Murray and Cartwright (1993) found that among women with a previous history of depressive disorder, delivery by forceps or caesarean section was associated with the occurrence of postpartum depression. O'Hara, Schlechte, Lewis, and Varner (1991) observed a similar finding: The joint presence of depression during pregnancy and relatively higher levels of obstetric stressors was a significant risk factor for postpartum depression. Other studies have found no association (Cox et al., 1982; O'Hara et al., 1984; Whiffen, 1988). Finally, there is almost no evidence that previous abortion or miscarriage increases risk for postpartum depression (Paykel et al., 1980; Kumar & Robson, 1984; Watson et al., 1984).

The variability in the outcomes of studies of the effects of obstetric stress may be, in part, a result of the various measures of stress that have been used. For example, some studies include a wide range of labor-relevant variables in their measure of obstetric stress (O'Hara, Schlechte, Lewis, & Varner, 1991). Other studies rate obstetric stress primarily on the basis of the type of delivery, caesarean section being regarded as the most stressful (Whiffen, 1988). The findings in this area do suggest that third variables, such as psychiatric history, may mediate the relation between obstetric stress and postpartum depression (Murray & Cartwright, 1993; O'Hara, Schlechte, Lewis, & Varner, 1991), and further research along these lines is clearly warranted.

✓ Stressful Life Events

Negative life events (e.g., serious illness in a family member and unemployment), which have been found to increase the likelihood of depression in nonpuerperal women (Brown & Harris, 1978), may also occur and raise the risk of depression during pregnancy and after delivery. Negative events might be especially potent during this period if they have implications for the woman's ability to properly care for her infant (e.g., severe financial reversal or abandonment by spouse). Not surprisingly, a number of studies have found that higher levels of stressful life events during pregnancy and after delivery were associated with an increased risk of postpartum depression (Martin, Brown, Goldberg, & Brockington, 1989; Paykel et al., 1980; O'Hara, 1986, 1994; O'Hara, Rehm, & Campbell, 1983) and higher risk for relapse after delivery among women with previous histories of affective disorder (Marks, Wieck, Checkley, & Kumar, 1992). However, there have been some failures to find the expected association between negative life events and depression (Pitt, 1968; Kumar & Robson, 1984; Hopkins, Campbell, & Marcus, 1987), although in one of these studies the investigators did find an association between infant postnatal complications and postpartum depression (Hopkins et al., 1987). Nevertheless, all these studies, taken as a whole, do suggest an important role for negative life events in postpartum depression.

✓ Marital Relationship

Probably no relationship is more important to a woman during the puerperium than that with her spouse. Many studies have found that postpartum depressed women report poor marital relationships after delivery (Campbell et al., 1992; Paykel et al., 1980; Cox et al., 1982; O'Hara, 1994; O'Hara et al., 1983). More important, several studies assessed the marital relationship during pregnancy and found that the poor marital relationship preceded the postpartum depression (Gotlib et al., 1991; Kumar & Robson, 1984; O'Hara, 1986; Robinson, Olmsted, & Garner, 1989; Watson et al., 1984; Whiffen, 1988). However, a few studies have found that marital distress during pregnancy did not predict postpartum depression (O'Hara et al., 1983) or depression relapse during the puerperium (Marks et al., 1992).

Parental Conflict

Few investigators have studied the effect of parental conflict and loss on the likelihood of postpartum depression. Kumar and Robson (1984) found that a poor relationship with the woman's own mother was associated with postpartum depression. In a more recent study, Gotlib et al. (1991) found that more negative perceptions, measured during pregnancy, of maternal and paternal caring during childhood were associated with diagnosis of postpartum depression. However, Paykel et al. (1980) found no association between parental conflict or childhood parental loss and postpartum depression. Similarly, Watson et al. (1984) found no association between childhood separation from parents and postpartum depression.

Social Support

Social support from spouse, family, and friends during times of stress (e.g., helping in household tasks or acting as a confidant) is thought to reduce the likelihood of depression (Mueller, 1980). The findings from research linking social support and postpartum depression have been rather consistent. Lack of spousal support has been found to be associated with increased levels of postpartum depression (Campbell et al., 1992; O'Hara, 1986; O'Hara et al., 1983); however, two major studies did not find this association (Hopkins et al., 1987; O'Hara, 1994). Other studies have found that lack of an adequate confidant or lower levels of support from a confidant are associated with postpartum depression (O'Hara et al., 1983; Paykel et al., 1980). Finally, Cutrona (1984) reported that several dimensions of perceived social support measured during pregnancy were associated with level of postpartum depression symptoms.

Personal and Family Psychopathology

Indices of depressive symptomatology, anxiety, and neurotic behavior during pregnancy have been consistently associated with level of postpartum depressive symptomatology and have been found to distinguish postpartum depressed and nondepressed women (Cutrona, 1983; Gotlib et al., 1991; O'Hara et al., 1984; O'Hara, Schlechte, Lewis, & Varner, 1991; Watson et al., 1984; Whiffen, 1988). Although the general pattern of these findings has been consistent and may indicate a continuity of psychological distress across pregnancy and the puerperium, a few studies have found little association between pre- and postpartum distress (e.g., Kumar & Robson, 1984).

Women who have experienced previous psychiatric disorder appear to be at risk for postpartum depression. Several studies have obtained data regarding previous psychiatric disturbance and found an association with postpartum depression (Campbell et al., 1992; O'Hara, 1994; O'Hara et al., 1983; Paykel et al., 1980; Watson et al., 1984). A recent study that included women with a previous history of bipolar disorder, schizoaffective disorder, or major depression found that 22 of the 43 women (51%) experienced a psychotic or nonpsychotic depression or mania (and, in a few cases, an anxiety disorder) after delivery (Marks et al., 1992). However, this general link between history of psychiatric disorder and postpartum depression has not always been found (Pitt, 1968; Kumar & Robson, 1984). In addition, O'Hara (1994) reported that in an earlier study (O'Hara, 1986) in which the number of previous episodes of depression were reported to be associated with risk for postpartum depression, the effect was largely due to one subject who had numerous episodes and the finding could not therefore be considered reliable.

Family history of psychopathology has also been studied as a predictor of postpartum depression. The findings from these studies, with one clear exception (Kumar & Robson, 1984), have largely supported an association between family psychopathology and postpartum depression (Campbell et al., 1992; O'Hara et al., 1984; Watson et al., 1984). Also, O'Hara (1994) reported that postpartum depressed subjects had a greater proportion of depressed mothers than did the postpartum nondepressed subjects. Nevertheless, a recent meta-analysis suggests that overall there may be little or no association between family history of psychopathology and postpartum depression (O'Hara & Swain, 1996).

Psychological Constructs

Several constructs derived from cognitive-behavioral theories of depression (Abramson, Seligman, & Teasdale, 1978; Rehm, 1977) have been tested as predictors of postpartum depression. The logic of these studies was that certain types of psychological vulnerability (e.g., dysfunctional attributional style or self-control attitudes or maladaptive cognitions) should increase a person's risk for depression in the context of a stressful life event (e.g., giving birth). Most of the positive or supportive findings in this work have been in the context of predicting level of depressive symptomatology rather than depression diagnosis. For example, O'Hara et al. (1982) and Cutrona (1983) found that attributional style (the types of causes women identify for good and bad events) (Abramson et al., 1978), measured during pregnancy, predicted level of postpartum depression symptoms. Studies attempting to predict postpartum depression diagnosis using these types of psychological constructs have been unsuccessful (O'Hara et al., 1984; O'Hara, Schlechte, Lewis, & Varner, 1991; Whiffen, 1988). The fact that several studies have found that these constructs are predictive of level of postpartum depressive symptomatology (Atkinson & Rickel, 1984; Cutrona, 1983; O'Hara et al., 1982, 1984) suggests that different causal factors may be important in the development of depressive symptoms versus the development of the syndrome of depression in childbearing women.

Summary of Causal Factors

None of the potential social and psychological causal factors in postpartum depression have been supported unambiguously in the literature. The pattern of results reviewed here suggests that gynecological and obstetric variables are not in themselves specifically related to postpartum depression. There is valid evidence that a woman's psychological adjustment before and during pregnancy is associated with the development of postpartum depression. Moreover, women who experience high levels of stress during pregnancy and after delivery, and women who lack a supportive spouse, appear to be particularly vulnerable to developing postpartum depression. These are psychosocial variables that figure prominently in models of the etiology of nonpostpartum depression (Depue, 1979). In fact, many recent investigators have assumed that the postpartum period is simply a high-risk time for depression and that it is an appropriate context in which to test etiological models developed to account for nonpostpartum depression (e.g., Atkinson & Rickel, 1984; Cutrona, 1983; Gotlib et al., 1991; O'Hara et al., 1984; Whiffen, 1988).

TREATMENT

In general, postpartum depressed women receive the same treatments that other depressed patients receive. However, because of the timing of postpartum depression, the possible role of reproductive hormones, and the special significance that many women and clinicians attach to depression during the postpartum period, specific treatments for postpartum depression have been developed. These treatments are of two general sorts: treatments given during pregnancy or early in the puerperium, often to at-risk women, designed to prevent the development of a postpartum depression, and treatments given to women after delivery who are already depressed.

Several prevention studies have been conducted and each of them involved a series of group sessions (two or more) that helped women (and sometimes their partners) prepare for the postpartum responsibilities (Elliott, Sanjack, & Leverton, 1988; Gordon & Gordon, 1960; Halonen & Passman, 1985). The targets of these preventive interventions varied from the practical (e.g., advice regarding the necessity of getting help during the postpartum period and identifying a pediatrician prior to delivery) to more therapeutic activities (e.g., learning to relax or simply discussing common concerns in a group setting). Overall, women receiving each of these interventions had better postpartum emotional adjustment than did women receiving a control intervention.

In a rather innovative study in South Africa, Wolman, Chalmers, Hofmeyr, and Nikodem (1993) evaluated the efficacy of providing companionship during labor to a group of women who had no companions of their own. The authors reasoned that labor was a time when women were especially vulnerable to losing confidence in their competence as mothers and that a feeling of incompetence as a mother was a causal factor in the development of postpartum depression. The provision of support during labor was hypothesized to increase women's confidence in their competence and to reduce depressive and anxious symptomatology during the postpartum period. This rather brief intervention during labor resulted in significantly greater levels of confidence and significantly lower levels of depressive and anxious symptomatology in the treated group relative to the untreated group.

The only published controlled study of the effects of a psychological intervention for postpartum depression involved brief treatment (using a Rogerian approach) by health visitors (in Scotland) over a period of 8 weeks (Holden, Sagovsky, & Cox, 1989). Depression remitted in a significantly greater proportion of the women exposed to the health visitor intervention (69%) than in the women who received no treatment (38%). Further, in an open clinical trial, Stuart and O'Hara (1995a, 1995b) reported success with interpersonal psychotherapy for postpartum depression. Two additional unpublished studies were conducted in Sweden (Johansson, 1993) and England (Cooper & Murray, 1994). Both studies found evidence of a significant effect of counseling relative to no treatment for postpartum depression, and one study found evidence of a significant effect of other forms of treatment, in particular cognitive-behavioral therapy and a dynamic psychotherapy (Cooper & Murray, 1994; see Cooper & Murray, Chapter 8, this volume). Finally, in a Canadian study, postpartum depressed women (based on self-report) received eight group sessions of social support group therapy or no treatment (Fleming, Klein, & Corter, 1992). There were no treatment effects with respect to depressive symptomatology; however, there was some evidence that the social support groups had a positive effect on mother–infant interaction.

Few controlled pharmacotherapy trials for postpartum depressed have been carried out. One British study evaluated the effects of transdermal estrogen in a double-blind, randomized, placebo-controlled study (Gregoire et al., 1996). Results suggested that women receiving 6 months of treatment with estradiol skin patches showed a more rapid and greater improvement in their depressive symptomatology than did women in the placebo condition.

Too little treatment research has been conducted to draw conclusions with any degree of confidence regarding the efficacy of various treatments of postpartum depression. Conventional treatments for depression appear to be effective for women experiencing a postpartum depression. However, caution is advised. For example, little is known about the extent to which women experiencing postpartum depression have been represented in therapy outcome studies. Given concerns about the effects of antidepressants in breast milk, it is unlikely that childbearing women have been included in general trials of antidepressants. The childbearing status of women in therapy outcome studies is rarely mentioned, so it is unclear whether depression in the puerperium is responsive to conventional pharmacotherapies and psychotherapies. Also, the clinician must remain sensitive to these women's needs as new mothers during the postpartum period. Medical centers are increasingly developing specialized units to treat women with postpartum mood disorders. In Great Britain, special mother–baby units have been developed to care for women who require hospitalization for depression or other psychiatric disorder after delivery (see Hipwell & Kumar, Chapter 11, this volume). These units allow the baby to stay with the mother so that development of the mother–infant relationship and the mother's parenting skills is disrupted as little as possible.

CONCLUSION

Depression is a serious and common problem for childbearing women. It is disruptive to their daily life and impairs their functioning in all domains. Although there may be a form of depression that is peculiar to the postpartum period, postpartum depressions share many characteristics, including risk factors, with depressions that occur at other times. Important new studies on both psychological and pharmacological preventive and treatment interventions for postpartum depression have recently been completed or are currently under way. These efforts are critical to prevent the negative consequences to the mother, family, and child associated with maternal depression.

REFERENCES

Abramson, L. Y., Seligman, M. E. P., & Teasdale, J. D. (1978). Learned helplessness in humans: Critique and reformulation. *Journal of Abnormal Psychology, 87,* 49–74.

American Psychiatric Association. (1980). *Diagnostic and statistical manual of mental disorders* (3rd ed.). Washington, DC: Author.

American Psychiatric Association. (1994). *Diagnostic and statistical manual of mental disorders* (4th ed.). Washington, DC: Author.

Atkinson, A. K., & Rickel, A. U. (1984). Postpartum depression in primiparous parents. *Journal of Abnormal Psychology, 93,* 115–119.

Ballinger, C. B., Kay, D. S. G., Naylor, G. J., & Smith, A. H. W. (1982). Some biochemical findings during pregnancy and after delivery in relation to mood change. *Psychological Medicine, 12,* 549–556.

Beck, A. T., Ward, C. H., Mendelson, M., Mock, J., & Erbaugh, J. (1961). An inventory for measuring depression. *Archives of General Psychiatry, 4,* 561–569.

Boyce, P. M., & Stubbs, J. M. (1994). The importance of postnatal depression. *Medical Journal of Australia, 161,* 471–472.

Brockington, I. F., Cernik, K. F., Schofield, E. M., Downing, A. R., Francis, A. F., & Keelan, C. (1981). Puerperal psychosis: Phenomena and diagnosis. *Archives of General Psychiatry, 38,* 829–833.

Brown, G. W., & Harris, T. (1978). *Social origins of depression: A study of psychiatric disorder in women.* New York: Free Press.

Campbell, J. L., & Winokur, G. (1985). Post-partum affective disorders: Selected biological aspects. In D. G. Inwood (Ed.), *Recent advances in post-partum psychiatric disorders* (pp. 19–40). Washington, DC: American Psychiatric Press.

Campbell, S. B., & Cohn, J. F. (1991). Prevalence and correlates of postpartum depression in first-time mothers. *Journal of Abnormal Psychology, 100,* 594–599.

Campbell, S. B., Cohn, J. F., Flanagan, C., Popper, S., & Meyers, T. (1992). Course and correlates of postpartum depression during the transition to parenthood. *Development and Psychopathology, 4,* 29–47.

Carroll, B. J., & Steiner, M. (1978). The psychobiology of premenstrual dysphoria: The role of prolactin. *Psychoneuroendocrinology, 3,* 171–180.

Cooper, P. J., Campbell, E. A., Day, A., Kennerley, H., & Bond, A. (1988). Non-psychotic psychiatric disorder after childbirth: A prospective study of prevalence, incidence, course and nature. *British Journal of Psychiatry, 152,* 799–806.

Cooper, P. J., & Murray, L. (1994, September). *Three psychological treatments for postnatal depression: A controlled treatment comparison.* Paper presented at the International Conference of the Marcé Society, Queens College, Cambridge University, England.

Cooper, P. J., & Murray, L. (1995). Course and recurrence of postnatal depression: Evidence for the specificity of the diagnostic concept. *British Journal of Psychiatry, 166,* 191–195.

Cox, J. L. (1986). *Postnatal depression.* Edinburgh: Churchill Livingstone.

Cox, J. L., Connor, Y., & Kendell, R. E. (1982). Prospective study of the psychiatric disorders of childbirth. *British Journal of Psychiatry, 140,* 111–117.

Cox, J. L., Holden, J. M., & Sagovsky, R. (1987). Detection of postnatal depression: Development of the 10-item Edinburgh Postnatal Depression Scale. *British Journal of Psychiatry, 150,* 782–786.

Cox, J. L., Murray, D., & Chapman, G. (1993). A controlled study of the onset, duration and prevalence of postnatal depression. *British Journal of Psychiatry, 163,* 27–31

Cox, J. L., Rooney, A., Thomas, P. F., & Wrate, R. W. (1984). How accurately do mothers recall postnatal depression? Further data from a 3 year follow-up study. *Journal of Psychosomatic Obstetrics and Gynaecology, 3,* 185–189.

Cutrona, C. E. (1983). Causal attributions and perinatal depression. *Journal of Abnormal Psychology, 92,* 161–172.

Cutrona, C. E. (1984). Social support and stress in the transition to parenthood. *Journal of Abnormal Psychology, 93,* 378–390.

Dalton, K. (1980). *Depression after childbirth.* Oxford, England: Oxford University Press.

Dean, C., & Kendell, R. E. (1981). The symptomatology of puerperal illnesses. *British Journal of Psychiatry, 139,* 128–133.

Dennerstein, L., Morse, C. A., & Varnavides, K. (1988). Premenstrual tension and depression—Is there a relationship? *Journal of Psychosomatic Obstetrics and Gynecology, 8,* 45–52.

Depue, R. A. (Ed.). (1979). *The psychobiology of the depressive disorders: Implications for the effects of stress.* New York: Academic Press.

Elliott, S. A., Sanjack, M., & Leverton, T. J. (1988). Parents groups in pregnancy: A preventive intervention for postnatal depression? In B. H. Gottlieb (Ed.), *Marshaling social support: Formats, processes, and effects* (pp. 87–110). Newbury Park, CA: Sage.

Fleming, A. S., Klein, E., & Corter, C. (1992). The effects of a social support group on depression, maternal attitudes and behavior in new mothers. *Journal of Child Psychology and Psychiatry, 33,* 685–698.

Gard, P. R., Handley, S. L., Parsons, A. D., & Waldron, G. (1986). A multivariate investigation of postpartum mood disturbance. *British Journal of Psychiatry, 148,* 567–575.

George, A. J., Copeland, J. R. M., & Wilson, K. C. M. (1980). Serum prolactin and the postpartum blues syndrome. *British Journal of Pharmacology, 70,* 102–103.

George, A. J., & Sandler, M. (1988). Endocrine and biochemical studies in puerperal mental disorders. In R. Kumar & I. F. Brockington (Eds.), *Motherhood and mental illness 2: Causes and consequences* (pp. 78–112). London: Wright.

Ghodsian, M., Zajicek, E., & Wolkind, S. (1984). A longitudinal study of maternal depression and child behavior problems. *Journal of Child Psychology and Psychiatry and Allied Disciplines, 25,* 91–109.

Gordon, R. E., & Gordon, K. K. (1960). Social factors in the prevention of postpartum emotional problems. *Obstetrics and Gynecology, 15,* 433–438.

Gotlib, I. H., Whiffen, V. E., Wallace, P. M., & Mount, J. H. (1991). Prospective investigation of postpartum depression: Factors involved in onset and recovery. *Journal of Abnormal Psychology, 100,* 122–132.

Greenwood, J., & Parker, G. (1984). The dexamethasone suppression test in the puerperium. *Australian and New Zealand Journal of Psychiatry, 18,* 282–284.

Gregoire, A. J. P., Kumar, R., Everitt, B., Henderson, A. F., & Studd, J. W. W. (1996). Transdermal oestrogen for treatment of severe postnatal depression. *The Lancet, 347,* 930–933.

Halonen, J. S., & Passman, R. H. (1985). Relaxation training and expectation in the treatment of postpartum distress. *Journal of Consulting and Clinical Psychology, 53,* 839–845.

Hamilton, J. A. (1962). *Postpartum psychiatric disorders.* St. Louis: C. V. Mosby.

Hamilton, J. A., & Harberger, P. N. (Eds.). (1992). *Postpartum psychiatric illness: A picture puzzle.* Philadelphia: University of Pennsylvania Press.

Handley, S. L., Dunn, T. L., Waldron, G., & Baker, J. M. (1980). Tryptophan, cortisol and puerperal mood. *British Journal of Psychiatry, 136,* 498–508.

Harris, B. (1993). Post-partum thyroid dysfunction and post-natal depression. *Annals of Medicine, 25,* 215–216.

Harris, B., Johns, S., Fung, H., Thomas, R., Walker, R., Read, G., & Riad-Fahmy, D. (1989). The hormonal environment of post-natal depression. *British Journal of Psychiatry, 154,* 660–667.

Harris, B., Othman, L., Davies, J. A., Weppner, G. J., Richards, C. J., Newcombe, R. G., Lazarus, J. H., Parkes, A. B., Hall, R., & Phillips, D. I. (1992). Association between postpartum thyroid dysfunction and thyroid antibodies and depression. *British Medical Journal, 305,* 152–156.

Holden, J. M., Sagovsky, R., & Cox, J. L. (1989). Counselling in a general practice setting: Controlled study of health visitor intervention in treatment of post-natal depression. *British Medical Journal, 298,* 223–226.

Hopkins, J., Campbell, S. B., & Marcus, M. (1987). The role of infant-related stressors in postpartum depression. *Journal of Abnormal Psychology, 96,* 237–241.

Johansson, B. (1993, November). *Postnatal depression: A screening and intervention study within the Swedish Child Health Care.* Paper presented at the International Conference of the Marcé Society, Eindoven, The Netherlands.

Johnson, J., Weissman, M. M., & Klerman, G. L. (1992). Service utilization and social morbidity associated with depressive symptoms in the community. *Journal of the American Medical Association, 267,* 1478–1483.

Jolivet, A., Blanchier, H., & Gautray, J. P. (1974). Blood cortisol variations during late pregnancy and labor. *American Journal of Obstetrics and Gynecology, 119,* 775–783.

Kendell, R. E., Chalmers, J. C., & Platz, C. (1987). Epidemiology of puerperal psychoses. *British Journal of Psychiatry, 150,* 662–673.

Kennerley, H., & Gath, D. (1989). Maternity blues I. Detection and measurement by questionnaire. *British Journal of Psychiatry, 155,* 356–362.

Kessler, R. C., McGonagle, K. A., Zhao, S., Nelson, C. B., Hughes, M., Eshleman, S., Wittchen, H. -U., & Kendler, K. S. (1994). Lifetime and 12-month prevalence of DSM-III-R psychiatric disorders in the United States: Results from the National Comorbidity Survey. *Archives of General Psychiatry, 51,* 8–19.

Kuevi, V., Causon, R., Dixson, A. F., Everard, E. M., Hall, J. M., Hole, D., Whitehead, S. A., Wilson, C. A., & Wise, J. C. M. (1983). Plasma amine and hormone changes in "post-partum blues." *Clinical Endocrinology, 19,* 39–46.

Kumar, R., & Brockington, I. F. (Eds.). (1988). *Motherhood and mental illness 2: Causes and consequences.* London: Wright.

Kumar, R., & Robson, K. M. (1984). A prospective study of emotional disorders in childbearing women. *British Journal of Psychiatry, 144,* 35–47.

Marks, M. N., Wieck, A., Checkley, S. A., & Kumar, R. (1992). Contribution of psychological and social factors to psychotic and non-psychotic relapse after childbirth in women with previous histories of affective disorder. *Journal of Affective Disorders, 29,* 253–264.

Martin, C. J., Brown, G. W., Goldberg, D. P., & Brockington, I. F. (1989). Psychosocial stress and puerperal depression. *Journal of Affective Disorders, 16,* 283–293.

Metz, A., Cowen, P. J., Gelder, M. G., Stump, K., Elliott, J. M., & Grahame-Smith, D. G. (1983). Changes in platelet alpha$_2$ adrenoceptor binding post-partum: Possible relation to maternity blues. *Lancet, ii,* 495–498.

Mueller, D. P. (1980). Social networks: A promising direction for research on the relationship of the social environment to psychiatric disorder. *Social Science and Medicine, 14a,* 147–161.

Murray, L., & Cartwright, W. (1993). The role of obstetric risk factors in postpartum depression. *Journal of Reproductive and Infant Psychology, 11,* 215–219.

Myers, J. K., Weissman, M. M., Tischler, G. L., Holzer, C. E., Leaf, P. J., Orvaschel, H., Anthony, J. C., Boyd, J. H., Burke, J. D., Kramer, M., & Stoltzman, R. (1984). Six-month prevalence of psychiatric disorders in three communities: 1980 to 1982. *Archives of General Psychiatry, 41,* 959–967.

Nott, P. N. (1987). Extent, timing and persistence of emotional disorders following childbirth. *British Journal of Psychiatry, 151,* 523–527.

Nott, P. N., Franklin, M., Armitage, C., & Gelder, M. G. (1976). Hormonal changes in mood in the puerperium. *British Journal of Psychiatry, 128,* 379–383.

Oakley, A. (1980). *Women confined—Towards a sociology of childbirth.* Oxford, England: Martin Robertson.

O'Hara, M. W. (1986). Social support, life events, and depression during pregnancy and the puerperium. *Archives of General Psychiatry, 43,* 569–573.

O'Hara, M. W. (1991). Postpartum mental disorders. In J. J. Sciarra (Ed.), *Gynecology and Obstetrics* (Vol. 6, pp. 1–17). Philadelphia: Harper & Row.

O'Hara, M. W. (1994). *Postpartum depression: Causes and consequences.* New York: Springer-Verlag.

O'Hara, M. W. (1995). Childbearing. In M. W. O'Hara, R. Reiter, S. Johnson, A. Milburn, & J. Engeldinger (Eds.), *Psychological aspects of women's reproductive health* (pp. 26–48). New York: Springer.

O'Hara, M. W., Neunaber, D. J., & Zekoski, E. M. (1984). A prospective study of postpartum depression: Prevalence, course, and predictive factors. *Journal of Abnormal Psychology, 93,* 158–171.

O'Hara, M. W., Rehm, L. P., & Campbell, S. B. (1982). Predicting depressive symptomatology: Cognitive-behavioral models and postpartum depression. *Journal of Abnormal Psychology, 91,* 457–461.

O'Hara, M. W., Rehm, L. P., & Campbell, S. B. (1983). Postpartum depression: A role for social network and life stress variables. *Journal of Nervous and Mental Disease, 171,* 336–341.

O'Hara, M. W., Schlechte, J. A., Lewis, D. A., & Varner, M. W. (1991). A controlled prospective study of postpartum mood disorders: Psychological, environmental, and hormonal variables. *Journal of Abnormal Psychology, 100,* 63–73.

O'Hara, M. W., Schlechte, J. A., Lewis, D. A., & Wright, E. J. (1991). Prospective study of postpartum blues: Biologic and psychosocial factors. *Archives of General Psychiatry, 48,* 801–806.

O'Hara, M. W., & Swain, A. M. (1996). Rates and risk of postpartum depression: A meta-analysis. *International Review of Psychiatry, 8,* 37–54.

O'Hara, M. W., & Zekoski, E. M. (1988). Postpartum depression: A comprehensive review. In R. Kumar & I. F. Brockington (Eds.), *Motherhood and mental illness 2: Causes and consequences* (pp. 17–63). London: Wright.

O'Hara, M. W., Zekoski, E. M., Philipps, L. H., & Wright, E. J. (1990). A controlled prospective study of postpartum mood disorders: Comparison of childbearing and nonchildbearing women. *Journal of Abnormal Psychology, 99,* 3–15.

Paykel, E. S., Emms, E. M., Fletcher, J., & Rassaby, E. S. (1980). Life events and social support in puerperal depression. *British Journal of Psychiatry, 136,* 339–346.

Philipps, L. H. C., & O'Hara, M. W. (1991). Prospective study of postpartum depression: 4½-year follow-up of women and children. *Journal of Abnormal Psychology, 100,* 151–155.

Pitt, B. (1968). "Atypical" depression following childbirth. *British Journal of Psychiatry, 114,* 1325–1335.

Playfair, H. R., & Gowers, J. I. (1981). Depression following childbirth—A search for predictive signs. *Journal of the Royal College of General Practitioners, 31,* 201–208.

Pop, V. J. M., de Rooy, H. A. M., Vader, H. L., van der Heide, D., van Son, M., Komproe, I. H., Essed, G. G. M., & de Geus, C. A. (1991). Postpartum thyroid dysfunction and depression in an unselected population. *New England Journal of Medicine. 324,* 1815–1816.

Purdy, D., & Frank, E. (1993). Should postpartum mood disorders be given a more prominent or distinct place in the DSM-IV? *Depression, 1,* 59–70.

Railton, I. E. (1961). The use of corticoids in postpartum depression. *Journal of American Medical Women's Association, 16,* 450–452.

Regier, D. A., Narrow, W. E., Rae, D. S., Manderscheid, R. W., Locke, B. Z., & Goodwin, F. K. (1993). The de facto US mental and addictive disorders service system: Epidemiologic Catchment Area prospective 1-year prevalence rates of disorders and services. *Archives of General Psychiatry, 50,* 85–94.

Rehm, L. P. (1977). A self-control model of depression. *Behavior Therapy, 8,* 787–804.

Robinson, G. E., Olmsted, M. P., & Garner, D. M. (1989). Predictors of postpartum adjustment. *Acta Psychiatrica Scandinavica, 80,* 561–565.

Schlesser, M. A. (1986). Neuroendocrine abnormalities in affective disorders. In A. J. Rush & K. Z. Altshuler (Eds.), *Depression: Basic mechanisms, diagnosis, and treatment* (pp. 45–71). New York: Guilford Press.

Singh, B., Gilhotra, M., Smith, R., Brinsmead, M., Lewin, T., & Hall, C. (1986). Post-partum psychoses and the dexamethasone suppression test. *Journal of Affective Disorders, 11,* 173–177.

Speroff, L., Glass, R. H., & Kase, N. G. (1989). *Clinical gynecologic endocrinology and infertility.* Baltimore: William & Wilkins.

Spitzer, R. L., Endicott, J., & Robins, E. (1978). Research diagnostic criteria: Rationale and reliability. *Archives of General Psychiatry, 36,* 773–782.

Stein, G. (1982). The maternity blues. In I. F. Brockington & R. Kumar (Eds.), *Motherhood and mental illness* (pp. 119–154). New York: Grune & Stratton.

Steiner, M. (1979). Psychobiology of mental disorders associated with childbearing. *Acta Psychiatrica Scandinavica, 60,* 449–464.

Stuart, S., & O'Hara, M. W. (1995a). Interpersonal psychotherapy for postpartum depression: A treatment program. *Journal of Psychotherapy Practice and Research, 4,* 18–29.

Stuart, S., & O'Hara, M. W. (1995b). Treatment of postpartum depression with interpersonal psychotherapy [Letter]. *Archives of General Psychiatry, 52,* 75–76.

Troutman, B. R., & Cutrona, C. E. (1990). Nonpsychotic postpartum depression among adolescent mothers. *Journal of Abnormal Psychology, 99,* 69–78.

Vemer, H. M., & Rolland, R. (1981). The dynamics of prolactin secretion during the puerperium in women. *Clinical Endocrinology, 15,* 155–163.

Watson, J. P., Elliott, S. A., Rugg, A. J., & Brough, D. I. (1984). Psychiatric disorder in pregnancy and the first postnatal year. *British Journal of Psychiatry, 144,* 453–462.

Weissman, M. M., & Paykel, E. S. (1974). *The depressed woman: A study of social relationships.* Chicago: University of Chicago Press.

Wells, K. B., Stewart, A., Hays, R. D., Burnam, M. A., Rogers, W., Daniels, M., Berry, S., Greenfield, S., & Ware, J. (1989). The functioning and well-being of depressed patients: Results from the Medical Outcomes Study. *Journal of the American Medical Association, 262,* 914–919.

Whiffen, V. E. (1988). Vulnerability to postpartum depression: A prospective multivariate study. *Journal of Abnormal Psychology, 97,* 467–474.

Whiffen, V. E., & Gotlib, I. H. (1993). Comparison of postpartum and nonpostpartum depression: Clinical presentation, psychiatric history, and psychosocial functioning. *Journal of Consulting and Clinical Psychology, 61,* 485–494.

Wolkind, S., Coleman, E., & Ghodsian, M. (1980). Continuities in maternal depression. *International Journal of Family Psychiatry, 1,* 167–182.

Wolman, W. L., Chalmers, B., Hofmeyr, G. J., & Nikodem, V. C. (1993). Postpartum depression and companionship in the clinical birth environment: A randomized, controlled study. *American Journal of Obstetrics and Gynecology, 168,* 1388–1393.

World Health Organization. (1992). *International classification of diseases and health related problems* (10th rev.). Geneva: Author.

Yalom, I. D., Lunde, D. T., Moos, R. H., & Hamburg, D. A. (1968). "Postpartum blues" syndrome. *Archives of General Psychiatry, 18,* 16–27.

II

THE ARCHITECTURE OF MOTHER–INFANT INTERACTIONS AND THE IMPLICATIONS FOR POSTPARTUM DEPRESSION

2

Fragile Aspects of Early Social Integration

Hanuš Papoušek
Mechthild Papoušek
University of Munich

In this chapter, we do not base our comments on interrelationships between postpartum depression and child development on a straightforward experimental or clinical approach to postpartum depression. Rather, they result from four independent sources of experimental and clinical experience: research on infant coping with problematic situations (Papoušek, 1967, 1969); research on early, preverbal communication between infants and caregivers (Papoušek & Papoušek, 1987); consulting services to mothers volunteering in long-term studies on infant mental development; and clinical services for families with disorders in preverbal social communication and integration (Papoušek, Hofacker, Malinowski, Jacubeit, & Cosmovici, 1994). In line with contemporary beliefs that the etiology of postpartum depression is still unclear but is obviously multifactorial (Hopkins, Marcus, & Campbell, 1984) and possibly linked to risk status in infants (Blumberg, 1980; Buxbaum, 1983; Murray, Stanley, Hooper, King, & Fiori-Cowley, 1996; O'Hara, Rehm, & Campbell, 1983; Sameroff & Chandler, 1975), interdisciplinary exchange of information and interactionistic interpretation of etiology may point toward diagnostic and therapeutic improvements.

With this in mind, a combination of experimental studies and clinical observations may be particularly helpful because factors disturbing mother–infant interactions can neither be included in experimental interventions in human subjects nor applied in animal models insofar as they concern species-specific forms of human interaction. Moreover, questionnaires or interviews cannot adequately replace direct observations because a large number of interactional behaviors, and communicative interchanges in particular, escape the conscious awareness of parents (Papoušek & Papoušek, 1987). Observations of parent–infant interactions have attracted increasing attention in recent years as a result of discoveries that improve interpretation and point toward effective, albeit insufficiently investigated, intrinsic motivators in the behavioral regulation of both mothers and infants.

A better understanding of the motivators involved in the behavioral regulation of mother–infant interactions is particularly desirable because of the relatively high incidence of dysphoric postpartum states—the maternity blues, postpartum depression, and postpartum affective psychosis, (O'Hara, Chapter 1, this volume). The number of women who, for various reasons, would have been restrained or eliminated from the process of reproduction in former times but who opt to have children nowadays has increased. Situational stressors that have been identified as potential risk factors for dysphoric postpartum states are still present and may even have increased, especially those due to unfavorable economic circumstances and/or destabilized family structures.

Two decades of neonatal research sharpened my (H. P.) attention to the course of maternal adjustment to biological, sociocultural, or psychodynamic changes accompanying the delivery of a child—that dramatic experience when the fetus, seemingly a part of the maternal body, starts functioning as a new, autonomic, and yet totally dependent personality. In addition, we gained experience with more than 300 mothers who spent several postpartum months in a lying-in unit for research on early infant development, and who were helped, in daily consultations, in their sometimes problematic efforts to identify their new roles and to understand their new psychological problems. Observational experience stimulated new types of analyses of parental competence (Papoušek & Papoušek, 1978, 1987) and, recently, verified certain interpretive concepts in the treatment of disorders in parent–infant interactions in families with excessively crying infants. Links between unfavorable behavioral deviations on the part of both mother and infant have emerged from several studies (Cox, Puckering, Pound, & Mills, 1987; Field, 1984; Murray, 1992; Murray & Trevarthen, 1985; Radke-Yarrow, Cummings, Kuczynski, & Chapman, 1985). Some data from these studies have been related to deviations in emotional attachment; other data have indicated involvement of communicative difficulties.

Functional analyses of early postpartum interactions between mothers and infants appear to be particularly relevant to the interpretation of behavioral regulation and the vicious circles that originate from inconspicuous deviations but lead to serious disorders. Therefore, we discuss these analyses in more detail in the next sections of this chapter, first in relation to maternal factors and then in relation to infant factors.

THE MATERNAL ROLE IN EARLY INTERACTIONS WITH INFANTS

Maternal caregiving competence has usually been viewed as a combination of biological predispositions and culture-dependent interventions. This view is problematic insofar as biological predispositions have often been limited to emotional bonding and culture-dependent interventions to rational and consciously controlled forms of behavior. Such a conceptual oversimplification may have been caused by a tendency to use experimental animal models for research on early social interactions, by an overestimation of the similarities between emotional bonding in humans and laboratory primates, and by insufficient interest in the differences between them. In contrast, comparative ethologists recommend that the focus should be on the differences between humans and other mammals to detect species-specific means of biological adaptation. Such means have commonly been selected during evolution on the basis of universal behavioral tendencies, and in combination with both strong intrinsic motivators and extrinsic supports, that have coevolved in the social environment.

It is true that human forms of maternal caregiving partly belong to a universal set of mammalian behaviors that have come about with the evolution of the old mammalian brain, according to McLean (1990), and include emotional bonding, breastfeeding, and vocal signaling, along with other forms of care for dependent progeny. However, emotional bonding is not what has made humans different from other mammals and primates. For example, von Bertalanffy (1968) argues that humans would be only a moderately social species if their instinctual equipment were not associated with the capacity for symbolic thinking and communication. Only this capacity has specifically evolved in humans as their most powerful means of biological adaptation and the basis for specific languages and cultures. It is the invention of a symbolic universe that made humans better and worse than other species with their innate drives and controls. Thus, the mother is merely mammalian in her love for her child; however, she is human in her ability to support the development of symbolic capacities in her child and to guide the child toward the acquisition of language and into human culture. To interpret the mother's most important role merely in terms of affective bonding, we must narrow down her functioning to values that are equaled, or even surpassed, by many other animal species (Papoušek & Papoušek, 1995).

Audiovisual microanalyses have detected new—intuitive—patterns in parental behaviors that have escaped scientific attention because parents themselves are not aware of them and, therefore cannot report on them in questionnaires or interviews. For example, mothers observe sleeping newborns from the reading distance of 40–50 cm but halve the distance (as appropriate for the newborn's vision) when newborns open their eyes; mothers then position themselves in the center of newborns' visual field, try to reach their visual attention in various ways, and reward achievement of visual attention with expressive greeting responses. They exhibit these patterns even if they strongly believe that newborns cannot yet see anything (Schoetzau & Papoušek, 1977).

It may in part be the case that intuitive forms of behavior have been neglected because they are seen as relics of animal behaviors, undesired in advanced human societies. Only recently have cognitive psychologists become aware of the significance and frequency of nonconscious processes of thought in the regulation of human behavior and begun to pay them necessary respect (Kihlstrom, 1987). Neurophysiologically, intuitive behaviors are faster and less strenuous than rationally controlled behaviors. Their latencies (intervals between stimulation and response) are usually within 200–400 ms; thus, they are longer than in simple innate reflexes (40–60 ms) but shorter than latent periods in rational decisions. Even simple sensory perception needs a longer stimulation to be consciously perceived; if the brain cortex is stimulated directly, a minimum of 500–600 ms stimulation is necessary for conscious perception (Vander, Sherman, & Luciano, 1990).

The evidence of intuitive tendencies in the repertoire of parental care for infants is interesting from the psychobiological point of view: It indicates predispositions for a significant means of adaptation that have been selected during the process of evolution. For example, infants obviously have to learn the language of their cultural niche; however, their caregivers are rarely able to explain in which ways, and indeed whether at all, they guide their infants toward so important an achievement. Until lately, the coevolution of social support for the development of typical human adaptive capacities—symbolic communication, thinking, and self-consciousness—belonged to unexplored aspects of parental competence. We (Papoušek & Papoušek, 1978) suggested and chose as a central research topic a new interpretation of the environmental support that is hidden in "intuitive" forms of parenting. It has been demonstrated that human intuitive parenting may also serve as a biological prototype of teaching competence (Papoušek & Papoušek, 1989); parents assess and modify the general state of infant alertness, structure "teaching materials" according to the contemporary level of infant learning abilities, and are sensitive to feedback cues on infant coping. Thus, they facilitate progress in learning and reward it with pleasurable affective displays.

For example, during interchanges with infants, parents observe infant attention to vocal or visual stimulation or try to open the infant's mouth or palm and find cues in infant responses for decisions about whether to amuse, feed, soothe, or lull the infant to sleep (Papoušek & Papoušek, 1984). In this way, parents test and influence infant behavior, with a tendency to maintain active waking states during interactions, to facilitate transitions to quiet sleep, and to minimize transitory behavioral states during which learning is most difficult. Visual cues, such as arm positions and hand gestures, in infants alone elicit appropriate parental interventions, as demonstrated in laboratory experiments (Kestermann, 1982). The universal tendency to display short, stereotypical, and repetitive behavioral patterns in infant-directed communication can be viewed as an adjustment to constraints in early cognitive capacities during the first months of life when infants need many trials to learn (Papoušek, 1967). Particularly meaningful are those patterns exhibited by parents in response to infant cues: They allow infants to detect contingencies and to learn how to control the partner's behavior (i.e., environmental events). Parents, for instance, not only draw the infant's visual attention to their face—a source of important messages—but also, and without conscious awareness, reward the infant for achieving visual contact with a "greeting response" that functions as one of the first postpartum contingencies.

Infant-directed speech is perhaps the best example of an intuitive support to early development of integrative and communicative capacities in infants. Microanalytical studies have revealed a series of adjustments corresponding astonishingly to those fundamental steps through which the infant gradually acquires the necessary skills for speech and verbal communication. Caregivers' infant-directed speech is categorically different from adult-directed speech, and its typical features are universal among caregivers across sex, age, culture, and even modalities insofar as they also characterize infant-directed signing (American Sign Language) in deaf mothers (Erting, Prezioso, & Hynes, 1990). These features are obviously based on biological predispositions as no cultural traditions or institutions have been known to consciously introduce and regulate them. With the infant's progress in communicative competence, caregivers readjust the structure and quality of infant-directed speech while leading the infant in the direction of the next developmental step (Papoušek & Papoušek, 1987).

As we explain in the next section, infants' first expression of noncry vocal communication comes with prolonging of vowel-like primary voicing and modulating its pitch. Caregivers support infants by displaying frequent, prolonged, and strikingly melodic vowels; they encourage imitation of their models and reward infants for successful imitation with expressions of pleasure. Melodic contours play a special role in early communication. In adult-directed speech, caregivers use them rather moderately for syntactic and semantic purposes and/or for emphasizing affective significance: Typically, they use them to give their sentences the meanings of statements, questions, warnings, and the like. In infant-directed speech, however, melodic contours acquire another significance, independent of the meaning of words and syntactic structure of sentences; they themselves become categorical messages, context-specific symbols, and precursors of abstract words (Papoušek, Papoušek, & Bornstein, 1985). For example, prototypical forms of melodic contours or their combinations can tell the infant to attend to the onset of important events, to reduce superfluous arousal in the presence of a helping caregiver, to continue ongoing activities as adequate, or to stop them as inadequate. Effects of "approving" or "disapproving" messages in the absence of lexical content were experimentally demonstrated in the coping behaviors of 4-month-olds (Papoušek, Bornstein, Nuzzo, Papoušek, & Symmes, 1990).

Thus, we can assume that the behavioral regulation on the part of the mother includes intrinsic motivators related to a remarkably adaptive function, namely, parental support of the progeny's early communicative and cognitive development. The intuitive character of this support, its universality, and the striking involvement of affective components indicate biological origins and a superior effectiveness in behavioral regulation—related either to rewarding experiences during successful coping with caregiving situations or to frustrations with potential pathogenetic consequences in opposite cases.

THE INFANT'S ROLE IN EARLY
INTERACTIONS WITH MOTHERS

Infants' competence for learning and cognitive processing of a perceived experience is known to function early and to be based on universal, vital capabilities of living organisms. It has been richly documented in the literature on infant development. However, few studies have focused on the course of infant learning or the circumstances necessary for it or that facilitate it, particularly in preverbal infants. Yet, developmental analyses of learning abilities have shown remarkable constraints in newborns and a rapid improvement during the first 3 months (Papoušek, 1967, 1977). Observation of facial and vocal expressions in those studies have also revealed behavioral cues that allow the observer or the caregiver to assess the course of learning processes, the degree of difficulty that may accompany coping with problematic learning situations, and, eventually, signs of pleasure on final success. Indirectly, such evidence indicates the participation of effective intrinsic motivators for learning and for activation of all the prerequisites for a successful integration of learning experience. These include, for instance, spatial orientation, exploration in available perceptual modalities, and energetic adjustments in the autonomic system, where the costs for integrative processes are far from negligible during the first months of postpartum life.

Thus, the integration of the first postpartum experiences represents relatively difficult and, in terms of metabolic adjustments, costly processes. Observable cue signals indicating changes in the infant's behavioral/emotional state, the course of coping with novel situations, and the limits of infant tolerance play a particularly important role in the care of young infants; they help caregivers to facilitate infant learning and to avoid interventions that might go beyond the limits of infant tolerance. Sir

Karl Popper's (1994) principle that all life is problem solving is certainly true about the very beginning of human postpartum life. In our interpretation of interrelationships between the course of integrative processes and the regulation of infant behavior, we (Papoušek & Papoušek, 1979a) have drawn attention to this aspect and described, among others, a "biological fuse" that protects young infants against the stress of difficult coping in the form of a sudden temporary reduction of responsiveness reminiscent of "playing possum."

In studies on infant learning, I (H. P.) have tried to design learning experiments parallel to the integration of everyday experience: In a special combination of instrumental learning and Pavlovian conditioning, infants have to detect a contingent event on the one hand and, at the same time, learn that they can control the event only in the presence of a conditioning signal (Papoušek, 1967). This design can be modified to reach various degrees of complexity, and it can also be used in preverbal infants for studies of concept formation, including numerical concepts at the age of 4–5 months (Papoušek, 1969). Thus, these studies have allowed an insight into the early development of integrative capacities and have shown that, with age, infant capacities improve not only as a result of maturation but also as a result of learning experience and environmental interventions in the form of suitable arrangements of experimental tasks (Papoušek & Papoušek, 1984). However, the complexity of early-life conditions is hard to model in laboratory experiments. The newborn infant has to cope with many novel circumstances, from the circadian periodicity and differences between intrauterine and extrauterine environments to the confrontation with a new social milieu and its challenging efforts to communicate.

Learning how to communicate represents perhaps the most important developmental process to take place during infancy. The process depends on innate predispositions, just as it does on sociocultural factors. It requires a complex orchestration of motor skills, physiological functions, and integrative capacities in the central nervous system. As shown in the aforementioned experimental studies, fundamental forms of infant learning function only under favorable conditions, such as an appropriate behavioral state, a relatively large number of repetitive learning trials, or the careful arrangement and display of learning episodes with respect to feedback cues indicating infant attention and tolerance.

During the initial absence of speech signals, any observable component of infant behavior may function as a communicative signal insofar as the caregiver is capable of processing it in this sense. At the same time, it may also serve as an intentional communicative signal as soon as the infant has detected its contingent effects on the caregiver and has learned the rules of its use. Although caregivers cannot explain anything about verbal communication to preverbal infants in words, infants typically demonstrate an evident tendency to detect the rules of communication and to imitate and learn a spoken language in speaking families or a sign language in signing families (for review, see Papoušek, 1994). The acquisition of verbal competence gives integrative processes new dimensions: fast and economic accumulation of information, the use of abstract and hierarchically structured symbolic thinking, the development of conscious self, and interactions with culture. Thus, integrative and communicative competence of human infants develop under a sociocultural guidance beyond the universal mammalian scope in the direction of human-specific forms of communication and cultural integration.

As explained in the preceding section of this chapter, infant predispositions for the acquisition of species-specific means of human communication function in an intimate interaction with parental predispositions for supporting this acquisition process in intuitive, didactically effective ways (Papoušek & Bornstein, 1992; Papoušek, 1992). However, if the communicative circumstances are defective or too difficult, they may surpass the limits of infant integrative capacities and cause behavioral disorders (Papoušek & Papoušek, 1992).

This conceptual framework concerning the infant's early mental and communicative abilities and the mother's support of them may differ from other interpretations in several respects. For example, infants' slow development in locomotion is not viewed as a general altricity; human infants are precocious in communication and symbolic thinking, and the development of these abilities may profit from the close contact with the caregiver (Papoušek & Papoušek, 1984). As another example, infant behaviors are not viewed as mere expressions of emotional feelings; as pointed out by Bühler (1935), they not only express internal feelings but also represent situational contexts and appeal to the social environment for responses. Intimate interrelationships between learning/cognitive processes and expressions of internal affects have been observed under experimental conditions (Papoušek, 1967).

IMMINENT VICIOUS CIRCLES

As we explained in preceding sections, mother–infant interactions in humans consist of substantially more than an exchange of expressions of affective bonding. Unlike the situation with all other animals, primates included, human parenting generally subserves the early development of highly effective means of species-specific adaptation—processing of symbolic information, speech, and cultural integration. Parents, mothers in particular under typical circumstances, guide infants toward these unique capacities along an avenue that is predetermined by biological predispositions during the preverbal period of development. The characteristics of these predispositions, universality, relative independence of conscious control, close relation to affects, indicate their significant position in behavioral regulation, as is typical for biologically relevant means of adaptation in general.

The interplay of infantile and parental predispositions is astonishingly harmonious and mutually rewarding for both partners as long as all prerequisites function smoothly and no unfavorable contextual factors intervene. Under such conditions, the course of pleasurable interactions can facilitate developmental processes in the infant as well as reinforce self-

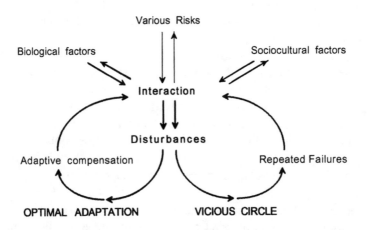

COURSE OF MOTHER - INFANT INTERACTIONS

FIGURE 2.1. A hypothetical model of interrelationships between the course of mother–infant interactions and various biological, sociological, or other risk factors. A twofold path of outcome is indicated: either a compensatory effect and strengthening of the dyad's resistance or a vicious circle that may lead to serious failures.

confidence and facilitate the display of intuitive interventions in the mother, as Figure 2.1 hypothetically suggests (according to Papoušek & Papoušek, 1979b). Such mother–infant dyads may cope easily with various difficulties and successfully resist environmental risk factors. By contrast, however, interactional disorders themselves may act as risk factors that are more dangerous, the more relevant the means of adaptation they concern. Minor initial deviations can elicit chains of secondary deteriorations and initiate vicious circles. Thus, difficulties in mother–infant communication can lead to serious interactional failures, including maternal rejection of the infant (MacCarthy & Booth, 1970; Winnicott, 1931) and child abuse (Kreisler, 1984).

Because of its adaptive significance in the human evolution, communication seems to play a central role among the factors that lend early mother–infant interactions the character of either an effective mechanism of reinforcement and compensation or an imminent vicious circle. The dual role of early communication in the environmental support to infant development should be kept in mind: It fortifies emotional bonding on the one hand and serves as a vehicle for didactic interventions that train learning and cognitive capacities in infants on the other hand (Papoušek & Papoušek, 1984, 1987). For this reason, the bilateral interrelationships between communicative failures and other disturbances in mental development are very close.

For instance, children have frequently been treated as mentally retarded or behaviorally disturbed, although the primary defect originally concerned only the production of speech sounds (Amorosa, 1992; Martin, 1981). In other cases, a primary muscular hypotonia with a decreased expressiveness in facial and vocal signaling can, secondarily, lead to communicative failures, parental neglect, and an impairment of originally normal intellect in infants. Hearing defects can cause social isolation and mental retardation because of the ineffective environmental support of infants' communicative and integrative capacities. This support can also be missing in otherwise healthy infants because of social deprivation or maternal rejection following an unwanted pregnancy.

Summarizing initial clinical evidence, we (Papoušek & Papoušek, 1992) have drawn attention to the following, particularly frequent, clinical combinations of communicative and integrative disorders:

1. *Missed experience in initial communication.* For various reasons, such as maternal separation due to perinatal complications, father's ab-

sence, or the isolation of premature newborns due to intensive medical care, parents miss the first chance of interacting with newborns and orchestrating intuitive predispositions for parenting in accordance with the newborn's individuality. Although most parents may overcome the effects of such disruptions, some parents may be discouraged or may misinterpret the lack of infant attention to them as their own incompetence. Similar situations may arise if parents adopt an older infant.

2. *Initial discouragement due to infant handicaps.* Infant initial responsivity and communicative expressiveness may temporarily decrease as a result of postpartum complications (e.g., muscular hypotonia or hyperbilirubinemic hypersomnia). Conversely, an increased irritability in hypoxic newborns may similarly complicate initial communication. Unsuccessful parental attempts to initiate interchanges, together with deviant or absent responses in infants, may inhibit intuitive predispositions in parents, and such an inhibition may persist beyond the infant's recovery.

3. *Mismatch between parental and infantile predispositions.* Occasionally, parental predispositions may become maladaptive because of contextual incongruences. For instance, perceptual thresholds may be elevated in an infant due to various nervous disorders. Such an infant would still respond to sufficiently intensive stimulations; however, his or her parents may act under the impression of being confronted with a sick and fragile infant and therefore may tend to use careful, tender stimulation that is too weak for the infant to perceive.

4. *Major prolongation in the need for preverbal forms of communication.* For various reasons, some children do not acquire speech during the first few years of life. In the meantime, they lose the features of babyishness that, along with behavioral cues, elicit intuitive support to speech acquisition. Although these children still need the kind of support that parents give to preverbal infants, they no longer elicit it in parents. Moreover, the parents' original competence may have been inhibited because of a lack of communicative success in previous efforts

Frequently, early communicative failures lead to excessive crying or behavioral disorders in infants and to the necessity on the parents' part to seek medical help for infants. However, a thorough examination often reveals primary causes of infantile difficulties in the marital or socioeconomic problems of the parents themselves. Unfortunately, some family physicians or pediatricians tend to medicate the infant with various sedative drugs rather than examining potential risk factors in the infant's environment. For this reason, I (M.P.) organized a special consulting service and a research center for families with excessively crying infants in Munich in 1990 (Papoušek et al., 1994). In close collaboration, pediatricians and psychologists specializing in developmental neurology, psychiatry, clinical psychology, and psychotherapy examine both infantile and environmental circumstances as thoroughly as possible and analyze parent–infant interactions with the help of audiovisual microanalyses (Papoušek & Papoušek, 1987) under laboratory conditions. In serious situations, infants together with the parents can be observed and/or treated in a lying-in department. Some cases illustrate close interrelationships between interactive or communicative failures and maternal postpartum depression (Table 2.1).

In 75 cases, families were referred to this center because of seemingly groundless crying in the infant that was hard to appease and tolerate and had mostly begun soon after the birth. Frequent periods of distress (in

TABLE 2.1. Mother's Psychological Condition, Infant Temperament, and Marital Dissatisfaction during the First 6-Postpartum Months

Infant groups	Low cry	Medium cry	High cry	ANOVA: F($df=2$)	p
Mean duration of crying/fussing (minutes per 24 hours)	62.4	110.9	295.0		
Edinburgh Postnatal Depression Scale (mothers above the cutoff value of 12)	4.0* 0.0	7.0* 5.0	10.5* 66.6	13.8	.0000
Maternal Child-Care Attitudes and Feelings (Engfer)					
Anxious Overprotection	16.8	18.5	21.5*	4.9	.01
Anger/Frustration	15.9*	19.4*	23.5*	15.3	.0000
Exhaustion/Overstrain	14.4*	20.4	20.9	16.0	.0000
Depressed Mood	14.9*	21.5	24.2	24.9	.0000
Self-Efficacy (Lips)	120.9*	109.0	108.2	10.4	.0001
Infant Characteristics Questionnaire (Bates)					
Difficulty	20.1*	28.7*	35.2*	40.6	.0000
Unpredictability	8.8	9.9	12.9*	8.2	.0007
Unadaptability	9.1*	11.6	12.8	5.5	.006
Marital Dissatisfaction (BELPAR)	5.8	8.9	13.4*	7.7	.0009
Social Provision Scale (SPS)	27.3	25.7	24.7	2.3	.10

Note. One-way analysis of variance (ANOVA).
*Duncan multiple-range test with significance level = .05.

52.9% of infants), sleep disorders (85.8%), feeding disorders (25.1%), and interactive irregularities (11.6%) characterized the infants, along with the excessive crying. Maternal pregnancy showed complications that were mild in 62% of cases, and serious in 29% of cases; in the newborns, mild neurological deviations were found in 35% of cases and serious deviations in 6% of cases. Psychosocial forms of stress appeared in 46% of families. Recurrent infections were reported in 29% of infants and various other pediatric complications in 17%.

As shown in Table 2.1, maternal depression—both in terms of the Edinburgh Postnatal Depression Scale (as modified for German samples) and Engfer's Scale for Maternal Child-Care Attitudes and Feelings—significantly correlated with the infant's duration of crying. Mothers were increasingly inclined to anxious overprotection, exhaustion, and frustration with the frequency of infant crying. In a similar correlation, they found their infants increasingly difficult, hard to predict, and insufficiently adapted, according to Bates's Infant Characteristics Questionnaire.

The frequency of marital dissatisfaction was significantly correlated with the number of infant crying episodes, whereas the role of social support, according to the Social Provision Scale, showed no significant influence. With respect to the approximative character of the scales applied, it should be noted that statistical criteria can serve as mere orientational indicators for clinical attempts to analyze complex interactional systems when exact measures of all involved factors and the application of nonlinear models are not yet thinkable.

The necessary clinical conclusion should be not to look for primary causes either in infants or in parents but to try to mitigate all risk factors in question in a complex therapeutic intervention. Acebo and Thoman (1992) similarly recommended that the social context should be taken into account for an infant's crying as a window on the nature of the mother–infant relationship. Maternal postpartum depression may represent another such window.

CONCLUSION

Mindful of the frequent dysphoric postpartum states in mothers, we have attempted to review our experiences from both experimental research and clinical observations and consider potential risk factors that are difficult to assess and often escape attention. Our considerations are based on the evidence that, from the very beginning of maternity, the mother–infant communication plays a crucial role in both the motivational systems controlling interactional behaviors and the pathogeny of mental or emotional disorders. This position of communication is based on the specific adaptive relevance of communication in human evolution.

Various factors connected with the constraints in integrative and communicative capacities in infants or with the lability of maternal attitudes and caregiving predispositions in mothers can disturb the complex interchanges between mothers and infants that would otherwise strengthen the resistance of the mother–infant system against unfavorable circumstances.

If the mother–infant communication does not develop adequately, its compensatory function fails, and vicious circles with serious consequences can develop as was evident in our clinical observations on the coincidence of excessive infant crying and maternal depression.

In our view, taking the functional involvement of communicative processes in the behavioral regulation into account helps elucidate the pathways between disorders in mother–infant interchanges and the pathogeny of postpartum depression in some clinical forms, at least.

Unfortunately, clinical assessment of the infantile or maternal factors concerned is not easy. The clinician should remember that both the infant constraints and the disturbances of maternal caregiving predispositions have been detected in elaborate experimental analyses of mother–infant interactions. Typically, the caregiving predispositions almost entirely escape the individual's conscious awareness. Therefore, detailed audiovisual analyses of mother–infant interactions cannot be replaced with interviews or questionnaires. Similarly, direct instructions on how to communicate with an infant cannot help the mother either; she cannot rationally and consciously control each of the hundreds of minute supportive interventions which she intuitively—and without any strain—displays in daily dialogues with the infant under normal circumstances.

Conversely, there are various forms of therapeutic intervention that can generally mitigate situational stressors and thus indirectly improve functioning of the specific caregiving predispositions. Obviously, in addition to medical help, adequate psychotherapeutic and social services should be available, based, of course, on the present understanding of the significance of mother–infant communication.

ACKNOWLEDGMENTS

The preparation of this chapter was kindly supported by the Alexander von Humboldt Foundation.

REFERENCES

Acebo, C., & Thoman, E. B. (1992). Crying as social behaviour. *Infant Mental Health Journal, 13*, 67–82.

Amorosa, H. (1992). Disorders of vocal signalling in children. In H. Papoušek, U. Jürgens, & M. Papoušek (Eds.), *Nonverbal vocal communication: Comparative and developmental approaches* (pp. 192–204). New York: Cambridge University Press.

von Bertalanffy, L. (1968). *General systems theory: Foundations, development, applications.* New York: Braziller.

Blumberg, N. J. (1980). Effects of neonatal risk, maternal attitude, and cognitive style on early postpartum adjustment. *Journal of Abnormal Psychology, 89,* 139–150.

Bühler, K. (1934). *Sprachtheorie.* Jena, Germany: Fischer.

Buxbaum, E. (1983). Vulnerable mothers—vulnerable babies. In J. D. Call, E. Galenson, & R. L. Tyson (Eds.), *Frontiers of infant psychiatry* (pp. 86–94). New York: Basic Books.

Cox, A. D., Puckering, C., Pound, A., & Mills, M. (1987). The impact of maternal depression in young children. *Journal of Child Psychology and Psychiatry, 28,* 917–928.

Erting, C. J., Prezioso, C., & Hynes, M. O. (1990). The interactional context of deaf mother–infant communication. In V. Volterra & C. Erting (Eds.), *From gesture to language in hearing and deaf children* (pp. 97–106). Berlin: Springer-Verlag.

Field, T. M. (1984). Early interactions between infants and their postpartum depressed mothers. *Infant Behaviour and Development, 7,* 517–522.

Hopkins, J., Marcus, M., & Campbell, S. B. (1984). Postpartum depression: A critical review. *Psychological Bulletin, 95,* 498–515.

Kestermann, G. (1982). *Gestik von Säuglingen: Ihre kommunikative Bedeutung für erfahrene und unerfahrene Bezugspersonen* [*Gesticulation in infants: Their communicative significance for experienced and inexperienced caregivers*]. Doctoral dissertation, University of Bielefeld, Germany.

Kihlstrom, J. F. (1987). The cognitive unconscious. *Science, 237,* 1445–1452.

Kreisler, L. (1984). Paediatric to psychosomatic economy: Fundamentals for a psychosomatic pathology of infants. In J. D. Call, E. Galenson, & R. L. Tyson (Eds.), *Frontiers of infant psychiatry* (Vol. II, pp. 447–454). New York: Basic Books.

MacCarthy, D., & Booth, E. M. (1970). Parental rejection and stunting of growth. *Journal of Psychosomatic Research, 14,* 259–265.

Martin, J. A. M. (1981). *Voice, speech, and language in the child: Development and disorder.* New York: Springer.

McLean, P. D. (1990). *The triune brain in evolution. Role in paleocerebral functions.* New York: Plenum Press.

Murray, L. (1992). The impact of postnatal depression on infant development. *Journal of Child Psychology and Psychiatry, 33,* 543–561.

Murray, L., Stanley, C., Hooper, R., King, F., & Fiori-Cowley, A. (1996). The role of infant factors in postnatal depression and mother–infant interactions. *Developmental Medicine and Child Neurology, 38,* 109–119.

Murray, L., & Trevarthen, C. (1985). Emotional regulation of interactions between two-month-olds and their mothers. In T. M. Field & N. A. Fox (Eds.), *Social perception in infants* (pp. 177–197). Norwood, NJ: Ablex.

O'Hara, M. W., Rehm, L. P., & Campbell, S. B. (1983). Postpartum depression: A role for social network and life stress variables. *Journal of Nervous and Mental Disease, 171,* 336–341.

Papoušek, H. (1967). Experimental studies of appetitional behaviour in human newborns and infants. In H. W. Stevenson, E. H. Hess, & H. L. Rheingold (Eds.), *Early behavior: Comparative and developmental approaches* (pp. 249–277). New York: Wiley.

Papoušek, H. (1969). Individual variability in learned responses during early post-natal development. In R. J. Robinson (Ed.), *Brain and early behaviour. Development in the fetus and infant* (pp. 229–252). London: Academic Press.

Papoušek, H. (1977). Entwicklung der Lernfähigkeit im Säuglingsalter [Development of learning abilities during infancy]. In G. Nissen (Ed.), *Intelligenz, Lernen und Lernstörungen* [*Intelligence, learning and learning disorders*] (pp. 89–197). Berlin: Springer-Verlag.

Papoušek, H., & Bornstein, M. H. (1992). Didactic interactions: Intuitive parental support of vocal and verbal development in humans. In H. Papoušek, U. Jürgens, & M. Papoušek (Eds.), *Nonverbal vocal communication: Comparative and developmental aspects* (pp. 209–229). Cambridge, England: Cambridge University Press.

Papoušek, H., & Papoušek, M. (1978). Interdisciplinary parallels in studies of early human behaviour: From physical to cognitive needs, from attachment to dyadic education. *International Journal of Behavioural Development, 1,* 37–49.

Papoušek, H., & Papoušek, M. (1979a). The infant's fundamental adaptive response system in social interaction. In E. B. Thoman (Ed.), *Origins of the infant's social responsiveness* (pp. 175–208). Hillsdale, NJ: Erlbaum.

Papoušek, H., & Papoušek, M. (1979b). Care of the normal and high risk newborn: A psychobiological view of parental behaviour. In S. Harel (Ed.), *The at risk infant* (International Congress Series No. 492, pp. 368–371). Amsterdam: Excerpta Medica.

Papoušek, H., & Papoušek, M. (1984). Learning and cognition in the everyday life of human infants. In J. S. Rosenblatt, C. Beer, M.-C. Busnel, & P. J. B. Slater (Eds.), *Advances in the study of behavior* (Vol. 14, pp. 127–163). New York: Academic Press.

Papoušek, H., & Papoušek, M. (1987). Intuitive parenting: A dialectic counter-part to the infant's integrative competence. In J. D. Osofsky (Ed.), *Handbook of infant development* (2nd ed., pp. 669–720). New York: Wiley.

Papoušek, H., & Papoušek, M. (1989). Intuitive parenting: Aspects related to educational psychology [Special issue]. *European Journal of Psychology of Education, 4*(2), 201–210.

Papoušek, H., & Papoušek, M. (1992). Beyond emotional bonding: The role of preverbal communication in mental growth and health. *Infant Mental Health Journal, 13,* 43–53.

Papoušek, H., & Papoušek, M. (1995). Intuitive parenting. In M. H. Bornstein (Ed.), *Handbook of parenting: Vol. II. Ecology and biology of parenting* (pp. 117–136). Hillsdale, NJ: Erlbaum.

Papoušek, M. (1992). Early ontogeny of vocal communication in parent–infant interactions. In H. Papoušek, U. Jürgens, & M. Papoušek, (Eds.), *Nonverbal vocal communication: Comparative and developmental aspects* (pp. 230–261). Cambridge, England: Cambridge University Press.

Papoušek, M. (1994). *Vom ersten Schrei zum ersten Wort: Anfänge der Sprachentwicklung in der vorsprachlichen Kommunikation* [*From the first cry to the first word: The beginnings of speech development in preverbal communication*]. Bern: Huber.

Papoušek, M., Bornstein, M. H., Nuzzo, C., Papoušek, H., & Symmes, D. (1990). Infant responses to prototypical melodic contours in parental speech. *Infant Behaviour and Development, 13,* 539–545.

Papoušek, M., Hofacker, V. N., Malinowski, M., Jacubeit, T., & Cosmovici, B. (1994). Münchener Sprechstunde für Schreibabys. Erste Ergebnisse zur Früherkennung und Prävention von Störungen der Verhaltensregulation und der Eltern-Kind-Beziehungen [The Munich Fussy Baby Program: The first data on early detection and prevention of disorders in behavioural regulation and parent–infant interaction]. *Sozialpädiatrie und Kinderärztliche Praxis, 16*(11), 680–686.

Papoušek, M., Papousek, H., & Bornstein, M. H. (1985). The naturalistic vocal environment of young infants: On the significance of homogeneity and variability in parental speech. In T. Field & N. Fox (Eds.), *Social perception in infants* (pp. 269–297). Norwood, NJ: Ablex.

Popper, K. R. (1994). *Alles Leben ist Problemlösen: Über Erkenntnis, Geschichte und Politik* [*All life is problem solving: On cognition, history and politics*]. Munich: Piper.

Radke-Yarrow, M., Cummings, E. M., Kuczynski, L., & Chapman, M. (1985). Patterns of attachment in two- and three-year olds in normal families and families with parental depression. *Child Development, 56,* 884–893.

Sameroff, A. J., & Chandler, M. J. (1975). Reproductive risk and the continuum of caretaking casuality. In F. P. Horowitz (Ed.), *Review of child development research* (Vol. 4, pp. 187–244). Chicago: University of Chicago Press.

Schoetzau, A., & Papoušek, H. (1977). Mütterliches Verhalten bei der Aufnahme von Blickkontakt mit dem Neugeborenen [Maternal behavior in relation to the achievement of visual contact with the newborn]. *Zeitschrift für Entwicklungspsychologie und Pädagogische Psychologie, 9,* 231–239.

Vander, A. J., Sherman, J. H., & Luciano, D. S. (1990). *Human physiology: The mechanisms of body functions* (5th ed.). New York: McGraw-Hill.

Winnicott, D. W. (1931). *Clinical notes on disorders of childhood.* London: Heinemann.

3

Depressed Mothers and Infants: Failure to Form Dyadic States of Consciousness

E. Z. Tronick
M. Katherine Weinberg
Harvard Medical School

Our primary aim in this chapter is to present a model of the process of infant emotional functioning and experience—the Model of Mutual Regulation—that in part accounts for the toxic effects of maternal depression on a child's social–emotional functioning and development. A consequence of successful mutual regulation, the creation of dyadic states of consciousness is presented as a way of explaining why humans so strongly seek states of intersubjectivity. To accomplish these aims, we summarize our work on microanalytic studies of normal interactions and our experimental perturbations of interactions in the Face-to-Face Still-Face Paradigm. We do not review the literature on maternal depressive effects, normal interactions, or intersubjectivity, much of which is available in other chapters of this volume.

Our research focuses on understanding normal interactions, including interactive errors and repairs, deviations, and disruptions. It also provides an understanding of the different emotional and social regulatory styles observed in the sons and daughters of depressed as well as normal mothers. Our hope is to understand why some children of depressed mothers develop behavioral disorders or even a pathology that is similar to their mother's pathology. We also recognize that many of these children develop normally. Thus an account of the development of children of depressed mothers must ipso facto account for a wide variety of outcomes including normalcy: a daunting task.

THE MUTUAL REGULATION MODEL

The Mutual Regulation Model (MRM) focuses on the joint or interactive nature of development. A critical assumption of the MRM is that the infant is motivated to communicate with people or, as we originally formulated, to establish intersubjective states (Tronick, 1980, 1989). This motivation is assumed to be a biological characteristic of our species, but see later for a systems-based interpretation. (Tronick, 1980; Bruner, 1995; Trevarthen, 1979, 1989a, 1990). The child also is inherently motivated to act on the world of objects. The accomplishment of motivated action on the inanimate world, however, depends on the establishment of intersubjective relationships. As is the case for adults, children can only create meanings in collaboration with others. Their understanding of the world of objects, no matter how primitive, depends on establishing intersubjective states with others and the mutual construction of meaning. Thus, the establishment of social relationships is the primary process of development and the understanding of the inanimate world is secondary to it. When the child successfully accomplishes communication with others which creates dyadic states of consciousness, normal development occurs. A child who does not engage the world in a culturally appropriate manner does not develop normally no matter what causes the failure—chronic or acute illness, congenital malformations, poor parenting, toxic exposures, or parental psychopathology.

Success or failure in accomplishing motivated intentions depends on at least three critical processes among others. The first is the integrity and capacity of the child's physiological systems and central nervous system to organize and control the child's physiological states and behavior. The second is the integrity of the infant's communicative system including the central nervous system centers that control and generate messages and meanings and the motor system that makes the messages manifest. The earliest and continuing function of the communicative system is to express the child's intention for action to the caregiver and to communicate the extent to which the infant is succeeding or failing in fulfilling his or her intentions or goals. The third process, reciprocal to the second, is the caretaker's capacity to read appropriately the child's communications and willingness to take appropriate action. Therefore, successful engagement with the world of people and things depends on the status and the effectiveness of the child–caretaker communicative system in facilitating the child's motivated intentions. These processes make up the process of mutual regulation: the capacity of each of the interactants, child and adult, to express their motivated intentions, to appreciate the intentions of the partner, and to scaffold their partner's actions so that their partner can achieve their goals.

THE WORKINGS OF MUTUAL REGULATION

How does the mutual regulatory process work? We focus on its workings from the child's perspective, but it should be obvious that the model applies to the adult as well. When infants are not in homeostatic balance (e.g., they are cold) or are emotionally dysregulated (e.g., they are distressed), they are at the mercy of these states. Until these states are brought under control, infants must devote all their regulatory resources to reorganizing them. While infants are doing that, they can do nothing else. Their engagement with people or things is preempted by their internal discordance and by the singular devotion of their capacities to overcome it. On the other hand, when their internal states are controlled, infants are free to take agency and act on the world. Their internal states become an organized background for foreground actions with people and things (Sander, 1983).

This account sounds like the precept of Claude Bernard—the maintenance of milieu interior is the organism's primary task. Bernard, however, failed to appreciate a critical feature of the homeostatic regulatory process for humans (and many other species as well). For humans, the maintenance of homeostasis is a dyadic collaborative process. Humans evolved in such a manner that they must collaborate with others to regulate their physiological states, emotional states, and external engagements with people and objects. Obviously, the infant is a bounded organism and the adult is external to that boundary. Nonetheless, the adult is a part of the infant's regulatory system, as much a part as any internal regulatory process.

What do we mean by this? We start with an example of Bernard's classic case of temperature regulation. Although Bernard did not see it, the regulation of the infant's core body temperature is a dyadic process. Infants may regulate their temperature by changing their posture and increasing their activity level. They may also be held against the caretaker's body. These processes, internal and external, are functionally equivalent processes for regulating the infant's temperature. Moreover, these regulatory processes involve communication among different components of the infant's regulatory system. Central and peripheral mechanisms, which respond to signals from central and peripheral sites, guide changes in metabolism. Active (e.g., crying) and passive (e.g., color changes) signals from the infant guide changes in the holding patterns of caretakers. Thus the infant's physiological state is dyadically regulated with the caregiver functioning as an external regulatory component of the infant's regulatory system. As we shall see, infant emotions are also regulated dyadically. The principal components are the infant's central nervous system (e.g., primarily the limbic system) and the behaviors it controls (e.g., facial and vocal emotional displays) and the caregiver's regulatory input (e.g., facial expressions). Communication between internal and external components (i.e., infant and caregiver) guides this dyadic collaborative regulatory system.

The animal as well as the human literature supports the idea of caregiver behavior as an external regulator of the infant's states. Hofer (1981, 1984) demonstrated that specific maternal stimuli modify a host of the immature offspring's physiological systems. Maternal body warmth affects the infant's neuroendocrine system, maternal touch affects growth hormone production, and maternal milk affects heart rate, B adrenergic systems, responsiveness to touch, and the production of growth hormone. Importantly, it is not just the body that is affected by caretaker behavior but the brain as well (Lester & Tronick, 1994). What we now know about brain development is a radical shift from the perspective that saw interactive experience as modifying only what an already formed brain learns or stores. We now know that the quality of caretaking affects the function, structure, and neurochemical architecture of the brain. For example, maternal touch affects hippocampal cell production and the production of neurotransmitters (Gunzenhauser, 1987; Spinelli, 1987).

In the following passage, pediatric neurologist Heinz Prechtl clearly expresses this view:

> The effects of selective pressure on the preprogrammed maturation of the nervous system [and related changes in behavior] should not be considered without taking into account the influence of the care-giver. There is an inevitable process of matching between the offspring and care-giver through mutual influences. Put differently, the young will only survive and grow and develop properly if the mothering and nursing repertory of the care-giver is precisely adapted to the properties of the young and vice versa. . . . [Thus] within limits, during normal development a biologically different brain may be formed given the mutual influence of maturation of the infant's nervous system and the mothering repertory of the caregiver (adapted from Prechtl; in Connelly & Prechtl, 1981, pp. 199, 212)

Prechtl's position is broad; nonetheless, he is specific that non-neurological factors such as the "mothering and nursing repertory" and caregiver's and infant's behavioral characteristics are among the primary forces shaping the organization of the infant's brain. These effects have lifetime consequences. For example, the increase in the proliferation of hippocampal cells associated with maternal touch in infancy has an effect on memory during senescence (Schore, 1994; Gunzenhauser, 1987). Thus, the critical nature of mutual regulation is clear—it shapes the behavior, the body, and the brain (Tronick & Morelli, 1991).

THE MUTUAL REGULATION OF INFANT–MOTHER (AND OTHER) SOCIAL INTERACTIONS

Research into social interactions between infants and parents began with Brazelton's pioneering study (Brazelton, Koslowski, & Main, 1974). Brazelton filmed the face-to-face interactions of mothers and infants and then coded the mothers' and infants' behavior on a second-by-second time base. Brazelton characterized the interaction as reciprocal, that is, infant and mother moving in synchrony from positive through negative behavioral states. The cycle was analogized to a sinusoid wave with "synchrony" requiring the matching of both positive and negative emotions. At about the same time, Condon and Sander (1974) described a phenomenon of microsynchrony between infant movement and the phoneme boundaries of the adult partner's speech. They professed that infant movements of a variety of limbs were coincident with the phoneme boundaries of speech. This coordination was too fast to take place on a contingent basis because movements take longer to organize than the duration of phoneme boundaries. Thus, Condon and Sander argued that there was a coordination of the biorhythms of speech and movement that accounted for the observed synchrony.

These two terms—"synchrony" and "reciprocity"—became the primary descriptors for normal mother–infant interactions. Synchrony was argued to be the optimal state of the interaction and to be nearly perfect over the course of the interaction (Condon & Sander, 1974). In addition, in the synchrony model, the interaction was seen as having high levels of positive emotions, little anger, sadness, or distress. Thus "optimal" mother–infant interactions were typically in "synch" and emotionally positive. Other features of the synchrony model included the characterization of the infant as diffusely organized. Therefore, the infant's behavior was unrelated to specific stimulation expressed by the adult. From this perspective the infant did not appreciate or respond to the mother's social affective behavior. Rather, the mother was the active interactant and she created the structure of the interaction. Thus, the interaction was seen as a "pseudo-dialogue" (Schaffer, 1977; Kaye, 1977). The mother structured the interaction and made the infant appear "as if" he was active. The "optimal" interaction was analogized to a synchronous dance with one partner fully in control; it was a unilaterally regulated system.

Based on the synchrony model, researchers developed clinical assessment scales that rated the interaction on a dimension of synchrony, attunement, or contingency (Massie, 1982). Underlying these scales was the widely accepted assumption that the more synchronous and contingent the interaction, the more positive the affect, the better the interaction, and the more optimal the outcome of the child. The synchrony model was a prototypical model and allowed for little variation and, like other categorical models, saw deviation from the prototype as (potentially) pathological.

The Failure of the Synchrony Model

Using the temporal microanalytical coding systems (Tronick & Cohn, 1989; Dowd & Tronick, 1986; Weinberg & Tronick, 1989, 1992, 1994, 1996; Cohn & Tronick, 1987, 1988, 1989; Mayer & Tronick, 1985; Tronick, 1985), we found that the synchrony model needed radical revision. We found that infants, mothers, and their interactions did not fit the model. We found that infants' communicative behavior was well organized and contingently related to maternal communicative behaviors (Weinberg & Tronick, 1994; Tronick & Cohn, 1989). Furthermore, we found little evidence for the synchrony described by Condon and Sander (Dowd & Tronick, 1986). We did find that infants, as well as their mothers, adjusted their behavior in relation to the behavior of their partner with some measurable temporal delay (Cohn & Tronick, 1988). Moreover, we found that the interactions of normal mothers and their infants were characterized at most by moderate levels of positive affect, by some negative affect, and by only moderate levels of synchrony (Tronick & Cohn, 1989; Cohn & Tronick, 1987).

Infant communicative behavior is hardly diffuse. Weinberg and Tronick (1994) found that infant affective behavior is organized into configurations of face, voice, gesture, and gaze. In one configuration, labeled social engagement, the infant looks at the mother, positively vocalizes, and smiles. Importantly, crying, looking away, and withdrawal behaviors are less likely to occur. In another configuration, active protest, the infant looks away from the mother, engages in active withdrawal behaviors, cries, and displays a facial expression of anger. In this configuration, smiles, and positive gestures and vocalizations are inhibited. There are two other configurations, object engagement and passive withdrawal, that also involve distinct combinations of expressive modalities. From our perspective, each of these configurations reflects a different state of brain organization that assembles distinctly different configurations of face, voice, and body. Such expressive configurations and brain organization shatter the idea that the infant is diffusely organized.

Each configuration clearly communicates the infant's affective state and evaluation of the interaction. The social engagement configuration functions to convey the message "I like what we are doing"; the active protest configuration tells the caregiver, "I don't like what is happening and I want it to change now"; the passive withdrawal configuration communicates such messages as "I don't like what is happening but I don't know what to do"; and the object engagement configuration conveys the message "Let's continue what we are doing, I like looking at this object." Thus the configurations regulate the behavior of the partner during the interaction by conveying information to the partner about the infant's immediate intentions and the infant's evaluation of the current state of the interaction. Nonetheless, as clearly defined as these configurations are, the interaction is neither always positive nor synchronous.

Normal Interactions, Boys and Girls, and Cultural Forms

In our studies of normal mother–infant face-to-face interactions, expressions of positive affect by either the mother or the infant occur, respectively, about 42% of the time for the mother and 15% of the time for the infant (Tronick & Cohn, 1989; Cohn & Tronick, 1987). A dramatic instance of normal variation is Weinberg's (1992; Weinberg & Tronick, 1992) finding of gender differences in the affective and regulatory behaviors of normal 6-month-old infants as well as differences in interactive coherence between mothers and sons and mothers and daughters (Tronick & Cohn, 1989; see also Hay, Chapter 4, this volume). Infant boys are more emotionally reactive than girls. They display more positive as well as negative affect, focus more on the mother, and display more signals expressing escape and distress and demands for contact than do girls. Girls show more interest in objects, a greater constancy of interest, and better self-regulation of emotional states. Girls also evidence greater stability of sadness over time than do boys. Sex differences in interactive coherence (i.e., synchrony) have also been demonstrated, with mother–son dyads evidencing more coherence than mother–daughter dyads (Tronick & Cohn, 1989). These gender differences reflect *normal* variants and highlight the range of affective expressiveness, regulatory behavior, and synchrony that occurs during normal interactions.

These findings speak strongly against hypotheses such as the synchrony model, which asserts that there is a single optimal form of interaction unless one is willing to assert that the interaction of boys (or girls) is more appropriate than the interaction of girls (or boys). The findings on differences in interactions in different communities also speak against optimization models of the mother–infant interaction. The structure of the interaction varies in different community settings where there are different emotional and interactive socialization goals for children. For example, Tronick and his colleagues (Keefer, Tronick, Dixon, & Brazleton, 1982) found that among the Gusii, an agricultural community in Western Kenya, mothers turn away from their infants just as their infants become most affectively positive and excited. Among the Gusii, this maternal behavior presages the socialization of later restrictions on the expression of positive affect among different individuals (e.g., younger individuals do not look directly at older individuals, especially when expressing strong affect). This looking-away pattern is normative for the Gusii but is quite different from that seen in the United States. American middle-income mothers respond to the infant's affective excitement with continued intense looking and heightened positive arousal.

Thus there is no singular universal optimal form of mother–child interaction in which deviations are considered pathological as implied by the synchrony model (but for an alternative view, see Trevarthen & Hubley, 1978; Trevarthen, 1990). Rather, interactions vary among individuals and across communities in regular and culturally meaningful ways. On a daily basis, infants repeatedly participate in interactive routines—routines with beginnings, middles, and ends—that eventually socialize the infant to appropriate culturally accepted social–emotional interactive practices. We can think of these interactive routines as having a narrative structure, even though it is a narrative of communicative action and not words (Bruner, 1983). Like a narrative, interactive routines serve as a meaning system for the child based on the sequencing of affective messages in the flow of social interaction. The child comes to "know" that "this is what is happening; this is what will happen; and this is how it will feel" (Bruner, 1995). This meaning system is established long before the child can engage in a narrative of words. In fact, we agree with Bruner (1983) that participation in this narrative of affective routines is a prerequisite for learning language. However, the unit of meaning is not primarily sensory–motor, although sensory–motor action in the form of affective communicative displays (e.g., facial expressions) is its manifest component (Cohen, 1988). The units of meaning (morphemes or, better yet, the sentences) are affective experiences (states of brain organization), and their sequencing in relation to external events, usually the communicative displays of others.

The analogy to narrative is limited. The interaction, as well as the affective meaning system, is jointly regulated and socially constructed by both the infant and the adult. Both partners appreciate and adjust their behavior in relation to their partner's behavior and the state of the interaction. In a series of papers, we have explored the contingencies and the structure of the interaction (Cohn & Tronick, 1987, 1988, 1989; Tronick, 1980; Tronick & Cohn, 1989). For example, episodes when the infant averts from the mother are prolonged by maternal elicitation and shortened when the mother watches and waits for the infant to look back at her (Cohn & Tronick, 1987).

Bidirectionality, Positive Affect, and Reparation

We have demonstrated this bidirectionality using time-series analyses of interactions at 3, 6, and 9 months of age (Cohn & Tronick, 1987; Tronick & Cohn, 1989; Mayer & Tronick, 1985). In these analyses, we found that the infant's and mother's behaviors are explained by two factors. The first is the infant's and the mother's own behaviors as measured by their autocorrelation. The autocorrelation measures how much of an individual's behavior can be accounted for by his or her own preceding behavior. The second component, as measured by the cross-correlation of the mother's and infant's behaviors after removal of the autocorrelation, indexes the degree of influence each partner has on the other. At 3 months of age, more than 50% of the mother's and 39% of the infant's behaviors were influenced by their partner's behaviors. This research indicates that a large proportion of mother–infant pairs are responding to and adjusting their affective behavior to the behavior of their partner. It is also of interest that the proportion of bidirectional pairs does not increase with infant age. Infants as young as 3 months appear to be as capable of making adjustments as are older infants. Perhaps this is a characteristic of the infant or of the dyad. Unfortunately, no research looking at the stability of bidirectionality has been carried out.

Despite the finding of bidirectionality, when we examined the proportion of time that mother and infant were in synchronous states, we found that synchrony occurred only a moderate proportion of the time (Tronick, Als, & Brazelton, 1980a). For example, matching of infant and mother social–affective states occurred only 24% of the time. In an alternative analysis of synchrony using time-series analysis, the coherence of the interaction accounted for only 17% of the variance of the interactions. Thus interactions are not as "synchronous" as predicted by the synchrony model. Rather, interactions move between matching/synchronous states and nonmatching/nonshared states, then back again to matching/synchronous states (Tronick & Cohn, 1989) (see Figure 3.1).

Based on these findings, Tronick (Tronick & Cohn, 1989) characterized the typical mother–infant interaction as one that moves from coordinated (or synchronous) to miscoordinated states and back again over a wide affective range (see Figure 3.2). The miscoordinated state is referred to as a normal interactive communicative error. The interactive transition from a miscoordinated state to a coordinated state is an "interactive repair." The process of reparation, like the dynamics of regulating

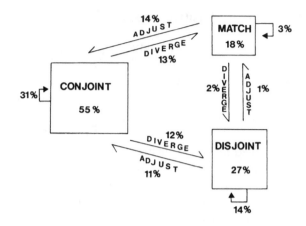

FIGURE 3.1. Movement of a 6-month-old mother–infant dyad among dyadically defined matching (e.g., mother and infant doing the same social–emotional actions at the same time), conjoint (e.g., mother and infant doing similar but not identical social–emotional actions at the same time), and disjoint (e.g., mother and infant engaging in different social emotional activities at the same time) states. "Adjust" is what is referred to in this chapter as reparation—that is, moving from less similar dyadic states to more similar states, whereas "diverge" is what is referred to here as an interactive error.

homeostatic states, is mutually regulated. The partners, infant and adult, signal their evaluation of the state of the interaction through their affective configurations. In turn, in response to their partner's signals each partner attempts to adjust his or her behavior to maintain a coordinated state or to repair an interactive error. Critically, successful reparations and the experience of coordinated states are associated with positive affective states whereas interactive errors generate negative affective states. Thus the infant's affective experience is determined by a dyadic regulatory process.

In normal dyads, interactive errors are quickly repaired. In studies of face-to-face interaction at 6 months of age, repairs occur at a rate of once every 3–5 seconds and more than one-third of all repairs occur by the next step in the interaction (Tronick & Gianino, 1980). Observations by Beebe (Beebe & Lachmann, 1994) and Isabella and Belsky (1991) replicate these findings and support the hypothesis that the normal interaction is a process of reparation. They found that maternal sensitivity in the midrange, rather than at the low or high end, typify normal interactions. Midrange sensitivity is characterized by errors and repairs as contrasted to interactions in which the mother is "never sensitive or always sensitive."

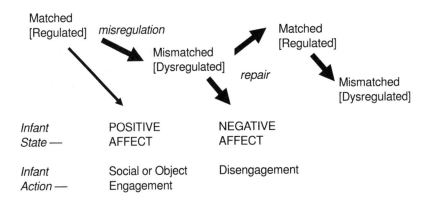

FIGURE 3.2. A schematic of the regulatory structure of the interaction. Matched or regulated states when misregulated change to mismatched states but reparation reachieves matched states. Matched states and reparation are associated with positive affect whereas mismatched states and interactive errors are associated with negative affect. Matching can either be purely social or focused on objects.

These researchers also found that midlevel sensitivity was associated with security of attachment.

The Functional Effects of Reparation and Reparatory Failure

It is our hypothesis that reparation of interactive errors is the critical process of normal interactions that is related to developmental outcome rather than synchrony or positive affect per se. That is, reparation, its experience and extent, is the "social–interactive mechanism" that affects the infant's development. In interactions characterized by normal rates of reparation, the infant learns which communicative and coping strategies are effective in producing reparation and when to use them. This experience leads to the elaboration of communicative and coping skills and the development of an understanding of interactive rules and conventions. With the experiential accumulation of successful reparations and the attendant transformation of negative affect into positive affect, the infant establishes a positive affective core (Emde, Kligman, Reich, & Wade, 1978; Gianino & Tronick, 1988). The infant also learns that he or she has control over social interactions. Specifically, the infant develops a representation of him- or herself as effective, of his or her interactions as positive and reparable, and of the caretaker as reliable and trustworthy. These representations are crucial for the development of a sense of self that has coherence, continuity, and agency and for the development of stable and secure relationships (Tronick, 1980; Tronick, Cohn, & Shea, 1986).

The functional consequences of reparation from the perspective of mutual regulation suggest that when there is a prolonged failure to repair communicative errors, infants initially attempt to reestablish the expected interaction, but when these reparatory efforts fail they experience negative affect. To evaluate this hypothesis, we created a prolonged mismatch by having the mother hold a still face and remain unresponsive to the infant (Tronick, Als, Adamson, Wise, & Brazelton, 1978). The mother fails to engage in her normal interactive behavior and regulatory role. The effect on the infant is dramatic. Infants almost immediately detect the change and attempt to solicit the mother's attention. Failing to elicit a response, most infants turn away only to look back at the mother again (see top part of Figure 3.3). This solicitation cycle may be repeated several times. But when infants' attempts fail to repair the interaction infants often lose postural control, withdraw, and self-comfort (see bottom part of Figure 3.3). The disengagement is profound even with this short disruption of the mutual regulatory process and break of intersubjectivity. The infant's reaction is reminiscent of the withdrawal of Harlow's isolated monkeys or of the infants in institutions observed by Bowlby and Spitz (Spitz, 1965; Bowlby, 1951, 1980). The still-faced mother is a short-lived, experimentally produced form of neglect.

Maternal Depression and Reparation

To examine the process of reparatory failure in natural settings we examined the interaction of infants with depressed mothers. We hypothesized that maternal depression, like the still face, disrupts the mutual regulatory process and constitutes a break in intersubjectivity. The break is brought about by the effects of depression on maternal affect and responsiveness. Depression compromises the mother's and eventually the dyad's capacity to mutually regulate the interaction (Cohn & Tronick, 1989; Gianino & Tronick, 1988; Tronick & Field, 1987; Weinberg & Tronick, 1994). However, we found that not all depressed mothers disrupt the interaction in the same fashion, and that depressed mothers with similar levels of depressive symptoms do not engage in the same interactive style (Cohn, Matias, Tronick, Connell, & Lyons-Ruth, 1986; Tronick, 1989). There are at least two interactive patterns (intrusiveness and withdrawal) and each disrupts the regulatory process. Importantly, each form has a different effect on the infant.

We found that "intrusive" mothers engaged in rough handling, spoke in an angry tone of voice, poked at their babies, and actively interfered with their infants' activities. Withdrawn mothers, by contrast, were disengaged, unresponsive, and affectively flat, and did little to support their infants' activities. As a striking demonstration of the sensitivity of the infant to affective displays, we found that infants of intrusive mothers

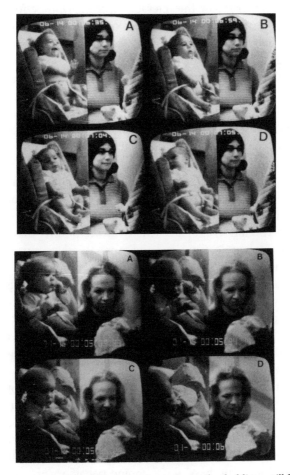

FIGURE 3.3. Sequences of two infants reacting to the mother holding a still face in Tronick's Face-to-Face Still-Face Paradigm.

(re)acted one way whereas infants of withdrawn mothers (re)acted another way. Infants of intrusive mothers spent most of their time looking away from the mother and seldom looked at objects. They cried infrequently. Infants of withdrawn mothers were more likely to protest and to be distressed than the infants of the intrusive mothers, suggesting that maternal withdrawal may be particularly aversive to young infants.

These differential infant reactions are expectable. The infants are reacting to and acting on different kinds of input (i.e., the affective reality they are regulating is different). Infants of withdrawn mothers are failing to achieve social connectedness because of the mothers' lack of response and their inability to repair the interaction. Initially, they may become angry. However, because they are unable to cope successfully or self-regulate this heightened negative state, they become dysregulated, fuss, and cry. This dysregulation, similar to the dysregulation associated with homeostatic failures, compels them to devote much of their coping resources to controlling their dysregulated affective state. With chronic exposure, they develop a disengaged and self-directed regulatory style characterized by self-comforting, self-regulatory behaviors (e.g., looking away, sucking on their thumb), passivity, and withdrawal as a way of coping with their state. To the extent that this coping style is successful in stabilizing their affective state, it is deployed automatically and becomes defensive. This self-directed style of coping is used in an effort to preclude anticipated negative emotions even in situations in which negative affect may not occur. This interpretation explains Tiffany Field's finding that infants of depressed mothers have less engaged and more negative interactions with a friendly stranger than do infants of nondepressed mothers (Field et al., 1988). The infants of the depressed mothers are utilizing this strategy automatically without evaluating whether it is warranted. Eventually, with the reiteration and accumulation of failure, these infants develop a negative affective core primarily characterized by sadness and anger, a representation of the mother as untrustworthy and unresponsive, and a representation of themselves as ineffective and helpless.

The infants of hostile intrusive mothers must cope with a different affective regulatory problem. The mother's behavior prevents reparation of the interaction because she consistently disrupts the infant's activities. These infants initially experience anger, turn away from the mother, push her away, or screen her out. However, unlike the failure experience of the infants of withdrawn mothers, these coping behaviors are occasionally successful in limiting the mother's intrusiveness. Thus these infants erratically experience reparation (i.e., a transformation of their anger into a more positive state). To the extent that these coping behaviors are successful in fending off the mother, these infants eventually internalize an angry and protective style of coping which is deployed defensively in anticipation of the mother's intrusiveness. We believe that infants are easily angered when interacting with their mother and others and more easily frustrated when acting on objects.

More speculatively, these differences in infant reactions to maternal withdrawal and intrusiveness suggest an interpretation of differential effects associated with parental neglect and abuse. Infant failure to thrive, withdrawal, and lack of motivation seen in situations of parental neglect probably result from the constant demands forced on the infant to self-regulate. The infant is continuously required to control his or her own physiological and affective states. This self-directed coping style compromises the infant's interchanges with the environment and motivation to engage with the world. By contrast, parental abuse leads to chronic physical defensiveness and anger as well as heightened vigilance and fear.

These observations need to take into account gender differences in infant regulatory and affective styles (Weinberg & Tronick, 1992; Weinberg, 1992). Boys are more affectively reactive and less able to self-regulate their affective states. We hypothesize that they may be particularly susceptible to the withdrawn style associated with depression because maternal withdrawal denies them the regulatory support they need. On the other hand, girls, who at 6 months are significantly more focused on objects than are boys, may be more vulnerable to the intrusive style of depression which interferes with their activities. Combined with the findings that girls show more stability of sadness than do boys, and boys show more stability of distancing and escape behaviors than do girls, we think these gender differences in regulatory styles may be the first signs presaging the differential proportion of depression in girls and hyperactivity and aggressiveness in boys. It is not that girls are inherently depressed and boys inherently hyperactive. Rather, each has different regulatory styles that in, interaction with different caregiving styles, make one or another outcome more likely.

Reparation, Conduct Disorders, and Anger

This perspective also has implications for the higher rates of conduct and delinquency disorders in boys. We know from the literature on juvenile delinquency that boys commit many more crimes than do girls. However, there is no adequate explanation for this phenomenon. Our research indicates that gender differences in infancy may already set the stage for this differential rate. The explanation, however, is not simply that boys are more aggressive than girls but, rather, that boys have greater difficulty controlling their emotional reactions. Because of this difficulty, they are more likely than girls to fail to accomplish their goals. This failure generates frustration and anger and may lead to aggression. This may be exacerbated in those situations in which parenting behavior is also compromised by, for example, depression.

The argument is as follows: Boys are more demanding and more reactive than girls and have a harder time controlling both their negative their positive emotional states. This makes it more difficult for parents to interact with them and sets the stage for later struggles and conflicts. There is also strong evidence indicating that boys continue to be more demanding and emotionally reactive as they grow up (Weinberg, 1992). During the preschool period, boys are more aggressive than girls and parents report having more difficulty disciplining them. It is also during the preschool period that we begin to see a surge in the number of boys seen in clinical settings who have conduct disorders. Children with conduct disorders, both during the school-age period and in adolescence, are characterized by acting-out behavior, destructiveness, impulsiveness, and an inability to control their emotions. Our hypothesis is that they have problems regulating their affective states and are therefore easily frustrated and angry. Failure to control emotional states interferes with the accomplishment of goals. During infancy, these goals revolve around the exploration of objects and social interaction. During adolescence, these goals include successful performance in school and interaction with peers. Failure to accomplish these goals leads to frustration, anger, and in some cases aggression, which may result in conduct disorders or delinquency. Thus it is not aggression per se that distinguishes boys from girls but their emotional regulatory differences.

There is a parental piece to the argument as well. During infancy and at later ages, parents help children modulate their emotional states. Parents play a crucial role in teaching their children how to talk about and cope with failure, anger, and frustration. They also teach their children how to channel these emotions into productive activities. If a parent is unable to provide the guidance children need because they are depressed, fatigued, physically ill, or simply not present in their children's lives, the stage is set for conflict and struggle with the child.

During infancy, parental unresponsiveness or inappropriate parenting dysregulates the infant, which prevents the infant from achieving his or her goals of social interaction and object exploration. This pattern leads to anger and a decrease in enjoyment. The infant learns that the parent is unreliable and unavailable. Most important, it also has the effect of interfering with the infant's development of a sense of mastery and control over events. That is, the infant fails to learn that he or she has the power to change things. Instead the infant develops a sense of helplessness and hopelessness. These developments may be more likely in boys because of their greater need for parental regulatory support.

These early processes may become more problematic during adolescence. Adolescence is a time of turmoil and change for both adolescents and parents. Normally, adolescence is a difficult time for boys, girls, and parents alike. An adolescent who has been chronically deprived of parental guidance, support, and involvement during infancy and childhood will not have had the opportunity to master the coping strategies necessary to successfully cope with the normal changes and pressures of adolescence. The child will also not have developed a sense of effectance or a sense that he or she has the power to change events in his or her life. Similarly, parents who have been chronically uninvolved with their child will not have learned how to help that child cope with the normal vicissitudes of life. Therefore, it is unlikely that these parents will suddenly be able to help the child cope with the normal tasks of adolescence. Again, failure to master the tasks of adolescence leads to frustration, anger, low self-esteem, and sometimes aggression. This aggression may lead to an affiliation with other children who have similar problems and propensities. Again, boys may experience these problems more acutely because of their early regulatory problems and the subsequent parenting they received.

In general, just as in the case of conduct disorders, the model of mutual regulation must be modified as the child gets older because of developmental changes. For example, around the end of the first year infants begin to develop an awareness of their own and their partners' intentions and affective states. This awareness was introduced by Tronick and named "intersubjectivity" (Tronick, Als, & Adamson, 1978). It has been adapted and elaborated by Trevarthen as secondary intersubjectivity and by Stern as attunement (Stern, 1977; Trevarthen, 1980, 1993). The developmental accomplishment of secondary intersubjectivity has important implications for the effects of maternal depression on the child.

THE FORMATION OF DYADIC STATES
OF CONSCIOUSNESS

With the development of secondary intersubjectivity in the older infant, infants of depressed mothers become increasingly aware that their mothers are angry, hostile, and/or sad. They no longer simply react to what the mother does. Rather, they are becoming aware of and react to her state of mind. This awareness is not necessarily conscious but takes the form of an apprehension of her mental state even when that state is not directly manifest in her behavior. However, it is also not a "magical nonmaterial" apprehension but one generated by the child's newly developed capacities for integrating past experiences. At this age, infants also become aware of their own feelings of sadness, helplessness, and anger. The awareness of their own negative feelings must be especially intolerable because it is associated with their mother and demands an enormous regulatory effort to control. It is our expectation that older infants become hypervigilant of their mother's emotional state to protect themselves from her state. They also monitor their own emotional reactions, especially their anger, and attempt to control it so as not to express it to their mother. An additional cost of this vigilance is that they need to limit their excited positive feelings because a high level of arousal, even if it is positive, might threaten their capacity to control their affective states. Thus they may become emotionally constricted. Osofsky (1992) presents findings that support this argument. She found that by the end of the first year, infants of depressed mothers express less intense affective reactions to stressful situations and are less emotionally responsive than are infants of nondepressed mothers.

Secondary Intersubjectivity and Psychopathology

A serious implication of the development of secondary intersubjectivity is that it may "enable" the infant to develop psychopathological states. With the development of secondary intersubjectivity, the infant's reaction is no longer determined simply by what he or she directly experiences in interaction with the mother. The infant's reaction increasingly becomes an integration of immediate events with self-reflective representational processes. With these developmental changes, distortions of reality become possible. For example, we would expect that when children become aware of their depressed mother's affective state (e.g., her anger and sadness apparently directed at them) and their own intolerable feelings of rage directed at her, children may develop a pathological form of coping—denial, detachment, repression, projection—in an attempt to control their awareness of these overwhelming feelings.

Representations take time to develop and have different forms during development. Early in development these representations are instantiated in patterns of action and emotion before they become representations incorporating elements of the self, cognition, and history. Critically, these representations are not simply stored information in a preformed or predetermined universal brain. Mutual regulatory experience is not simply the storage of material (e.g., the filing of information in some area of the brain dedicated to the storage of information) that can be accessed for present use. Rather, mutual regulation is one of the processes that shapes the brain itself. Thus the brain, like emotional experience, is jointly created. Or, to invert the idea, the human brain is inherently dyadic and is created through interactive interchanges.

Dyadic States of Consciousness and Systems Coherence

Until now, we, like others (Emde et al., 1978; Trevarthen, 1993; Tronick, 1980), have assumed that the motivation for intersubjectivity is an inherent, biologically given characteristic of our species. This assumption has its rationale in the evolution of our species as a social species, in our use of language, in the collaborative nature of meaning making, and in relational theories of the formation of attachments and the self (Tronick, 1980; Tronick, Morelli, & Winn, 1987; Stern, 1985; Bowlby, 1980; Trevarthen, 1989b). However, although the assumption is reasonable, it is a de facto assumption, making it less satisfying. It assumes the phenomenon we want to explain: Why do we seek (choose the term) "connectedness," "social contact," "intersubjectivity," "attunement," "emotional synchrony"? We would like to advance the dyadic consciousness (DC) hypothesis, which may offer a way out of this conundrum. The DC hypothesis explains the centrality of intersubjectivity in terms of principles borrowed from systems theory. Furthermore, the DC hypothesis moves away from the strictly behavioral account offered previously to a more mindful account of social–emotional development that provides a richer understanding of depression and its effects.

A first principle of systems theory is that open biological systems, such as humans, function to incorporate and integrate information into increasingly coherent and complex states. This incorporative process is paradoxical. On the one hand, more information is integrated into the system, making it more complex; on the other hand, to the extent that a more coherent state is formed, the new organization with its greater amount of information is simpler. This process is often thought of as a self-generated characteristic of open systems. However, it is can also be a dyadic process—a process involving two minds.

Self-Organization and Dyadic Organization

The infant is able to endogenously (self-) organize a coherent affective state. This state can be thought of as a state of consciousness, or, if one prefers, a state of brain organization. The state of consciousness is isomorphically manifest in the infant's affective configurations of face, body, voice, gaze, and gesture. The state incorporates a certain amount of information—perceptual input, motor output, representations, information feedback and feed forward, plans, intentions, reentry information, and much more (Edelman, 1987; Stern, 1985; Weinberg & Tronick, 1994). Constraints on the complexity of this self-generated state are determined by the limits of the infant's central nervous system (speed of information processing, channel capacities of different sensory modalities, motor control limitations, etc.) (Aronson & Tronick, 1971). However, the complexity of the infant's state of consciousness does not solely depend on processes endogenous to the infant. As an open system, the complexity of the infant's state is expandable with input from an external source—the caregiver.

The caregiver provides the infant with regulatory input that can expand the complexity and coherence of the infant's state of consciousness. This expansion of consciousness is an emergent property of the mutual microexchange of affective information. During an interaction, information about the infant's state of consciousness (e.g., intentions, affective states, and arousal level) is conveyed through affective configurations that are apprehended by the mother. In response to this information about the infant's state of consciousness, the mother provides the infant with regulatory support that permits the infant to achieve a more complex state of organization. For example, the caregiver, by giving the infant postural support in response to the infant's frustration vocalizations because he cannot "free" his arms and control his posture at the same time, facilitates the infant's

ability to employ gestural communication during social interaction—
a complex action beyond the infant's own ability. At the same time, the
infant's state of consciousness gains coherence and complexity beyond the infant's endogenous capacities. Bullowa (1979) emphasized
this phenomenon when she documented the greater complexity of the
infant's behavior in the presence of others compared to the infant's
behavior when alone.

The Emergence of Dyadic States of Consciousness

There is a critical and emergent property of this collaboration—the creation of single dyadic state of consciousness. This dyadic state organization
is bounded and has more components—the infant and the mother—than
the infant's (or mother's) own state of consciousness. Thus this dyadic
system contains more information and is more complex and coherent
than either the infant's (or the mother's) endogenous state of consciousness alone. When infant and mother mutually create this dyadic state, they
fulfill the system's principle of gaining greater complexity and coherence.
Thus, the mother-held infant performs an action—gesturing—and experiences the state of consciousness associated with gesturing that is an
emergent property of the dyadic system. Both the behavior and the state
of consciousness occur because the infant and mother are related to the
other as components of a dyadic, mutually regulated system.

Creation of this dyadic system necessitates that the infant and
mother apprehend elements of the other's state of consciousness. If
they did not, it would not be possible to create a dyadic state. For
example, if the mother's apprehension of the infant's state of consciousness is that the infant intends to reach for a ball when in fact the
infant intended to stroke her face, a dyadic state will not be created.
The two systems—infant and mother—will remain separate and un-
coordinated. Thus a principle governing the human dyadic system is
that successful mutual regulation of social interactions requires a mutual mapping of (some of) the elements of each interactant's state of
consciousness into each of their brains. This mutual mapping process
may be a way of defining intersubjectivity. In the young infant the
process is one of emotional apprehension of the other's state, referred
to as primary intersubjectivity (Campos, Barrett, Lamb, Goldsmith, &
Stenberg, 1983; Tronick, Als, & Brazelton, 1980b). In the older infant,
the process is one of secondary intersubjectivity. The infant becomes

aware of his or her apprehension of the other's state. In older children and adults, the process may be what is called empathy—a state that contains an awareness of the other's state and a paradoxical awareness of the differentiation between one's own state and the state of the other.

To restate the DC hypothesis, each individual is a self-organizing system that creates its own states of consciousness—states of brain organization—which can be expanded into more coherent and complex states in collaboration with another self-organizing system. When the collaboration of two brains is successful, each fulfills the systems principle of increasing its coherence and complexity. The states of consciousness of the infant and the mother are more inclusive and coherent at that moment when they form a dyadic state that incorporates elements of the state of the other.

Thus, to return to the original question: What is it about intersubjectivity that makes it so critical to human experience and to development? The answer suggested by the DC hypothesis is that the "fulfilling" of the principle of systems theory for increased complexity and coherence is the motivation of social engagement. Fulfillment of this principle is what gives social interaction its critical experiential value. At the moment the dyadic system is created, both partners experience an expansion of their own state of consciousness. The boundary surrounding their own system expands to incorporate elements of consciousness of the other in a new and more coherent form. In this moment of dyadic consciousness, and for the duration of its existence, there must be something akin to a powerful experience of fulfillment as one paradoxically becomes larger than oneself.

CONCLUSION: DYADIC CONSCIOUSNESS
AND PSYCHOLOGICAL TOXICITY

An important consequence of the DC hypothesis relates to how the toxic effects on the infant of maternal depression, whichever its manifest style, come about. As we have demonstrated, maternal depression disrupts the establishment of a dyadic infant–mother system. The infant is deprived of the experience of expanding his or her states of consciousness in collaboration with the mother. This deprivation limits the infant's experience and forces the infant into self-regulatory patterns that eventually compromise the child's development. The DC hypothesis suggests another more insidious possibility. Given that the infant's system functions to expand its complexity, one way that the infant of the depressed mother can accomplish this expansion is to take on elements of the mother's state of consciousness. These elements are likely to be negative—sad and hostile affect, withdrawal, disengagement. However, by taking them on, the infant and the mother form a larger dyadic system. Intersubjectivity is established and with it the infant's state of consciousness is expanded. Thus, in the service of becoming more complex and coherent, the infant incorporates a state of consciousness that mimics the depressive elements of the mother. That this intersubjective state contains painful elements does not override the "need" for expansion. Critically, when the infant comes to other relationships, the only way he or she has learned and has available to expand the complexity of his or her states is by establishing intersubjective states around the depressive features of consciousness that were first established with the mother. Thus we see in some individuals the reiterated and often debilitating attachment to and seeking of negative relational experiences.

In sum, the process of mutual regulation, whether at the level of social emotional exchanges or at the level of states of consciousness and intersubjectivity, determines much of the emotional, social, and representational course of the infant, including the formation of the infant's brain. When regulation goes well, development proceeds apace. Increasingly complex tasks are approached and resolved, not by the child alone but by the child in collaboration with others. The child, as a system and as a component of a dyadic system, expands and becomes more coherent. When failures take place, development gets derailed and the child's complexity (and we expect the complexity of the child's partners as well) is limited or even reduced. The effect is in the child, but the failure is a joint failure. With continued, chronic failure and the structuring that goes on around that failure, affective disorders and pathology may result.

ACKNOWLEDGMENTS

This work was supported by grants from the National Science Foundation (BNS 85-06987) and the National Institute of Mental Health (RO1 MH 45547, RO1 MH 3398, and RO3 MH 52265). We wish to acknowledge Karen Olson, Marjorie Beeghly, Henrietta Kernan, Yana Markov, Flavia Teixeira, and all the mothers, fathers, and infants who participated in our studies.

REFERENCES

Aronson, E., & Tronick, E. Z. (1971). Perceptual capacities in early infancy. In J. Eliot (Ed.), *Human development and cognitive processes* (pp. 216–224). New York: Holt, Rinehart & Winston.

Beebe, B., & Lachmann, F. M. (1994). Representation and internalization in infancy: Three principles of salience. *Psychoanalytic Psychology, 11,* 127–165.

Blumberg, N. J. (1980). Effects of neonatal risk, maternal attitude, and cognitive style on early postpartum adjustment. *Journal of Abnormal Psychology, 89,* 139–150.

Bowlby, J. (1951). *Maternal care and mental health* (World Health Organization, Monograph Series No. 2) Geneva: World Health Organization.

Bowlby, J. (1980). *Attachment and loss: Vol. 1. Attachment.* New York: Basic Books.

Brazelton, T. B., Koslowski, B., & Main, M. (1974). The origins of reciprocity: The early mother–infant interaction. In M. Lewis & L. A. Rosenblum (Eds.), *The effect of the infant on its caregiver* (pp. 49–76). New York: Wiley.

Bruner, J. (1983). *Child's talk.* New York: Norton.

Bruner, J. (1995). *Acts of meaning.* Cambridge, MA: Harvard University Press.

Bullowa, M. (1979). Prelinguistic communication: A field for scientific research. In M. Bullowa (Ed.), *Before speech: The beginning of interpersonal communication* (pp. 1–62). Cambridge, England: Cambridge University Press.

Campos, J. J., Barrett, K. C., Lamb, M. E., Goldsmith, H. H., & Stenberg, C. (1983). Socioemotional development. In P. H. Mussen (Ed.), *Handbook of child psychology* (Vol. 2, pp. 783–915). New York: Wiley.

Cohen, J. (1988). *Statistical power analysis for the behavioral sciences.* Hillsdale, NJ: Erlbaum.

Cohn, J. F., Matias, R., Tronick, E. Z., Connell, D., & Lyons-Ruth, K. (1986). Face-to-face interactions of depressed mothers and their infants. In E. Z. Tronick & T. Field (Eds.), *Maternal depression and infant disturbance* (pp. 31–46). San Francisco: Jossey-Bass.

Cohn, J. F., & Tronick, E. Z. (1987). Mother–infant face-to-face interaction: The sequence of dyadic states at 3, 6, and 9 months. *Developmental Psychology, 23,* 68–77.

Cohn, J. F., & Tronick, E. Z. (1988). Mother–infant face-to-face interaction: Influence is bidirectional and unrelated to periodic cycles in either partner's behavior. *Developmental Psychology, 24,* 386–392.

Cohn, J. F., & Tronick, E. Z. (1989). Specificity of infants' response to mothers' affective behavior. *Journal of the American Academy of Child and Adolescent Psychiatry, 28,* 242–248.

Condon, W. S., & Sander, L. W. (1974). Neonate movement is synchronized with adult speech: Interactional participation and language acquisition. *Science, 183,* 99–101.

Connelly, K. J., & Prechtl, H. F. R. (1981). *Maturation and development: Biological and psychological perspectives.* Philadelphia: Lippincott.

Dowd, J., & Tronick, E. Z. (1986). Temporal coordination of arm movement in early infancy: Do infants move in synchrony with adult speech? *Child Development, 66,* 1714–1719.

Edelman, G. M. (1987). *Neural Darwinism: The theory of neuronal group selection.* New York: Basic Books.

Emde, R. N., Kligman, D. H., Reich, J. H., & Wade, T. D. (1978). Emotional expression in infancy: I. Initial studies of social signaling and an emergent model. In M. Lewis & L. A. Rosenblum (Eds.), *The development of affect* (pp. 125–148). New York: Plenum Press.

Field, T., Healy, B., Goldstein, S., Perry, S., Bendell, D., Schanberg, S., Zimmerman, E. A., & Kuhn, C. (1988). Infants of depressed mothers show "depressed" behavior even with nondepressed adults. *Child Development, 59,* 1569–1579.

Gianino, A., & Tronick, E. Z. (1988). The mutual regulation model: The infant's self and interactive regulation, coping, and defense. In T. Field, P. McCabe, & N. Schneiderman (Eds.), *Stress and coping* (pp. 47–68). Hillsdale, NJ: Erlbaum.

Gunzenhauser, N. (Ed.). (1987). *Infant stimulation: For whom, what kind, when, and how much?* Safe Harbor, CT: Johnson & Johnson.

Hofer, M. A. (1981). Parental contributions to the development of their offspring. In D. Gubernick & P. Klopfer (Eds.), *Parental care in mammals* (pp. 77–111). New York: Plenum.

Hofer, M. A. (1984). Relationships as regulators: A psychobiologic perspective on bereavement. *Psychosomatic Medicine, 46,* 183–197.

Isabella, R., & Belsky, J. (1991). Interactional synchrony and the origins of mother–infant attachment: A replication study. *Child Development, 62,* 373–384.

Kaye, K. (1977). Toward the origin of dialogue. In H. R. Schaffer (Ed.), *Studies in mother–infant interaction* (pp. 89–118). New York: Academic Press.

Keefer, C. H., Tronick, E. Z., Dixon, S., & Brazleton, T. (1982). Specific differences in motor performance between Gusii and American newborns and a modification of the Neonatal Behavioral Assessment Scale. *Child Development, 53,* 754–759.

Lester, B. M., & Tronick, E. Z. (1994). The effects of prenatal cocaine exposure and child outcome. *Infant Mental Health Journal, 15,* 107–120.

Massie, H. N. (1982). Affective development and the organization of mother–infant behavior from the perspective of psychopathology. In E. Z. Tronick (Ed.), *Social interchange in infancy: Affect, cognition and communication* (pp. 161–182). Baltimore: University Park Press.

Mayer, N., & Tronick, E. Z. (1985). Mother's turn-giving signals and infant turn-taking in mother–infant interaction. In T. Field & N. Fox, (Eds.), *Social perception in infants* (pp. 199–216). Norwood, NJ: Ablex.

Osofsky, J. D. (1992). Affective development and early relationships: Clinical implications. In J. W. Barron, M. N. Eagle, & D. L. Wolitzky (Eds.), *Interface of psychoanalysis and psychology* (pp. 233–244). Washington DC: American Psychological Association.

Sander, L. W. (1983). A twenty-five-year follow-up of the Pavenstedt Longitudinal Research Project: Its relation to early intervention. In J. D. Call, E. Galenson, & R. L. Tyson (Eds.), *Frontiers of infant psychiatry* (pp. 225–230). New York: Basic Books.

Schaffer, H. R. (1977). Early interactive development. In H. R. Schaffer (Ed.), *Studies in mother–infant interaction* (pp. 3–18). New York: Academic Press.

Schore, A. N. (1994). *Affect regulation and the origin of self: The neurobiology of emotional development.* Hillsdale, NJ: Erlbaum.

Spinelli, D. N. (1987). Plasticity triggering experiences, nature, and the dual genesis of brain structure and function. In N. Gunzenhauser (Ed.), *Infant stimulation: For whom, what kind, when, and how much?* (pp. 21–29). Safe Harbor, CT: Johnson & Johnson.

Spitz, R. (1965). *The first year of life.* New York: International Universities Press.

Stern, D. (1977). *The first relationship.* Cambridge, MA: Harvard University Press.

Stern, D. (1985). *The interpersonal world of the infant.* New York: Basic Books.

Trevarthen, C. (1979). Communication and cooperation in early infancy: A description of primary intersubjectivity. In M. M. Bullowa (Ed.), *Before speech: The beginning of interpersonal communication* (pp. 321–349). New York: Cambridge University Press.

Trevarthen, C. (1980). The foundations of intersubjectivity: Development of interpersonal and cooperative understanding in infants. In D. Olsen (Ed.), *The social foundations of language and thought: Essays in honor of J. S. Bruner* (pp. 316–342). New York: Norton.

Trevarthen, C. (1989a). Development of early social interactions and the affective regulation of brain growth. In C. von Euler, H. Lagercrantz, & H. Forssberg (Eds.), *The neurobiology of early infant behavior* (pp. 191–216). New York: Macmillan.

Trevarthen, C. (1989b). Signs before speech. In T. A. Sebeok & J. Umiker-Sebeok (Eds.), *The semiotic web* (pp. 689–755). Berlin: Mouton de Gruyter.

Trevarthen, C. (1990). Growth and education of the hemispheres. In C. Trevarthen (Ed.), *Brain circuits and functions of the mind* (pp. 334–363). Cambridge, England: Cambridge University Press.

Trevarthen, C. (1993). The function of emotions in early infant communication and development. In J. Nadel & L. Camaioni (Eds.), *New perspectives in early communicative development.* London: Routledge.

Trevarthen, C., & Hubley, P. (1978). Secondary intersubjectivity: Confidence, confiding and acts of meaning in the first year. In A. Lock (Ed.), *Action, gesture and symbol: The emergence of language* (pp. 183–229). New York: Academic Press.

Tronick, E. Z. (1980). The primacy of social skills in infancy. In D. B. Sawin, R. C. Hawkins, 2nd, L. O. Walker, & J. H. Penticuff (Eds.), *The exceptional infant* (pp. 144–157). New York: Brunner/Mazel.

Tronick, E. Z. (1985). Stress and coping in young infants. In T. Field, P. McCabe, & N. Schneiderman (Eds.), *Stress and coping* (Vol. 2). Hillsdale, NJ: Erlbaum.

Tronick, E. Z. (1989). Emotions and emotional communication in infants. *American Psychologist, 44,* 112–119.

Tronick, E. Z., Als, H., & Adamson, L. (1978). Structure of early face-to-face communicative interactions. In M. Bullowa (Ed.), *Before speech: The beginning of interpersonal communication.* Cambridge, England: Cambridge University Press.

Tronick, E. Z., Als, H., Adamson, L., Wise, S., & Brazelton, T. B. (1978). The infant's response to entrapment between contradictory messages in face-to-face interaction. *Journal of American Academy of Child Psychiatry, 17,* 1–13.

Tronick, E. Z., Als, H., & Brazelton, T. B. (1980a). Monadic phases: A structural descriptive analysis of infant–mother face-to-face interaction. *Merrill–Palmer Quarterly, 26,* 3–13.

Tronick, E. Z., Als, H., & Brazelton, T. B. (1980b). The infant's communicative competencies and the achievement of intersubjectivity. In M. R. Key (Ed.), *The relationship of verbal and nonverbal communication* (pp. 261–274). The Hague: Mouton.

Tronick, E. Z., & Cohn, J. F. (1989). Infant–mother face-to-face interaction: Age and gender differences in coordination and the occurrence of miscoordination. *Child Development, 60,* 85–92.

Tronick, E. Z., Cohn, J., & Shea, E. (1986). The transfer of affect between mother and infants. In T. B. Brazelton & M. W. Yogman (Eds.), *Affective development in infancy* (pp. 11–25). Norwood, NJ: Ablex.

Tronick, E. Z., & Field, T. (1987). *Maternal depression and infant disturbance.* San Francisco: Jossey-Bass.

Tronick, E. Z., & Gianino, A. (1980). An accounting of the transmission of maternal disturbance to the infant. *New Directions for Child Development.*

Tronick, E. Z., & Morelli, G. A. (1991). Foreword: The role of culture in brain organization, child development, and parenting. In J. K. Nugent, B. M. Lester, & T. B. Brazelton (Eds.), *The cultural context of infancy: Multicultural and interdisciplinary approaches to parent-infant relations* (2nd ed., pp. ix–xiii). Norwood, NJ: Ablex.

Tronick, E. Z., Morelli, G. A., & Winn, S. (1987). Multiple caretaking of Efe (Pygmy) infants. *American Anthropologist, 89,* 96–106.

Weinberg, M. K. (1992). *Sex differences in 6-month-old infants' affect and behavior: Impact on maternal caregiving.* Unpublished manuscript.

Weinberg, M., Gianino, A. F., & Tronick, E. Z. (1989, April). *Facial expressions of emotion and social and object oriented behavior are specifically related in 6-month-old infants.* [Abstract]. Poster session presented at the biannual meeting of the Society for Research in Child Development, Kansas City, KS.

Weinberg, M. K., & Tronick, E. Z. (1992). Sex differences in emotional expression and affective regulation in 6-month-old infants. [Abstract]. *Society for Pediatric Research, 31*(4), 15A.

Weinberg, M. K., & Tronick, E. Z. (1994). Beyond the face: An empirical study of infant affective configurations of facial, vocal, gestural, and regulatory behaviors. *Child Development, 65,* 1495–1507.

Weinberg, M. K., & Tronick, E. Z. (1996). Infant affective reactions to the resumption of maternal interaction after the still-face. *Child Development, 67,* 905–914.

III

~

COMPARATIVE STUDIES OF THE IMPACT OF POSTPARTUM DEPRESSION ON CHILD DEVELOPMENT

4

_∼_

Postpartum Depression
and Cognitive Development

Dale F. Hay
University of Cambridge

The study of the effects of postpartum illness on cognitive development falls squarely in the tradition within developmental psychology of looking at the long-term impact of infants' earliest experiences on later development. In this chapter, I propose that the mother's postpartum illness permanently affects some children's cognitive abilities. In setting forth that hypothesis, I draw on the general developmental literature on early cognitive development and on the results of several key studies of postpartum depression. I then speculate about a developmental pathway from early problems in attention and emotion regulation to later cognitive deficits that is exacerbated by postpartum depression. The evidence I review here has important implications for a general understanding of the development of intelligence, and in particular the role of the social environment in shaping children's learning and attainments. It also has important implications for clinical practice in terms of the treatments that may be offered depressed mothers and the stimulation that needs to be provided to their children.

Before evaluating the claim that postpartum depression stunts children's intellectual development, it is important to consider current thinking about intelligence and about the contributions of early experiences to intellectual development. We must begin with a general consideration of those factors that influence intellectual development.

THE ORIGINS OF INTELLIGENCE

Throughout this century, developmental theory and research have been bedeviled by the nature–nurture issue, and in no domain has this been more apparent than the study of intelligence (for recent contributions to the debate, see Cairns, McGuire, & Gariepy, 1993; Ceci, Baker-Sennett, & Bronfenbrenner, 1994; Herrnstein & Murray, 1994; Moffitt, Caspi, Harkness, & Silva, 1993; Plomin, 1994; Scarr, 1992). The pendulum swings from decade to decade and currently the statement that intelligence is substantially heritable receives much support. For example, Scarr (1992) has claimed that, within ordinary, expectable environments, environmental input makes very little difference to a child's intellectual abilities:

> Feeding a well-nourished but short child will not give him the stature of a basketball player. Feeding a below-average intellect more and more information will not make her brilliant. . . . The child with a below-average intellect and the shy child may gain some specific skills and helpful knowledge of how to behave in specific situations, but their enduring intellectual and personality characteristics will not be fundamentally changed. (p. 16)

In her review of the behavioral genetics literature, Scarr (1992) estimates the heritability of intelligence to be $h^2 = .70$; in other words, 70% of the variance in IQ scores would be due to genetic differences. Furthermore, attempts to map the human genome have provided evidence for two DNA markers (out of 40 tested) associated with differences between individuals of high and low intellectual ability (Plomin et al., 1994).

In a classic article on the nature-nurture debate, Lehrman (1970) noted that in addition to heritability, developmental fixity is the criterion most often used to defend the "innateness" of a trait. Hence there is considerable interest in the stability of IQ scores over the life span (e.g., McCall, Appelbaum, & Hogarty, 1973). Recently, Moffitt et al. (1993) examined the evidence for stability and change in IQ scores obtained at 7, 9, 11, and 15 years of age in a large, representative sample of New Zealand children. They discovered that change in IQ scores for the majority of the sample was no greater than would be expected on the basis of measurement error; only for a minority of children (14%) were there levels of change that exceeded expectations based on measurement error. However, most of the change detected in the latter group of children was fluctuating change rather than being cumulative and sequential. Moffitt et al. (1993) concluded that *"there is very little measurable naturalistic change in IQ across middle childhood and early adolescence. Moreover, the reliable change that does take place appears to be idiosyncratic; it is not systematically associated with environmental changes"* (p. 499, italics in original). These data do not, however, exclude the possibility of substantial changes in IQ scores prior to the age of 7.

So, in the contemporary literature, many theorists see intelligence as a trait of individuals showing high heritability and developmental fixity (Lehrman, 1970), that is, innate and relatively impervious to experience. Against this intellectual background of emphasis on the heritable features of intelligence, how are we to examine the effects of experience? It is conceded that gross environmental deprivation is associated with intellectual deficits (see Rutter, 1991; Scarr, 1992), but the effect of environmental variation within the normal range is seen as much less important. Behavioral geneticists have noted that for populations reared in ordinary, species-appropriate environments, variation in intelligence tends to be associated with unique experiences impinging on individuals, not with broader environmental features shared by all members of a family (Plomin & Daniels, 1987; Scarr, 1992). Thus, in attempting to examine the contributions of experience to a child's intellectual attainment, it behooves us to consider influences that impinge directly on that individual child, not on his or her brothers or sisters.

One way to identify unique experiences is to map the child's actual environment. Chipuer and Plomin (1992) attempted to do so by examining items on the HOME inventory, a checklist that classifies the physical and social features of children's homes (Caldwell & Bradley, 1984). As part of a longitudinal study of adoptive and biological siblings, the HOME inventory was administered when each sibling was 12 and 24 months of age. Thus it was possible to determine which features of the environment present when a younger child was a certain age had also been provided when an older sibling had been that same age.

In Chipuer and Plomin's (1992) study, a number of dimensions of the environment were not shared across siblings, including the mother's provision of affection, her disciplinary style, and the nature of books and toys provided. Thus, mothers do not necessarily interact with two siblings in the same way, even when the children are at comparable ages, although it is not clear from these data whether the mothers' differential behavior is associated with differences in the siblings' cognitive attainments. Such differential treatment may derive from the individual demands and characteristics of the different children in a family, but it may also be a function of the mother's mental state at different times in her own life.

In this chapter, I extend the concept of nonshared experiences by adopting an explicitly developmental perspective. I propose that some experiences that seem to be common to two siblings are not in fact shared because one of the siblings may be more vulnerable developmentally than the other. In other words, experiences impinging on the family as a whole may catch one of its members in a "sensitive period," and it is that developmentally vulnerable individual who may be most strongly affected. Hence the behavioral geneticists' concern with nonshared environments (Dunn & Plomin, 1990; Plomin & Daniels, 1987) must be integrated with the older literature on the impact of experience during sensitive periods in development (see Bateson, 1979; MacDonald, 1985; Thompson & Grusec, 1970).

EARLY EXPERIENCE, INTELLIGENCE, AND EMOTIONALITY

The proposal that experiences early in life have profound effects on development is found in a number of theoretical traditions, including embryology (e.g., Gottlieb, 1991), ethology (Lorenz, 1935/1970) and psychoanalysis (e.g., Freud, 1938). Perhaps the most familiar human example of a sensitive-period effect is in the realm of visual development—if a squint is left uncorrected past 2 years of age, a child cannot achieve binocular vision.

Within the realm of socioemotional development, the concern with early experience is most closely associated with attachment theory, as set forth by Bowlby (1958) and Ainsworth (1969). Within the realm of intellectual development, the importance of early experience was emphasized in Hebb's (1949) theoretical account of the development of the nervous system and was addressed in practical terms in the literatures on institutionalization and early educational interventions (see Clarke & Clarke, 1976; Hunt, 1961; Rutter, 1991). The two literatures are rarely, if ever, integrated; however, as we shall see, the early experience of one's mother's postpartum illness may have important consequences for emotional and intellectual development.

Initial formulations of the early experience hypothesis made reference to "critical periods" (e.g., Beach & Jaynes, 1954; Hess, 1959), but current theorists employ the term "sensitive periods," which conveys the notion of less abrupt temporal boundaries (see MacDonald, 1985). There is still, however, an assumption that the nervous system is increasingly less plastic as the young organism matures (Kuo, 1967). In any case, the actual boundaries of a sensitive period may be expected to vary depending on the intensity of the stimulation provided (see Schneirla, 1957): Experience at a given level of intensity may have effects at one age but not at another (Denenberg, 1968). The boundaries of a sensitive period also depend on the organism's degree of maturation. Infants must be mature enough to encode and store the experience yet young enough to be affected by it (Thompson & Grusec, 1970).

As with the nature–nurture issue, concern with sensitive periods goes in and out of fashion, and the concept certainly has received much criticism (e.g., Clarke & Clarke, 1976). Nonetheless, the fact that plasticity varies with age is well documented in a number of species (MacDonald, 1985), as has been the occurrence of permanent nervous system change as a function of early social experiences (e.g., Horn, 1993). Thus there is reason to entertain the hypothesis that intellectual development in humans is similarly more or less vulnerable to experience at different times in the child's life. Therefore, age-related vulnerability of the child may account for some of the nonshared environmental effects noted in the behavioral genetic studies (see Scarr, 1992).

However, it is not completely clear whether, for intellectual development, the period of infancy is especially sensitive. Some investigators have argued instead that the first year of life is relatively *insensitive* to the effects of experience, showing great canalization of development (Waddington, 1957). In this view, most infants in ordinary environments would be following along a narrow canal in which few individual differences would be apparent and their progress would be unlikely to be disrupted by particular experiences (see McCall, 1981).

In contrast to Waddington's view that intellectual development is highly canalized during infancy, I propose a model of early intellectual development that more closely resembles another classic account, Hebb's (1949) speculations about the developing nervous system. Hebb held that the infant's early perceptual learning experiences fundamentally changed the organization of the nervous system—which he described in terms of "cell assemblies" and "reverberating circuits." Hebb believed that the adult's capacity for learning thus depended critically on the infant's early perceptual learning. Although Hebb's particular characterization of the nervous system has yielded to new discoveries in the neurosciences, his claim that early perceptual experiences underlie subsequent intellectual development is still worthy of serious investigation.

I follow Plato (cited in Sternberg, 1990) and Hebb (1949) in identifying intelligence as the capacity to learn. In all that follows, I assume that standardized tests of intelligence represent an imperfect but partial measure of that capacity. I argue that social experiences that interfere with the infant's developing ability to attend to the environment result in decreased intellectual abilities and capacity for learning later in childhood.

As well as speculating about the role of early perceptual learning in development, Hebb (1946) also stressed the role of early experiences in emotional development, particularly with respect to the development of fear. Other investigators of early experience effects similarly underscored the importance of emotional factors (see Thompson & Grusec, 1970). These formulations are well in line with contemporary accounts of children's cognitive development, which stress the interplay between affect and cognition and the role of emotional factors in information processing (Bugental, Blue, Cortez, Fleck, & Rodriguez, 1992; Dodge, 1991). In the model I develop in this chapter, I propose that the two major developmental tasks of early infancy are the regulation of attention and emotion (see Cicchetti, Ganiban, & Barnett, 1991; Sigman & Mundy, 1993). Early social experiences that prevent the infant from learning how to regulate attention and emotion will have deleterious effects on cognitive as well as social development.

I argue further, in contrast to Scarr (1992), that early social experiences may have a critical impact on the developing infant in ordinary, not grossly deprived environments—in particular, when infants are reared at home, not in institutions but by caregivers who are depressed. Before presenting my developmental model, however, I review the evidence for links between maternal depression early in life and children's cognitive abilities.

LINKS BETWEEN MATERNAL DEPRESSION AND CHILD COGNITION

Evidence for an Association

Much attention has been directed in recent years to the impact of a mother's depression on her child's development and well-being (for a review, see Kumar & Hipwell, 1993; chapters in this volume). Many investigators have focused on socioemotional outcomes for the child, in particular guilt, poor self-esteem, and the child's own vulnerability to depressive illness (e.g., Zahn-Waxler, Cole, & Barrett, 1991). However, there are also indications of cognitive problems in the offspring of depressed parents. In particular, the children of depressed women have been reported to show attentional deficiencies (e.g., Weissman, Leckman, Merikangas, Gammon, & Prusoff, 1984; Winters, Stone, Weintraub, & Neale, 1981), reading problems (Stevenson & Fredman, 1980), and failures of social problem solving (Hay, Zahn-Waxler, Cummings, & Iannotti, 1992).

Effects on Early Perceptual Learning

I have proposed, following Hebb (1949), that maternal depression in the first year of life disrupts the infant's emerging abilities to regulate its attention and emotion and thus perceptual learning. Some evidence for this proposition is found in a community sample of depressed mothers and their infants. Murray (1992) undertook a detailed examination of the effect of a mother's depression on intellectual development in the first year of life, using as outcome measures not only standardized assessments of development and language but also observations of the infant's accomplishments of one of the major cognitive tasks in infancy, the understanding of object permanence. She focused on a community sample of women on the postnatal wards of the Cambridge maternity hospital who were screened at 6 weeks postpartum with the Edinburgh Postnatal Depression Scale and then interviewed to confirm the presence of either current or previous depression according to research diagnostic criteria. The screening and interview procedures yielded a subsample of 113 women who either had or had not had a history of major depression and experienced or did not experience depression following the birth of the focal child.

Those infants whose mothers experienced postnatal depression were reliably more likely than other infants to fail the object permanence tasks at 9 and 18 months of age. Infants whose mothers had a history of depression prior to the birth but had not experienced postnatal illness were not reliably different from the children of well women. At the earlier age, infants of the women who were experiencing depression for the first time in their lives were especially likely to do badly on the object permanence tasks. The difference between them and the infants of postnatally depressed women with a previous history was no longer statistically reliable at the 18-month assessment.

In contrast to the object permanence tasks, the mother's postnatal illness did not have a main effect on the infants' performance on the standardized assessments of mental development and language: Both were primarily influenced by the family's social class. However, the early experience of the mother's illness appeared to potentiate the social-class effects. Social class was reliably related to the infant's score on these tasks only in the presence of postnatal depression.

A follow-up of this sample at the age of 5 years indicated that these early differences on object permanence tasks and Bayley scores were not mirrored by reliable differences in standardized tests of cognitive ability (Murray, Hipwell, Hooper, Stein, & Cooper, in press). The follow-up analyses showed that the Cambridgeshire children's scores on the McCarthy Scales of Children's Abilities did not show a reliable effect of the mother's postnatal depression, even when taking social class into account. In two other samples with which I have worked, however, depression in the first year was found to have a reliable effect on 4-year-olds' cognitive abilities (Hay & Kumar, 1995; Sharp et al., 1995).

The North London Sample

Cognitive deficits in the 4-year-old children of women who were depressed postnatally were reported in a follow-up study of antenatal patients from a teaching hospital in North London (Cogill, Caplan, Alexandra, Robson, & Kumar, 1986). I conducted further analyses on those data to clarify the original findings and to determine whether the link between the mother's illness and the child's outcome could be explained by other factors (Hay & Kumar, 1995).

One-hundred nineteen women were selected for study from a population of 147 consecutive, unselected women expecting their first babies and attending clinics at the teaching hospital. About three-quarters were upper or middle class as judged by their partners' occupations. The women were repeatedly interviewed during pregnancy and the child's first year. At the time of the child's fourth birthday, 94 children were tested, using the McCarthy Scales of Children's Abilities, which yields an overall score, the General Cognitive Index (GCI), as well as scores on five subscales. The initial report (Cogill et al., 1986) was based on the sample of 94 children; however, inspection of the data indicated the presence of two outliers, children with GCI scores less than 50. One of these children had been diagnosed with autism. In the reanalyses, the outliers were excluded from the sample, thus reducing power and providing a more conservative test of the association between postnatal illness and the child's cognitive outcome.

The average GCI score in the North London sample was 110.9. Despite the removal of the outliers, the reanalyses confirmed the earlier finding that children of mothers who were depressed in the first year had reliably lower GCI scores than did children whose mothers were not ill at that time. However, additional multivariate analyses showed that the impact was greatest on the perceptual and performance scale—that is, on those aspects of intelligence that might most greatly depend on the perceptual learning taking place during the months when the mother was ill (Hebb, 1949). Depression during pregnancy or at the time of the follow-up did not affect the children's McCarthy scores.

Some investigators have claimed that apparent links between a mother's postnatal illness and deleterious outcomes for her child are actually mediated by vulnerability factors *within the child* that independently provoke depression in the mother and later problems in the child. For example, newborns whose mothers subsequently become depressed already show dysregulated levels of activity and a failure to regulate their own arousal (Field et al., 1988; Murray, Stanley, Hooper, King, & Fiori-Cowley, 1996; Sameroff, Seifer, & Zax, 1982). Cicchetti et al. (1991) suggested that a mother's unipolar depression might be associated with problems in the infant's neuroregulatory systems already present at birth. The reanalyses of Cogill et al.'s findings showed that the impact of the mother's illness on the children's intellectual test performance was still apparent when measures of prenatal and perinatal risk were included in the model. However, it did appear that low birthweight potentiated the risk. When birthweight was entered into the model as a categorical variable (low vs. normal weight), the effect of depression disappeared. This might be seen as supporting the claim made by Cicchetti and his colleagues, especially as the child's low birthweight was one of the factors observed to predict the mother's likelihood of becoming depressed in this sample (Kumar & Robson, 1984). However, when the six low-birthweight babies were removed from the sample, the effect of depression on the children's GCI scores remained a reliable one.

If low birthweight places the infants of depressed mothers at additional risk for cognitive problems, the mother's own level of education appears to protect them. The sample was divided into the 50 women who had obtained qualifications past national examinations given at 16 years of age in the United Kingdom (O-levels) and the 42 who had not; both maternal education and experience of depression in the first postnatal year had independent main effects on the children's GCI scores. There was no interaction between maternal education and illness in the first year; however, planned contrasts showed that the difference between the children of depressed and well mothers was only reliable when the mothers themselves were less well educated. It would seem that the mother's level of education had a specific protective effect beyond its association with the family's overall status. Social class as judged by the father's occupation did not affect GCI scores in this sample (which was, of course, biased toward the upper and middle classes).

In general, then, our reanalyses of Cogill et al.'s original findings confirmed the link between the mother's postpartum illness and the child's cognitive outcome, as measured by the GCI of the McCarthy Scales. However, the impact of the mother's illness seemed to be developmentally specific, affecting most strongly those components of intellectual skill that were developing at the time. Furthermore, low-birthweight infants seemed especially vulnerable whereas the infants of more highly educated mothers were protected.

The South London Sample

The results of our reanalyses of the North London study might be seen as having limited generalizability, given the overrepresentation of middle- to upper-class families in the sample. It was not at all clear that postnatal depression would yield similar effects in a less affluent sample. Furthermore, the observation that maternal education appeared to be a protective factor suggested that those children who might be most at risk from the effects of their mothers' illness were those living in more deprived circumstances in which mothers had not had as many educational opportunities. To address these issues, we conducted a follow-up study of another community sample of antenatal patients, this time women registered at two general practices in two relatively deprived areas of South London (Sharp, 1993).

Two hundred fifty-two women were recruited into the study during the first trimester of pregnancy, with 204 available for follow-up at 3 months postpartum. The Clinical Interview Schedule (CIS) was administered during pregnancy and at 3 and 12 months postpartum, and caseness for depression judged using research diagnostic criteria. One hundred seventy families were included in a follow-up study when the children were 46 months of age (Sharp et al., 1995). The McCarthy Scales of Children's Abilities were again administered, which provides comparability with both the North London and the Cambridgeshire samples. At the time of the follow-up, the mothers were administered the SADS-L. Women were considered to have been depressed in the first year if they had been judged to be cases on the CIS *or* if they recalled being depressed during the first year on the SADS. Women were considered to have been free of depression in that year only if they were judged not to be cases on both the CIS *and* the SADS.

In this more deprived sample, the average GCI score was 97.5 (*SD* = 15.4) and well below the means of the other two samples. Once again there was an overall main effect of the mother's postpartum illness; however, in this sample, it was bound up in an interaction with the child's gender. Sons of mothers who were depressed in the first year obtained GCI scores that were almost a standard deviation below those for the sons of women who had been well at that time (depressed mothers' sons *M* = 86.1, *SD* = 18.1). The decrement in McCarthy performance was shown equally by boys whose mothers had recovered from their postnatal depression and those whose mothers continued to be depressed in the subsequent years. A comparable effect was not found for the daughters of depressed women, whose GCI scores were slightly above those for the children of well mothers.

Multivariate analyses showed that, once again, the Perceptual and Performance subscale of the McCarthy was especially sensitive to the impact of the mother's illness; in this sample, however, verbal performance was also clearly affected. For this chapter, I conducted further analyses of the particular items comprising the GCI in an effort to determine what the specific nature of the deficit might be. Discriminant analyses indicated that the two items that were most sensitive to the effects of the mother's illness were both indexes of abstract intelligence: *reasoning about opposites and analogies* and the *draw-a-child* task, which is sometimes used to estimate general intelligence in very young children.

Analyses of covariance indicated that the impact of the mother's illness on boys' GCI scores could not be accounted for by coexisting behavioral problems, birthweight, associations with the mother's or father's own IQ scores, the marital relationship, or the harmony of mother–child interaction at the time of follow-up. However, planned contrasts indicated that, in this sample, the effect was only discerned in children whose families were judged to be working class. In this sample, in which few women obtained educational qualifications beyond the basic examinations at age 16, maternal education was not found to be a protective factor.

In general, then, in this larger, less affluent sample, maternal depression in the first year again exerted a deleterious effect on children's cognitive performance, but, in this case, the effect was primarily seen with boys, not girls, and it was not limited to perceptual abilities. Boys from working-class families were especially at risk. This risk seems to have translated into specific school-related problems. In a further follow-up (D. Sharp, personal communication, October 1994), reception-class teachers who knew nothing about the mother's experience of postnatal illness rated the children's settling into school. Boys whose mothers were depressed in the first year postpartum were having reliably more difficulties adjusting to their reception classes than were other children in the sample, and these difficulties were mediated by the boys' cognitive scores at 4 years of age.

PATHWAYS TO COGNITIVE PROBLEMS: SOME POSSIBLE MECHANISMS

A Comparison of Previous Findings

Existing studies demonstrate links between maternal depression in the first year of life and children's cognitive abilities, but there are many inconsistencies in the available data. For example, Murray's Cambridgeshire sample demonstrates the clear effects of the mother's postpartum illness on object permanence performance in the infancy period itself, but no reliable differences in McCarthy performance at 5 years (Murray, 1992; Murray et al., 1996). The absence of an effect in the preschool years might be attributed to the high proportion of middle-class families in Murray's sample; yet, in Kumar's equally middle-class sample in North London, researchers observed a strong main effect of the mother's postpartum illness. In Sharp's South London sample, which was characterized by higher levels of social adversity, postpartum illness was again associated with lower McCarthy scores in the preschool years, but this time the deficit was noted only for boys, particularly those in working-class homes.

Direct comparison of these findings is limited by the fact that potential risk and protective factors, such as gender, birthweight, and maternal education, are unequally distributed across the comparison groups in the different samples. For example, consider maternal education, which appeared to be a protective factor in the North London sample. In Murray's Cambridgeshire sample, 52% of the women who had been depressed in the postpartum period had attained A-levels (passed the advanced national examinations given to 18-year-olds in the United Kingdom) or higher qualifications; only 40% of the women in the control group had done so (Murray, Kempton, Woolgar, & Hooper, 1993). Although this is not a statistically significant confound, the slightly differential attainments of the two groups of women might serve to mute any differences linked to depression. Similarly, in the North London sample itself, maternal education was reliably confounded with gender; the mothers of sons were reliably more likely to have attained A-levels or higher qualifications than were the mothers of daughters. Thus, in that sample, boys were more likely to be afforded the protective factor of maternal education than were girls, which may have obscured any gender difference in that sample.

It has become clear that although all three of the studies just discussed represent careful, prospective analyses of community samples, and the sample sizes are respectable, the actual subsamples that are compared, particularly when examined in interaction with potential risk and protective factors, are very small. It is necessary to seek confirmation of these possible links between postpartum depression and children's cognitive problems in a much larger, representative sample. At the same time, however, such an effort must be grounded in theory. We must not simply look for any possible effects of the mother's postpartum illness at various ages of childhood, but, rather, we must attempt to trace developmental pathways and identify mediating mechanisms at key stages in the progression. Thus I have sketched out the following model of possible pathways from postpartum illness to cognitive deficits based on the clues and suggestions in the available literature. This model could then be used to direct further research in larger and more representative populations.

Dysregulated Arousal and Attention in Infancy

It seems clear that the infants of postnatally depressed women show patterns of dysregulated attention and arousal in infancy, which may be seen as an early outcome of the mother's illness or a vulnerability factor within the infant that might provoke the mother's depression (see Cicchetti et al., 1991; Murray & Cooper, Chapter 5, this volume). It is perhaps best to think of these associations between infant dysregulation and maternal illness as synergistic (for a discussion of synergistic causal models, see Pickles, 1993). For example, the infants of mothers who are depressed are more likely to have sleep problems (Murray, 1992). It is possible that this sleep disturbance reflects some problems in self-regulation by the infants that predated the mother's illness but must surely exacerbate it. It is also possible that depressed women whose own arousal systems and sleep patterns are disrupted are more likely to react to small murmurings and fussings of their half-waking babies. A view of the depressed mother and her infant as a dyad with dysregulated arousal and affect provides a starting point for a pathway to later problems (see Tronick & Weinberg, Chapter 3, this volume).

The clearest evidence for cognitive problems in the period of infancy itself comes from Murray's (1992) detailed examination of infants' performance on object permanence tasks. These deficits themselves can be characterized as a form of dysregulated attention. The infant's demonstration of an understanding of the permanence of objects has been described by many theorists as the ability to search—that is, to direct one's attention to cues in the environment in the effort to find invisible or partially visible objects (see Harris, 1983). As such, individual differences in the ability to regulate and direct attention would play a considerable role in the passing or failing of object permanence tasks such as those administered by Murray.

Infants' performance in experimental situations such as the object permanence tasks is not an ephemeral phenomenon with no sequelae. Rather, direct measures of attentional ability and recognition memory in infancy, as opposed to standardized developmental assessments such as the Bayley Scales, have been found to predict IQ scores in later childhood (see Bornstein & Sigman, 1986; McCall & Carriger, 1993). The association between the experimental assessments of attention and later IQ scores is indeed higher for high-risk samples than in populations not at risk for developmental problems (McCall & Carriger, 1993).

The association between attentional measures in infancy and later IQ, coupled with Murray's (1992) demonstration that infants of depressed mothers perform poorly on search tasks, suggests that the experience of the mother's depression in the first months of life may disrupt naturally occurring social processes that entrain and regulate the infant's developing capacities for attention. We may thus ask, first, how postnatally depressed women interact with their infants, and, second, how such interactions might be expected to constrain the infant's capacities for further learning. I hypothesize that two aspects of the regulation of attention may be affected by the mother's postpartum illness: (1) awareness of contingencies in the social and nonsocial environment and (2) ability to modulate one's own emotional state while processing information.

Awareness of Contingencies

Under normal circumstances, infants' abilities to pay attention to and learn about objects and events are sharpened by species-typical interactions with caregivers, often their mothers. Caregivers' naturally occurring ministrations maintain their infants in a state of alert, organized attention to the environment, which may easily deviate to one extreme or the other of sleep or distressed overexcitement (see Stern, 1977). The species-typical gazing and vocal games that mothers and other adults play with infants—in which mothers interpret and make consistent responses to the infant's own randomly occurring looks, smiles, and vocalizations—shape the infant's own behavioral regularities into the rhythms of dialogue and conversation. From such interactions with their caregivers, as well as their own exploration of the physical world, infants begin to attend to contingencies in the environment: things that reliably happen when the infant acts in a certain way.

To detect contingencies, infants must encounter events that occur regularly and close in time to the infant's own actions. For example, young infants cannot detect an association between two events if more than 5 seconds elapse between them (Finkelstein & Ramey, 1977). Lack of contingent stimulation may have adverse effects on infants' abilities to grasp order in their worlds: Experimental studies have shown that experience with noncontingently responding adults actually disrupts infants' future performance on nonsocial learning tasks (Dunham, Dunham, Hurshman, & Alexander, 1989; Dunham & Dunham, 1990). Infants of depressed mothers are certainly more likely than other infants to experience noncontingent interaction. Observational studies of mothers suffering from postpartum illness show that the ill mothers are often distracted and preoccupied with their own thoughts and respond to their infants in a more sluggish, less immediate manner (Campbell, Cohn, Flanagan, Popper, & Meyers, 1992; Field, 1992; Murray, Fiori-Cowley, Hooper, & Cooper, 1996).

In the course of her prospective study of the effects of postpartum illness on infant development, Murray categorized the nature of the speech produced by depressed and well mothers while interacting with their 2-month-old infants (Murray et al., 1993). An important distinction was the extent to which the speech was focused on the infant as opposed to the mother's own concerns and preoccupations; furthermore, infant-focused speech included explicit statements in which the infant's own actions were commented upon, as in " 'You're trying to kick your legs there' " (Murray et al., 1993, p. 1088). Clearly, infant-focused speech was much more likely to be contingent upon the infant's own state or actions, and descriptions of what the infant was doing at the moment would obviously be contingent. Mothers who were depressed in the postpartum period were less likely to use infant- as opposed to mother-focused speech and less likely to describe the infant as an agent. (Group differences in the latter, lower-frequency category only approached statistical significance.)

Murray's data provide suggestions of particular links between the mothers' contingent speech and the infants' cognitive abilities. Regardless of maternal diagnosis, infant-focused speech predicted better performance on the tests of object permanence at 9 months of age and better performance on the standardized Bayley Scales at 18 months. These findings suggest that when depressed mothers focus their attention on their infants, the infants do not show deficits in cognitive abilities. Thus, it may be a particular mode of interaction, rather than the mother's illness per se, that places infants at risk for cognitive problems.

Mothers' tendencies to focus on their infants' activities may be complemented by the infants' own willing engagement in interaction with their mothers. In the Cambridgeshire sample, the infant's own active engagement in interaction reliably predicted cognitive attainments 5 years later, whether or not the mother was depressed postnatally (Murray et al., 1996; Murray & Cooper, Chapter 5, this volume). This association is an important one as it identifies particular interactive processes that may be associated with depression but may also occur without it and thus raises possibilities for effective intervention based on the qualities of mother–child interaction, not mother's mental state alone (see Cooper & Murray, Chapter 8, this volume).

As infants grow older, their attention to the environment is shaped not only by their direct, one-to-one interactions with their mothers but also by their observations of the mother's encounters with the environment. An infant observes what the mother sees and finds of interest in her world and may come to regulate his or her own attention accordingly (see Bindra, 1974). For example, newly locomoting 9- to 12-month-old infants who followed their mothers around a novel environment were likely to discover hidden toys and, furthermore, to apply what they had learned to a new situation, discovering hidden toys in a different but similar environment. However, this was not true for infants who explored the first environment while their mothers remained seated, in the fashion of a "secure base," or if the mothers simply carried the infants around the first environment (Hay, 1977). Both infants and mothers had to be active explorers if learning was to occur.

This process of learning by following the mother and observing her interactions with the world may be much more difficult for the children of depressed women. For example, when mothers and toddlers were exploring a new environment together, depressed women were more likely than other mothers to show abrupt shifts in their own attention to the objects provided: They paid attention to more things for less time than did the well mothers (Breznitz & Friedman, 1988). This choppy attentional pattern was mirrored in the children of the depressed women, who similarly paid attention to more objects but for shorter periods of time than did the children of women who had not been depressed.

Emotional Regulation and Information Processing

Another factor that might constrain intellectual development for infants of depressed women is the experience of acute and chronic distress on the parts of both mothers and children. Depressed women are more likely to show negative affect than are other mothers (Campbell et al., 1992; Field, 1992; Murray et al., 1993; Murray, Fiori-Cowley, et al., 1996), and so are their children (Field, 1992). Furthermore, the infants of depressed women show higher rates of negative affect even when they are interacting with other, nondepressed adults (Field et al., 1988).

Exposure to negative affect and one's own distress impede learning. Experimental studies have shown that children's own dysregulated affect interferes with their abilities to process information (e.g., Bugental et al., 1992). In particular, infants' own negative affect interferes with learning and increases the likelihood that infants will forget what they have learned (Fagen, Ohr, Fleckenstein, & Ribner, 1985; Singer & Fagen, 1992).

Taken together, these findings suggest not only that the infants of depressed women receive less contingent stimulation from their mothers, but also that because of their dysregulated affect and their generalized, negative approach to social situations, they would be less able to profit from time spent with other persons who are not depressed. Moreover, the infants' acquired characteristics may disrupt such potentially compensatory encounters (Field et al., 1988): When 3- to 6-month-old infants of depressed mothers were tested with nondepressed nursery nurses, the infants' negative mood persisted. Even more disturbingly, the nondepressed nursery nurses themselves began to show flatter affect and lower rates of activity when interacting with these infants (Field et al., 1988). This social contagion of the infants' own affect may limit possibilities for effective intervention.

In tracing links between a mother's postpartum illness and outcomes for her child, it is important to remember that cognitive development is interwoven with emotional development and with the establishment of important personal relationships throughout the life span. In particular, the cognitive problems shown by some children of depressed women may need to be examined in the context of the mother–child attachment relationship, which is rather more likely to be insecure when the mother has been depressed (DeMulder & Radke-Yarrow, 1991; Murray, 1992). Insecure attachment is often thought to derive from insensitive mothering in the early months of life, with mothers not reacting promptly and sensitively to infants' overtures and expressions of need (see Belsky & Cassidy, 1994; Waters, Hay, & Richters, 1986). Thus the noncontingent, self-preoccupied behavior of depressed women may simultaneously promote insecure attachment and problems in learning. To the extent that insecure attachment is accompanied by overt behavioral problems and failures of self-regulation (see Turner, 1991; Waters et al., 1986), children's capacities to learn from persons other than their mother, such as nursery school teachers, may be further disrupted. Thus, by the years of childhood, we would expect to see not just a straightforward link between the mother's early illness and cognitive deficits but also a network of associations with the child's personal relations and behavioral difficulties. It is at this point, if not before, that we may discern separate pathways for girls and boys.

The Role of Gender

The available literature on links between postpartum depression and children's cognitive development indicates that girls and boys are affected in different ways. In the South London sample (Sharp et al., 1995), postpartum illness was associated with lower cognitive scores for boys but not for girls. In the North London sample, no such gender difference was apparent (Hay & Kumar, 1995), but in that sample boys were more likely to be protected by maternal education than were girls. Confirmation of a general difference between girls and boys awaits analysis of data in a larger, representative sample.

There are reasons to believe, however, that boys might be more greatly affected by mothers' noncontingent responsiveness and negative affect in infancy than are girls. On average, male infants are developmentally delayed in comparison to their female counterparts and may have particular problems in the regulation of arousal and emotion. For example, male, as opposed to female, infants spend more time expressing both positive and negative affect (see Tronick & Weinberg, Chapter 3, this volume). Some research on nonhuman primates has suggested that increased emotional reactivity in male infants derives from an immature organization of the cerebral hemispheres; females of the same age have achieved a more mature degree of hemispheric regulation (Hopkins & Bard, 1993). Cross-hemispheric integration has been implicated in human children's regulation of emotion (see Cicchetti et al., 1991). Thus, boys, as opposed to girls, may be in special need of external aid in the achievement of self-regulation and may suffer more if that aid is not forthcoming (see Tronick & Weinberg, Chapter 3, this volume).

It is also clear that boys, as opposed to girls, are more likely to develop insecure attachments (e.g., McCarthy, 1991; Murray, 1992; Murray, Fiori-Cowley, et al., 1996). To the extent that insecure attachment impedes social competence and fosters the development of behavioral problems, boys may be less likely than girls to profit from compensatory stimulation in later childhood. More windows may open up for girls in the second and third years of life, even if they had been adversely affected by their experiences in infancy. For example, in Murray's longitudinal observations, as mentioned earlier, a clear link was established between infant-focused speech at 2 months of age and the infant's ability to pass tests of object permanence at 9 months of age (Murray et al., 1993). The daughters and sons of depressed women were equally likely to fail such tests at 9 months, in contrast to infants whose mothers had not been depressed. However, when tests of object permanence were administered again at 18 months of age, achievement at 9 months predicted performance at 18 months, but girls showed greater improvement than boys between 9 and 18 months.

This suggests that the boys' performance was constrained by their earlier achievements, which in turn were linked directly to early interactive experiences with the mother. For girls, some sources of influence between 9 and 18 months led to improvement; it is not unlikely that attachment-related developments may be involved.

Most contemporary theorists of early experience believe that the effect of early experiences is mediated by an individual's current circumstances (see Nash & Hay, 1993; Rutter, 1991). To the extent that girls and boys find themselves in different social circumstances throughout life, they may be more or less likely to experience relationships and events that compensate for their early deprivation. Any attempt to test hypotheses about the effects of early contingency learning and dysregulated affect on the development of intelligence must take into account the new circumstances in which children find themselves.

CONCLUSION

There is reason to worry about the intellectual development of children whose mothers experience postpartum depression. Cognitive problems have been observed in all three of the community samples reviewed in this chapter, although those problems differ in kind and duration from sample to sample. There is also reason to think about prevention and intervention programs from the point of view of protecting children's intellectual development as well as alleviating mothers' symptoms. At the same time, however, we must be cautious before adopting an overly simplistic early-experience model to account for the links that have been observed. It is possible that there are some vulnerability factors in children, such as, in some circumstances, low birthweight, that make their mothers more likely to become depressed in the first place but also make the children more likely to experience problems if the mothers do become depressed (Cicchetti et al., 1991). It is also possible that the children of well-educated mothers are ultimately protected, though they may be even more greatly affected during the period of infancy itself (see Murray, 1992). It is possible that, in the presence of postpartum illness, gender is a risk factor for boys and a protective factor for girls.

All these possibilities need to be tested in further work with an explicit focus on social processes, not simple contrasts of static diagnostic categories. For example, Murray's most recent work has moved beyond a simple comparison of depressed and nondepressed women to identify particular patterns of early interaction that predict later cognitive performance (Murray et al., 1993; Murray, Fiori-Cowley, et al., 1996; Murray, Hipwell, et al., in press). These analyses are important for developmental theories of intelligence, because they show how early maternal inputs actually lower the association between the child's initial cognitive attainments and later outcomes. Thus, stability in cognitive performance, which has been taken as evidence of the heritability of intelligence (Moffitt et al., 1993), is itself sensitive to the impact of early social experiences. Further process-oriented research will be most welcome.

For the time being, however, the available data remind us that intelligence is in essence both a social skill and a social product. Our means of testing intelligence in childhood, using such procedures as the McCarthy Scales, rely on social interactions between children and testers. It is hardly surprising that early social experiences, perhaps those that impinge uniquely on children who are at particularly vulnerable stages in their own development, constrain the intellectual achievements that our standardized assessments manage to measure.

REFERENCES

Ainsworth, M. D. S. (1969). Object relations, dependency, and attachment: Theoretical review of the infant–mother relationship. *Child Development, 40,* 969–1025.

Bateson, P. P. G. (1979). How do sensitive periods arise and what are they for? *Animal Behavior, 27,* 470–486.

Beach, F. A., & Jaynes, J. J. (1954). Effects of early experience upon the behavior of animals. *Psychological Bulletin, 51,* 239–263.

Belsky, J., & Cassidy, J. (1994). Attachment: Theory and evidence. In M. Rutter & D. F. Hay (Eds.), *Development through life: A handbook for clinicians* (pp. 373–402). Oxford, England: Blackwell Scientific.

Bindra, D. (1974). A motivational view of learning, performance, and behavior modification. *Psychological Review, 81,* 1–26.

Bornstein, M., & Sigman, M. D. (1986). Continuity in mental development from infancy. *Child Development, 57,* 251–274.

Bowlby, J. (1958). The nature of the child's tie to his mother. *International Journal of Psycho-Analysis, 39,* 350–373.

Breznitz, Z., & Friedman, S. L. (1988). Toddlers' concentration: Does maternal depression make a difference? *Journal of Child Psychology and Psychiatry, 29,* 267–279.

Bugental, D. B., Blue, J., Cortez, V., Fleck, K., & Rodriguez, A. (1992). Influence of witnessed affect on information processing in children. *Child Development,* *63,* 774–786.

Cairns, R. B., McGuire, A. M., & Gariepy, J.-P. (1993). Developmental behavior genetics: Fusion, correlated constraints, and timing. In D. F. Hay & A. Angold (Eds.), *Precursors and causes in development and psychopathology* (pp. 87–122). Chichester, England: Wiley.

Caldwell, B., & Bradley, R. (1984). *HOME observation for measurement of the environment.* Little Rock: University of Arkansas.

Campbell, S. B., Cohn, J. F., Flanagan, C., Popper, S., & Meyers, T. (1992). Course and correlates of postpartum depression during the transition to parenthood. *Development and Psychopathology, 4,* 29–47.

Ceci, S., Baker-Sennett, J., & Bronfenbrenner, U. (1994). Psychometric and everyday intelligence: Synonyms, antonyms, and anonyms. In M. Rutter & D. F. Hay (Eds.), *Development through life: A handbook for clinicians.* Oxford, England: Blackwell Scientific.

Chipuer, H. M., & Plomin, R. (1992). Using siblings to identify shared and non-shared HOME items. *British Journal of Developmental Psychology, 10,* 165–178.

Cicchetti, D., Ganiban, J., & Barnett, D. (1991). Contributions from the study of high-risk populations to understanding the development of emotion regulation. In J. Garber & K. Dodge (Eds.), *The development of emotion regulation and dysregulation.* Cambridge, England: Cambridge University Press.

Clarke, A. M., & Clarke, A. D. B. (1976). *Early experience: Myth and evidence.* London: Open Books.

Cogill, S., Caplan, H., Alexandra, H., Robson, K., & Kumar, R. (1986). Impact of postnatal depression on cognitive development in young children. *British Medical Journal, 292,* 1165–1167.

DeMulder, E., & Radke-Yarrow, M. (1991). Attachment with affectively ill and well mothers: Concurrent behavioral correlates. *Development and Psychopathology, 3,* 227–242.

Denenberg, V. H. (1968). A consideration of the usefulness of the critical period hypothesis as applied to the stimulation of rodents in infancy. In G. Newton & S. Levine (Eds.), *Early experience and behavior: The psychobiology of development.* Springfield, IL: Thomas.

Dodge, K. A. (1991). Emotion and social information-processing. In J. Garber & K. A. Dodge (Eds.), *The development of emotion regulation and dysregulation* (pp. 159–181). Cambridge, England: Cambridge University Press.

Dunham, P. J., & Dunham, F. (1990). Effects of mother–infant social interactions on infants' subsequent contingency task performance. *Child Development, 61,* 785–793.

Dunham, P. J., Dunham, F., Hurshman, A., & Alexander, T. (1989). Social contingency effects on subsequent perceptual-cognitive tasks in young infants. *Child Development, 60,* 1486–1488.

Dunn, J. F., & Plomin, R. (1990). *Separate lives: Why siblings are so different.* New York: Basic Books.

Fagen, J. W., Ohr, P. S., Fleckenstein, L. K., & Ribner, D. R. (1985). The effect of crying on long-term memory in infancy. *Child Development, 56,* 1584–1592.

Field, T. (1992). Infants of depressed mothers. *Development and Psychopathology, 4,* 49–66.

Field, T., Healy, B., Goldstein, S., et al. (1988). Infants of depressed mothers show 'depressed' behaviour even with nondepressed adults. *Child Development, 59,* 1569–1579.

Finkelstein, N. W., & Ramey, C. T. (1977). Learning to control the environment in infancy. *Child Development, 48,* 806–819.

Freud, S. (1938). *An outline of psychoanalysis.* London: Hogarth.

Gottlieb, G. (1991). Experiential canalization of behavioral development: Theory. *Developmental Psychology, 29,* 4–13.

Harris, P. L. (1983). Infant cognition. In P. H. Mussen (Ed.), *Handbook of child psychology* (Vol. 2, pp. 689–782). New York: Wiley.

Hay, D. F. (1977). Following their companions as a form of exploration for human infants. *Child Development, 48,* 1624–1632.

Hay, D. F., & Angold, A. (Eds.). (1993). *Precursors and causes in development and psychopathology.* Chichester, England: Wiley.

Hay, D. F., & Kumar, R. (1995). Interpreting the effects of mothers' postnatal depression on children's intelligence: A critique and reanalysis. *Child Psychiatry and Human Development, 25,* 165–181.

Hay, D. F., Zahn-Waxler, C., Cummings, E. M., & Iannotti, R. J. (1992). Young children's views about conflicts with peers: A comparison of the daughters and sons of depressed and well women. *Journal of Child Psychology and Psychiatry, 33,* 669–683.

Hebb, D. O. (1946). On the nature of fear. *Psychological Review, 3,* 49–50.

Hebb, D. O. (1947). The effects of early experience on problem-solving at maturity. *American Psychologist, 2,* 306–307.

Hebb, D. O. (1949). *Organisation of behaviour.* New York: Wiley.

Herrnstein, R. J., & Murray, C. (1994). *The bell curve: Intelligence and class structure in American Life.* London: Free Press.

Hess, E. H. (1959). Imprinting. *Science, 130,* 133–141.

Hopkins, W. D., & Bard, K. A. (1993). Hemispheric specialization in infant chimpanzees (*Pan troglodytes*): Evidence for a relation with gender and arousal. *Developmental Psychobiology, 26,* 219–235.

Horn, G. (1993). Brain mechanisms of memory and predispositions: Interactive studies of cerebral function and behavior. In M. Johnson (Ed.), *Brain development and cognition: A reader* (pp. 481–509). Oxford, England: Blackwell Scientific.

Hunt, J. McV. (1961). *Intelligence and experience.* New York: Ronald.

Kumar, R., & Robson, K. (1984). A prospective study of emotional disorders in childbearing women. *British Journal of Psychiatry, 144,* 35–47.

Kuo, Z.-Y. (1967). *The dynamics of behavioral development.* New York: Random House.

Lehrman, D. S. (1970). Semantic and conceptual issues in the nature–nurture problem. In L. A. Aronson, E. Tobach, D. S. Lehrman, & J. Rosenblatt (Eds.),

Development and evolution of behavior: Essays in memory of T. C. Schneirla (pp. 17–52). San Francisco: Freeman.

Lorenz, K. (1970). Companions as factors in the bird's environment. In K. Lorenz (Ed.), *Studies on animal and human behavior* (Vol. 1, pp. 101–258). Cambridge, MA: Harvard University Press. (Original work published 1935)

MacDonald, K. (1985). Early experience, relative plasticity, and social development. *Developmental Review, 5,* 99–121.

McCall, R. B. (1981). Nature–nurture and the two realms of development: A proposed integration with respect to mental development. *Child Development, 52,* 1–12.

McCall, R. B., Appelbaum, M. I., & Hogarty, P. S. (1973). Developmental changes in mental performance. *Monographs of the Society for Research in Child Development, 38*(Serial No. 150).

McCall, R. B., & Carriger, M. (1993). A meta-analysis of infant habituation and recognition memory performance as predictors of later IQ. *Child Development, 64,* 57–79.

McCarthy, G. (1991). *Attachment relationships in the preschool years.* Unpublished doctoral dissertation, University of London.

Moffitt, T. E., Caspi, A., Harkness, A. R., & Silva, P. A. (1993). The natural history of change in intellectual performance: Who changes? How much? Is it meaningful? *Journal of Child Psychology and Psychiatry, 34,* 441–453.

Murray, L. (1992). The impact of postnatal depression on infant development. *Journal of Child Psychology and Psychiatry, 33,* 543–561.

Murray, L., Fiori-Cowley, A., Hooper, R., & Cooper, P. J. (1996). The impact of postnatal depression and associated adversity on early mother infant interactions and later infant outcome. *Child Development, 67,* 2512–2526.

Murray, L., Hipwell, A., Hooper, R., Stein, A., & Cooper, P. (in press). The cognitive development of five-year-old children of postnatally depressed mothers. *Journal of Child Psychology and Psychiatry.*

Murray, L., Kempton, C., Woolgar, M., & Hooper, R. (1993). Depressed mothers' speech to their infants and its relation to infant gender and cognitive development. *Journal of Child Psychology and Psychiatry, 34,* 1083–1101.

Murray, L., Stanley, C., Hooper, R., King, F., & Fiori-Cowley, A. (1996). The role of infant factors in postnatal depression and mother–infant interactions. *Developmental Medicine and Child Neurology, 38,* 109–119.

Nash, A., & Hay, D. F. (1993). Relationships in infancy as precursors and causes of later relationships and psychopathology. In D. F. Hay & A. Angold (Eds.), *Precursors and causes in development and psychopathology* (pp. 199–232). Chichester, England: Wiley.

Pickles, A. (1993). Stages, precursors and causes in development. In D. F. Hay & A. Angold (Eds.), *Precursors and causes in development and psychopathology* (pp. 23–49). Chichester, England: Wiley.

Plomin, R. (1994). *Genetics and experience: The interplay between nature and nurture.* Thousand Oaks, CA: Sage.

Plomin, R., et al. (1994). DNA markers associated with high versus low IQ: The IQ Quantitative Trait Loci (QTL) Project. *Behavior Genetics, 24,* 107–118.

Plomin, R., & Daniels, D. (1987). Why are children in the same family so different from each other? *Behavioral and Brain Sciences, 10,* 1–16.

Plomin, R., De Fried, J. C., & Fulker, D. W. (1988). *Nature and nurture during infancy and early childhood.* Cambridge, England: Cambridge University Press.

Rutter, M. L. (1991). A fresh look at "maternal deprivation." In P. Bateson (Ed.), *The development and integration of behaviour* (pp. 331–374). Cambridge, England: Cambridge University Press.

Sameroff, A. J., Seifer, R., & Zax, M. (1982). Early development of children at risk for emotional disorder. *Monographs of the Society for Research in Child Development, 50*(Serial No. 199).

Scarr, S. (1990). Developmental theories for the 1990s: Development and individual differences. *Child Development, 63,* 1–19.

Schneirla, T. C. (1957). The concept of development in comparative psychology. In D. B. Harris (Ed.), *The concept of development.* Minneapolis: University of Minnesota. Reprinted in L. R. Aronson, E. Tobach, J. S. Rosenblatt, & D. S. Lehrman (Eds.), *Selected writings of T. C. Schneirla* (pp. 259–294). San Francisco: Freeman.

Sharp, D. (1993). *Childbirth-related emotional disorders in primary care: A longitudinal prospective study.* Unpublished doctoral dissertation, London University.

Sharp, D., Hay, D. F., Pawlby, S., Schmucker, G., Allen, H., & Kumar, R. (1995). The impact of postnatal depression on boys' intellectual development. *Journal of Child Psychology and Psychiatry, 36,* 1315–1336.

Sigman, M. D., & Mundy, P. (1993). Infant precursors of childhood intellectual and verbal abilities. In D. F. Hay & A. Angold (Eds.), *Precursors and causes in development and psychopathology* (pp. 123–144). Chichester, England: Wiley.

Singer, J. M., & Fagen, J. W. (1992). Negative affect, emotional expression, and forgetting in young infants. *Developmental Psychology, 28,* 43–57.

Stern, D. (1977). *The first relationship.* Cambridge, MA: Harvard University.

Sternberg, R. J. (1990). *Metaphors of mind: Conceptions of the nature of intelligence.* Cambridge, England: Cambridge University Press.

Stevenson, J., & Fredman, G. (1980). The social environmental correlates of reading abilities. *Journal of Child Psychology and Psychiatry, 31,* 681–698.

Thompson, W. R., & Grusec, J. E. (1970). Studies of early experience. In P. H. Mussen (Ed.), *Carmichael's manual of child psychology* (Vol. 1, pp. 565–654). New York: Wiley.

Turner, P. (1991). Relations between attachment, gender and behavior problems with peers in preschool. *Child Development, 62,* 1475–1488.

Waddington, C. H. (1957). *The strategy of the genes.* London: Allen.

Waters, E., Hay, D. F., & Richters, J. (1986). Infant–parent attachment and the origins of prosocial and antisocial behavior. In D. Olweus, J. Block, & M. Radke-Yarrow (Eds.), *Development of antisocial and prosocial behavior: Research, theories, and issues* (pp. 97–125). New York: Academic Press.

Weissman, M. M., Leckman, J. F., Merikangas, K. R., Gammon, G. D., & Prusoff,

B. A. (1984). Depression and anxiety disorders in parents and children. *Archives of General Psychiatry, 41,* 845–851.

Winters, K. C., Stone, A. A., Weintraub, S., & Neale, J. M. (1981). Cognitive and attentional deficits in children vulnerable to psychopathology. *Journal of Abnormal Child Psychology, 9,* 435–453.

Zahn-Waxler, C., Cole, P., & Barrett, K. (1991). Guilt and empathy: Sex differences and implications for the development of depression. In J. Garber & K. Dodge (Eds.), *The development of emotion regulation and dysregulation* (pp. 234–272). Cambridge, England: Cambridge University Press.

5

~

The Role of Infant
and Maternal Factors
in Postpartum Depression,
Mother–Infant Interactions,
and Infant Outcome

Lynne Murray
Peter J. Cooper
University of Reading

Research on early social development has demonstrated a remarkable sensitivity in infants to the quality of their interpersonal environment from the first days of life. The evidence of neonatal imitation of facial movements and expressions (Maratos, 1973, 1982; Meltzoff & Moore, 1977, 1983; Kugiumutzakis, 1985, 1993), the selective responsiveness to human over nonhuman stimuli (Fantz, 1963; Goren, Sarty, & Wu, 1975; Friedlander, 1970; Eisenberg, 1975; Leslie, 1984), and the rapid development of preferences for the particular characteristics of persons involved in infant care (Field, 1985; De Casper & Fifer, 1980; McFarlane, 1975; Bushnell, Sai, & Mullin, 1989; Cernoch & Porter, 1985; Hepper, Scott, & Shahidullah, 1993) together attest to a preadaptation in the newborn to an environment of consistent interpersonal engagements. In infants of 2 months, the microanalytical study of naturalistic face-to-face engagements reveals a capacity to interact with others with complex and well-organized repertoires of gesture and facial expression that appear responsive to the form and timing of adult communication (Brazelton, Koslowski, & Main, 1974; Stern, 1974; Trevarthen, 1979; Tronick, Als, & Adamson, 1979).

In addition to research on infant social development, which employs naturalistic observations of parent–infant interactions, a substantial body of experimental work has examined the infant's response to episodes of disrupted or perturbed maternal communication. This work has been particularly fruitful in elucidating the nature of the infant's sensitivity to the quality of interpersonal engagements (Brazelton, Tronick, Adamson, Als, & Wise, 1975; Papoušek & Papoušek, 1975; Tronick, Als, Adamson, Wise, & Brazelton, 1978; Murray & Trevarthen, 1985). Two conclusions can be drawn from the accounts of infant responses to the wide variety of perturbations to maternal communication employed in these different studies. First, not only do infants appear equipped to detect alterations to single physical parameters of adult behavior (e.g., pitch of voice, direction of gaze, and degree of contingency), but they are capable of coordinating these different parameters to apprehend directly different personal and affective states. Second, infant protest and distress in the face of experimentally arranged maternal unresponsiveness indicate a motivation to achieve particular forms of interpersonal engagement. Part of the significance of these capacities is in their underpinning of the subsequent achievement, evident toward the end of the first year, of common understandings or the sharing of meaning, a process essential to the infant's integration into the wider social world of interpersonally constructed values (Richards, 1974; Tronick et al., 1979; Trevarthen & Hubley, 1978; Tronick & Weinberg, Chapter 3, this volume).

The findings of this research with normal populations, and particularly those on the infant's response to experimentally perturbed communication, have clear clinical implications. If infants are so sensitive to the quality of their interpersonal environment when it is disrupted experimentally in brief and mild ways, the question naturally arises as to what the consequences might be of the infant's exposure to an interpersonal environment more seriously disrupted for a longer period. Such disruption might be expected when the mother is depressed, because depression is associated with such interactional deficits as a slowed rate of speech

(Teasdale, Fogarty, & Williams, 1980) and a reduction in eye contact (Hinchcliffe, Lancashire, & Roberts, 1971) and emotional expressiveness and responsiveness (Lewinsohn, Weinstein, & Alper, 1970; Libert & Lewinsohn, 1973), the very parameters of human communication to which young infants are so sensitive. Indeed, one of the first studies to address the question whether maternal depression has an impact on mother–infant interactions, that of Cohn and Tronick (1983), employed the principal perturbation used in the experimental studies, the "still-face" paradigm, explicitly as a simulation of a depressed style of maternal communication. This report was followed by a number of studies that directly examined maternal communication in the context of depression and its effects on the infant's behavior in the interaction. As might be expected, the early work in this area demonstrated that infants who were exposed to disturbed patterns of communication in the context of depression, such as withdrawn and unresponsive maternal behavior or intrusive and hostile interactions (Field, 1984; Field et al., 1985; Cohn, Matias, Tronick, Connell, & Lyons-Ruth, 1986; Field et al., 1988; Field, Healy, Goldstein, & Guthertz, 1990), themselves showed signs of disturbance, with raised levels of distress, protest, and avoidance (Cohn et al., 1986; Field et al., 1990; Tronick & Weinberg, Chapter 3, this volume).

The accounts outlined here of the development of early interpersonal relationships, as well as those of the nature of depressed mother–infant interactions, were based on an essentially normative view of the infant and on the assumption that any divergence in developmental trajectories was largely a function of differences in parenting. Thus, although this literature did full justice to the remarkable capacities of the infant to engage in complex interpersonal exchanges, there was little discussion of individual differences between infants and of the impact such differences might exert on the process of communication with the caretaker and on infant outcome. In fact, a number of early studies suggested that individual infant characteristics were important in influencing the quality of parental engagements. These characteristics included infant constitutional factors (Brazelton, 1961; Yarrow, 1963; Schaffer & Emerson, 1964; Bell, 1968; Crockenberg, 1981) as well as more transient qualities such as physiological state (Levy, 1958). Consistent with these findings was evidence suggesting that in attempting to understand associations between parenting behavior and eventual child outcome, it is essential to take such individual differences into account (Bernal, 1974).

Evidence of an infant contribution to the quality of mother–infant interactions in general clearly raises the issue of the possible contribution of infant factors to the patterns of communication occurring between depressed mothers and their infants. It also complicates the interpretation of any adverse outcome in the offspring of postnatally depressed populations: It is possible that infant factors contribute to the onset of maternal depression, and the adverse infant outcome in the context of the maternal mood disorder arises not so much because the disturbances in parenting drive the course of infant development but because individual infant differences are themselves directly related to the adverse outcome. Alternatively, it may be the case that individual infant differences elicit particular styles of behavior in caretakers which themselves then go on to influence the subsequent course of child development.

The following sections of this chapter examine the relative contributions of infant and maternal factors to development in the context of postnatal depression by describing the findings of a research strategy that combines prospective examination with direct assessments of infant functioning, both independent of the mother and in the context of interactions with her. First, this chapter addresses the possible contribution of infant factors to the onset of postnatal depression itself. We then consider the role of infant and maternal factors in contributing to the quality of face-to-face interactions in depressed and well groups. Finally, we consider the relative contributions of maternal and infant factors to infant and child cognitive and emotional outcome in the context of maternal depression.

THE ROLE OF INFANT FACTORS
IN POSTNATAL DEPRESSION

On the whole, as described earlier, most studies assessing the infants of postnatally depressed mothers have done so in the context of interactions with the mother. Three studies have, however, examined independent infant functioning. Cutrona and Troutman (1986) found an association between mothers' level of depressed mood (assessed using the Beck Depression Inventory [BDI]) and the presence of difficult behavior in the infants at 3 months, as assessed by direct observations of infant crying, as well as by maternal crying records and reports. Similarly, Whiffen and Gotlib (1989), who assessed the 2-month-old infants of 25 women who were depressed and 25 well women, found that compared to the infants of well women, the infants of depressed mothers were more tense and less content and deteriorated more rapidly under the stress of developmental testing. Finally, Field et al. (1988) observed 40 infants of depressed mothers (defined by a BDI score > 12) and 34 infants of well women (BDI scores < 9) during interactions both with their mothers and with nondepressed adults at 3–6 months postpartum. In both conditions the infants of depressed women were rated worse on measures of state, physical activity, facial expressions, vocalizations, and fussing. The results of these studies are clearly consistent with the hypothesis that infant factors have an impact on maternal mental state, with difficult or irritable behavior in the infant contributing to the occurrence or the persistence of maternal depression. Indeed, such an inference would be in line with models of depressive mood disturbance which emphasize the role of aversive and uncontrollable events (in this case difficult infant behavior) in creating a sense of helplessness (Seligman, 1975). Nevertheless, because in each of these studies the infant assessments were conducted concurrently with those of maternal mental state, it is equally plausible that the findings reflect the impact of the maternal mood disorder on the infant.

The Cambridge Study of Infant Factors

A strict test of the role of infant factors requires an evaluation of infant functioning in the neonatal period before the onset of maternal depression. Until recently this has not been practicable because the incidence of depression is only around 10% in the first 2 months postpartum, and a full population screen of neonates would therefore entail the collection of a large amount of redundant data. However, the development of a predictive index for postnatal depression (Cooper, Murray, Hooper, & West, 1996) has facilitated the necessary prospective investigation by permitting the antenatal recruitment of a high-risk population of women: The infants of these women could be assessed in the neonatal period before the onset of the maternal mood disorder (Murray, Stanley, Hooper, King, & Fiori-Cowley, 1996). The predictive index comprises a range of personal and social factors which are implicated in the development of postnatal depression. Principally, these factors concern the mother's experience of the pregnancy (e.g., whether it was planned, her initial reaction, and her subsequent emotional state); the previous occurrence of affective disorder; and the quality of the mother's current relationships (e.g., the extent of friction with her partner and the presence of other confiding relationships). Using this index, a consecutive series of primiparous women attending the 32-week antenatal clinics at the Cambridge (England) maternity hospital was screened. Subsequently, those women who were identified as being at high risk for depression and who delivered full-term healthy infants were approached on the postnatal wards for recruitment. Of the 238 women eligible for inclusion in the study, 188 (79%) agreed to participate. In addition, to determine whether maternal risk status itself influenced neonatal functioning, and to examine whether there was any difference in the effects of infant variables on maternal mental state according to risk status, a smaller number of women at low risk for depression were recruited (43 out of the 46 who were approached agreed to participate). Because infant functioning in the days immediately following birth is influenced by the nature of the labor and delivery, and particularly the medication administered to the mother (Lester, Als, & Brazelton, 1982), the assessment of the neonate was delayed until 10 days postpartum. To take into account any influence on infant functioning of the mother's emotional state in the puerperium and her feelings of confidence and efficacy in relation to the infant, mothers completed the Maternity Blues Scale (Kennerly & Gath, 1989) and the Mother and Baby Scale (St. James Roberts & Wolke, 1988) in the first postpartum week. The latter scale concerns maternal perceptions of unsettled and irregular infant behavior, irritability and alertness during feeds, and overall impressions of infant difficulty, as well as maternal self-confidence.

At 10 days postpartum a trained researcher administered the Neonatal Behavioural Assessment Scale (NBAS; Brazelton, 1984) to the infants in their home, and the assessment was repeated at 15 days. The NBAS is a standardized assessment in which neonatal behavior is elicited in relation to a range of environmental stimuli, yielding scores on measures of orientation, motor behavior, the range and regulation of state, autonomic stability, reflexes, and irritability. The researcher also examined the infants to establish that no neurological abnormalities were present. Once the neonate was assessed, the researcher interviewed the mother using the Structured Clinical Interview for DSM-III-R (Spitzer, Williams, Gibbon, & First, 1989) to establish whether she had already become depressed. This applied to eight women from the high-risk sample and one from the group of mothers at low risk for depression, and these women were excluded from further participation in the study.

At 8 weeks postpartum the women were seen again at home by a second researcher who was unaware of all previous assessments, and their psychiatric state was once more systematically assessed. At this point, 32% of the high-risk sample had become depressed, as had 19% of the low-risk group (an unusually high rate for the low-risk sample in this maternity population).

Two neonatal characteristics were found to be strongly predictive of maternal mental state at 2 months. First, poor motor functioning, whether shown in hypo- or hyperaroused behavior, significantly increased the risk of the mother's becoming depressed. This applied to women from the high- and low-risk samples alike. Second, neonatal irritability (manifest, for example, in the infant's immediate and distressed response to mild stimulation and failure to be readily soothed by adult interventions) also increased the chances that the mother would become depressed, but this applied only within the high-risk group. The impact of these aspects of infant functioning on the risk of depression in the high-risk group is shown in Table 5.1. It is apparent that when both poor motor behavior and irritability were present, the great majority of mothers became depressed, whereas in the absence of these difficulties just under a fifth of high-risk women were depressed at 2 months.

Investigation of obstetric records provided no evidence that some third factor (e.g., maternal hypertension) could have accounted for both the neonatal behavior and later maternal depression. In addition, a number of findings indicated that the association between neonatal behavior and maternal mental state could not be explained by the impact on neonatal behavior of aspects of maternal caretaking associated with incipient depression. First, the rates of neonatal irritability and poor motor functioning did not vary as a function of maternal risk status. Second, infant irritability and motor behavior improved between 10 and 15 days postpartum, and the extent of improvement was comparable in infants of

TABLE 5.1. Proportions of High-Risk Women Who Became Depressed by Infant Performance on the NBAS

	Poor motor behavior	
Irritability	High	Low
High	80% (N = 10)	45% (N = 22)
Low	41% (N = 29)	19% (N = 119)

women who did and who did not go on to become depressed. Finally, neonatal functioning was unrelated to maternal mood and level of self-confidence in the period shortly before the infant assessment. These latter maternal factors were, as might be expected, predictive of later mental state, with increasing scores on the Blues scale as well as feelings that the infant's behavior was unpredictable and unsettled being associated with an increased likelihood of depression. However, it is striking that the effects of these maternal variables were not as marked as those of the neonatal factors, as is evident from Table 5.2, which shows the independent influences of all these variables on the risk of depression. It can be seen that the risk of depression increased almost fivefold in the context of poor infant motor behavior and around three and a half times when the infant was irritable.

It is not surprising that irritable infant behavior, being both distressing and relatively unamenable to parental ministrations, increased the risk of depression in women who were already vulnerable to affective disorder. Such an effect is entirely consistent with diathesis–stress models of depressive mood disorder in which stressful events precipitate episodes in those already at risk (Brown & Harris, 1978). However, less expected was the fact that poor motor functioning, even within a neurologically normal sample, had a significant impact on maternal mental state. Unlike irritability, which has long been identified as a possible source of parenting difficulties (Crockenberg, 1981, 1986), poorly regulated motor behavior has not generally been thought to influence maternal mood. In this study, however, its impact was even more marked than that of irritability, and similarly so in both the high- and low-risk groups. The design of the study does not permit the mechanisms involved in the association between poor motor behavior and mater-

TABLE 5.2. Effects of Neonatal Behavior and Maternal Factors Assessed in the Puerperium on Maternal Depression: Multivariate Logistic Regression

Effect	Estimated contribution to log odds	SD	Wald statistic	p	Multiplicative effect on risk
Poor motor behavior	1.59	0.49	3.22	<.005	4.88
Irritability	1.22	0.51	2.40	<.05	3.38
Maternal perception of unsettled/irregular behavior	0.79	0.47	1.67	<.10	2.19
Blues (each 5 points on scale)	0.50	0.18	2.79	<.01	1.65

Note: From Murray, Stanley, Hooper, King, and Fiori-Cowley (1996). Copyright 1996 by Mac Keith Press. Reprinted by permission.

nal depression to be identified, but a number of processes are possible. First, the infant's behavior may simply reduce the opportunity for interpersonal engagement. Thus, it is likely that ordinary caretaking activities, such as feeding or bathing the infant, may place considerable demands on the parents of infants with poor motor control, and these demands may limit the time available for more satisfying psychological contacts. A second possibility is that even when the parent's attention is not taken up with practical aspects of caretaking, the absence of well-coordinated behavioral patterns in the neonate means that some of the basis for experiencing a sense of relatedness or sympathy with the infant is missing. This suggestion is supported by two recent reports of an association between the development of motor control and the achievement of eye-to-eye contact in face-to-face interactions (van Wulfften Palthe & Hopkins, 1993; van Beek, Hopkins, Hoeksma, & Samsom, 1994). A third possibility is that the presence of behavior that is poorly organized and manifest in either jerky and tremulous movements or flat and sluggish activity may be intrinsically disturbing. This interpretation is consistent with the finding that during the first year, when infant behavior becomes temporarily disorganized, parents experience as distressing and difficult periods of developmental transition (van de Rijt-Plooij & Plooij, 1992).

It is striking that the impact on the mother of having an infant with poor motor behavior is profoundly emotional in nature. Thus, although previous research that has shown infant characteristics elicit a wide range of parental behavior (Bradley & Trevarthen, 1978; Murray & Trevarthen, 1986; Papoušek & Papoušek, Chapter 2, this volume), relatively little attention has been paid to the affective components of such responses. They do, however, complement the results of studies of the impact on the infant of perturbations to parental communication, where the infant's strong emotional reaction has been consistently documented. Together these findings attest to a parent–infant system, mutually organized from the first weeks of life, in which affective components have a core place in the regulation of interpersonal contacts.

Summary and Clinical Implications

A range of maternal factors can be identified antenatally that contribute to the occurrence of postnatal depression. These concern the mother's previous psychiatric history, her experience of pregnancy, and the quality of her current relationships. Nevertheless, in spite of the fact that evidence for such factors was derived from two large-scale predictive studies (Cooper et al., 1996; Appleby, Gregoire, Platz, Martin, & Kumar, 1994), the possibility of detecting women who are at high risk for postpartum depression on the basis of antenatal questionnaire data alone is limited. In the study of Cooper et al. (1996), in which more than 6,000 women were assessed in pregnancy and their mental state assessed at 2 months postpartum, the positive predictive value of scores above a threshold that could identify at least two-thirds of those who went on to experience an episode of depression was only 25%. However, when such antenatal data are considered together with information on neonatal functioning, considerable improvement can be achieved. From the current study we can estimate that, at least within the high-risk group, infant factors were likely to have accounted for a full 34% of depressive episodes. Some routine assessment of neonatal functioning, in addition to antenatal screening, may therefore be of considerable benefit to health care workers in identifying women at risk for depression. It may also be of direct benefit to mothers, if supportively included in the infant assessment (Nugent & Brazelton, 1989), because they may be helped to see that it is not their own mishandling that is causing difficult infant behavior and encouraged to devise more adaptive strategies for managing the infant.

THE RELATIVE CONTRIBUTION OF INFANT AND MATERNAL FACTORS TO THE QUALITY OF FACE-TO-FACE INTERACTIONS

We have already noted that, at the time when most episodes of depression arising in the first year postpartum are evident (i.e., around 6 to 12 weeks postpartum), and long before infants are able to manipulate objects or move about independently, infants are adept social partners and one can readily see periods of conversation-like interchange between parents and their offspring. For a number of reasons, such interactions have been regarded as important by researchers concerned with the possible impact of maternal depression on the child. Thus, these interactions are an arena in which the infants are able to express themselves actively, and where they manifest a sensitivity to disrupted behavior in the adult. Furthermore, unlike the case in which parents perform practical caretaking tasks, these interactions represent a situation that is likely to elucidate difficulties as well as strengths in parental interpersonal skills (Tronick et al., 1979).

They are also a context relevant to the infant's later development: Several studies have shown that the quality of these early interactions is predictive of cognitive functioning toward the end of the first year. To investigate the relative contributions of infant and maternal factors to such interchanges in the context of postnatal depression, we consider evidence from two Cambridge cohorts.

The Role of Infant Factors

Prospective Data

The study on the role of infant factors in the onset of postnatal depression enabled us to investigate prospectively whether infant characteristics influenced the quality of infant and maternal behavior in their interactions at 2 months. At the outset of this study it was anticipated that neonatal irritability would pose particular difficulties for the mother. For this reason a stratified sampling procedure was adopted and all those whose infants were classified as irritable in the neonatal period were invited to take part in a second phase of the study investigating the nature of face-to-face interactions (32 of 34 women accepted). Of the remaining mothers of nonirritable infants, a one-in-three random sample of women was asked to participate (all 45 of whom agreed). When the mother's psychiatric state was assessed at 2 months postpartum, a face-to-face interaction was video-recorded in the mother's home. When the infant was alert and not distressed, the mother was asked to play with the infant without the use of toys, for a 5-minute period. The videotapes were scored by a researcher who was unaware of the results of both the neonatal and the maternal assessments. Maternal communication was rated on a scale of sensitivity and on a dimension of intrusive to withdrawn behavior. Infant behavior was rated for the degree of active engagement with the mother and on a dimension of fretful to inert behavior (Murray, Fiori-Cowley, Hooper, & Cooper, 1996). First, the infant's behavior during the 2-month face-to-face interaction was considered in relation to the results of the neonatal assessment. Both those aspects of infant functioning on the Neonatal Behavioural Assessment Scale that predicted maternal depression (i.e., irritability and poor motor behavior) were associated with lower levels of infant communicative effort and attention to the mother during the interaction. In each case, however, the association, although statistically significant, was weak, the correlations being only .21 and .19 for irritability and motor functioning, respectively. Because the behavior of the two partners in face-to-face interactions on these measures is generally found to be highly correlated, it was not altogether surprising to find that maternal communication was even less clearly influenced by the infant's performance in the neonatal period: Neither irritability nor poor motor functioning at 10 days predicted the quality of the mother's engagement with the infant at 2 months.

Contemporaneous Data

The finding that individual neonatal characteristics may bear some, albeit weak, relation to the quality of the infant's behavior in later social interactions, but no relation to maternal communication, does not, however, rule out the possibility that individual differences between infants may play a key role in shaping the nature of mother–infant engagements. This is because the relevant intrinsic variables may become manifest and exert an impact on the environment only at a later stage of development. It is, thus, important in addressing the issue of the role of infant factors in face-to-face interactions to obtain information about contemporaneous infant functioning that is also assessed independently of communication with the mother.

The Cambridge Longitudinal Study of the Effects of Postnatal Depression on Infant Development

The contribution of infant factors was addressed in a second, longitudinal, study (Murray, Hipwell, Hooper, Stein, & Cooper, 1996) involving a representative low risk community sample of primiparous women recruited on the postnatal wards of the Cambridge maternity hospital and screened at 6 to 8 weeks postpartum with the Edinburgh Postnatal Depression Scale (Cox, Holden, & Sagovsky, 1987). Maternal mental state was confirmed by means of the Standardized Psychiatric Interview (Goldberg, Cooper, Eastwood, Kedward, & Shepherd, 1970), modified to give conformity with research diagnostic criteria for depressive disorder (minor definite or major) (Spitzer, Endicott, & Robins, 1978). The final study sample comprised 58 women who experienced an episode of depression after delivery, and 42 well women randomly selected from the same postnatal population. Half the study sample (29 postnatally depressed and 20 nondepressed mothers and their infants) was seen for assessment of face-to-face interactions at 2 months postpartum. On this occasion, as well as being video-recorded in interaction with the mother, the infant was filmed with a female researcher, the same researcher interacting with all infants. The mothers brought their infants to research rooms in the university and when the infant was alert and not distressed, both were filmed. Filming took place over three 5-minute episodes: First the infant was videotaped in face-to-face play with the mother, the infant was subsequently occupied with a toy, and finally the female researcher engaged the infant in face-to-face interaction. By using the same researcher as a partner for the infants at this early age, before such motivational states as fear of strangers or separation anxiety might be expected to swamp responses to the novel adult, we aimed to gain a standard measure of individual infant characteristics independent of communication with the mother. If infant factors are of key importance in influencing the quality of maternal communication, it should be possible, it was argued, to predict the quality of the mother's engagement with the infant from the nature of infant communication in the standard situation with the researcher. Maternal and infant behavior was scored by a researcher, unaware of maternal mental state, using the rating scheme described previously. Table 5.3 shows the association between maternal communication and infant behavior with the mother and the researcher.

It is apparent from the table that although there was some similarity in infant behavior in the two interactions in terms of the degree of active engagement, there was no evidence of an impact of infant characteristics on maternal communication: no association was found between the nature of infant behavior with the stranger and the degree of the mother's sensitivity or the extent to which she was either intrusive or withdrawn.

TABLE 5.3. Relationship between the Infant's Interaction with the Mother and with the Researcher

		Infant interaction with the researcher	
Mother–infant interaction		Active engagement	Inert–fretful
Mother:	Sensitivity	.12	.07
	Intrusive–remote	−.21	.07
Infant:	Active engagement	.50*	−.10
	Inert–fretful	.01	.11

Note. Pooled correlations, 19 controls and 26 cases. (Because of fatigue, four infants were not available for the interaction with the researcher.)

*$p < .05$.

The findings from these two studies concerning the role of infant characteristics in the quality of mother–infant interactions are remarkably consistent. Both the prospective and the contemporaneous data suggest that intrinsic infant factors are, to some extent, evident in the quality of the infant's engagement with the mother. Both suggest, however, that such individual differences are of little relevance to the mother's interactive style. What, then, are the principal determinants of maternal communication?

The Influence of Maternal Mental State and Adversity on Mother–Infant Interactions

As well as comparing the interactions of well and postnatally depressed women, the Cambridge longitudinal study of infant development involved an investigation of the impact of personal and social adversity on the quality of the mother's interactions with her infant. This was investigated using the Life Events and Difficulties Schedule (Brown & Harris, 1978). This interview yields valid and reliable assessments of stressful events and difficulties that are independent of subjective responses and mental state.

Maternal mental state was found to have a marked impact on the quality of the mother's engagement during the 5-minute sequence of face-to-face interaction at 2 months postpartum. Compared to well women, depressed mothers were rated as less sensitively focused on their infants' experience and were found to make more responses that were rejecting or affectively discordant with the infant's behavior (Murray, Kempton, Woolgar, & Hooper, 1993; Murray, Fiori-Cowley, et al., 1996). These negative responses appeared to arise as a function of the depressed mothers' selective sensitivity to signs of distressed or negative behavior in the infant. Those infants whose mothers were depressed were far more likely than control group infants to show abrupt breaks in their attention and engagement in the interaction. Microanalysis of infant and maternal behavior revealed that insensitive and rejecting responses by the mother precipitated these disruptions in the organization of infant behavior and attention (Murray, Fiori-Cowley, et al., 1996) (see Figure 5.1).

The presence of adversity during pregnancy and the first 2 months postpartum showed precisely the same relation to the quality of maternal and infant communication as did depression (Murray, Fiori-Cowley, et al., 1996). Depression and adversity were, unsurprisingly, associated with each other, but even in the absence of depression, women who experienced difficult circumstances showed the same patterns of interactive impairment with their infants as did depressed mothers. It appears that to be sensitively responsive to the infant, therefore, the mother needed to be free from preoccupations with other problems, as well as free from depressive disorder.

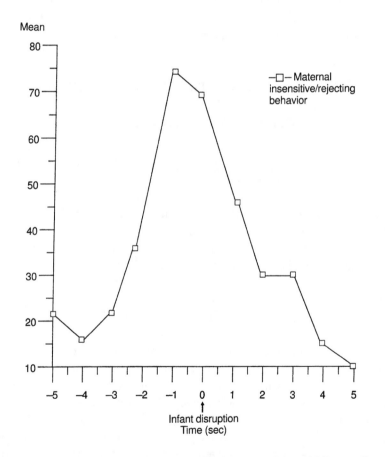

FIGURE 5.1. The proportion of 1-second time intervals preceding and following disruptions in infant attention and engagement in which insensitive/rejecting maternal behavior occurs.

Summary

Although infant characteristics appear to exert a significant influence on the occurrence of depression, by 2 months postpartum individual infant factors seem to have little direct relationship to the quality of mother–infant interactions. Thus, although the infant's behavior in the interaction is, to some extent, associated with independent assessments of his or her functioning, maternal behavior in the interaction is principally influenced by whether or not the mother is depressed and by the presence of adversity. The significance of individual infant characteristics at this stage is, therefore, that they may provoke conditions that themselves go on to influence the subsequent quality of the infant's interpersonal environment.

THE RELATIVE CONTRIBUTION OF INFANT AND MATERNAL FACTORS TO CHILD OUTCOME IN THE CONTEXT OF POSTNATAL DEPRESSION

Intrinsic factors might be expected to play a particularly important role in two child outcomes associated with the occurrence of postnatal depression: the presence of behavior problems (Murray, 1992) and cognitive deficits (Cogill, Caplan, Alexandra, Robson, & Kumar, 1986; Murray, 1992; Sharp et al., 1995). In the case of behavioral disturbance, it might be thought, for example, that the difficulties observed in infants of 18 months (manifest, principally, in terms of sleeping, feeding, and separation problems, and temper tantrums) may simply represent a more developmentally advanced version of those neonatal problems in behavioral regulation that are predictive of postnatal depression. In the case of poor cognitive outcome, the considerable literature on the prediction of later cognitive functioning from measures of infant attention (Slater, 1995) might lead one to suppose that the degree to which infant attention and engagement in early face-to-face interactions, which as noted earlier shows a moderate degree of consistency across interactions with mother and a stranger, would be an important factor driving later infant cognitive outcome. Similarly, research showing that infant distress in response to the violation of expected contingency is associated with poor long-term recall (Fagen, Ohr, Fleckenstein, & Ribner, 1985) suggests that assessment of this aspect of infant functioning may also elucidate the role of infant factors in cognitive outcome in the context of postnatal depression.

Behavioral Disturbance

A sample of 70 infants assessed as neonates, again stratified to include all available irritable neonates, were reassessed at 18 months. At that time, the mothers were interviewed about the presence of behavioral difficulties, using the Behaviour Screening Questionnaire (Richman & Graham, 1971) modified for infants (Murray, 1992). The interviewer was unaware of the results of the neonatal assessment and of maternal postpartum mental state. None of the neonatal measures, including general irritability, was found to be associated with behavioral problems at 18 months. Behavioral problems were, however, significantly predicted by the occurrence of postnatal depression ($Z = 2.93, p < .005$), as was previously found (Murray, 1992). These findings, together with the fact that a brief psychological treatment for postnatal depression was associated with a significant reduction in the rate of behavioral problems (see Cooper & Murray, Chapter 8, this volume), suggest that the infant characteristics we assessed are of little relevance to the occurrence of infant behavioral disturbance, maternal factors being of primary significance.

Cognitive Functioning

Two British cross-sectional studies of the cognitive development of 4-year-old children (Cogill et al., 1986; Sharp et al., 1995) have found significant deficits in performance on the McCarthy Scales of Children's Abilities when the mother experienced depression in the first postnatal year (see Hay, Chapter 4, this volume for a detailed discussion of these studies). In the Cambridge longitudinal study of the effects of postnatal depression on child development, 98 of the 100 mother–infant pairs recruited at 2 months postpartum were assessed at 18 months; of these, 95 were followed up again at 5 years. At 18 months, compared to infants of well women, those whose mothers had been depressed in the postnatal period were more likely to fail on stage V of Piaget's object concept tasks (Murray, 1992). On the more general measure of infant cognitive development, the Bayley Scales, although postnatal depression was not associated with reduced cognitive scores overall, there was, as in the study of Sharp et al. (1995), an interaction between postnatal depression and infant gender: The boys of postnatally depressed women performed poorly (Murray et al., 1993; Murray, Fiori-Cowley, et al., 1996).

In considering the possible contribution of infant characteristics to cognitive outcome, the infant's behavior during interaction with the researcher at 2 months was once again used to provide a standard assessment of the infant's capacity for sustained attention and engagement and the extent to which the infant was prone to be fretful or distressed. These two measures of infant behavior were analyzed in relation to the infant's performance on the Bayley Scales, but neither was found to be predictive (the R2 value for both these aspects of infant behavior considered together was only .08). In contrast to these findings, however, infant performance on the Bayley Scales was significantly related to the quality of the early mother–infant interaction (Murray et al., 1993; Murray, Fiori-Cowley, et al., 1996). Of particular importance was the mother's role in focusing on infant experience and actively sustaining the infant's attention in the interaction. Disruptions in the infant's attention were, as noted earlier, highly sensitive to the form of maternal behavior. It was not surprising, therefore, that, although the infant's behavior with the mother was, when considered alone, predictive of cognitive performance at 18 months, once the quality of the early maternal communication was taken into account, the contribution of the infant's behavior to outcome was no longer significant. Indeed, in the regression model, neither infant gender nor maternal depression was related to cognitive performance once the impact of maternal communication was entered.

Cognitive functioning was assessed again at 5 years, using the McCarthy Scales (Murray, Hipwell, et al., 1996). The children were tested in university research rooms by a researcher who was unaware of all previous assessments. In this low-risk sample, postpartum depression was no longer associated with poor cognitive functioning; however, it was again the case that the quality of mother–infant interactions at 2 months postpartum was predictive of cognitive outcome. Here, as at 18 months, it was the extent to which the infant had been actively engaged in communication with the mother that was predictive of the child's later cognitive functioning. Analysis of the children's performance at 5 years revealed, furthermore, that the impact of the early mother–infant engagements on cognitive performance seemed to have been effected by 18 months: When the infant's performance on the Bayley Scales at this age was taken into account, the association between 5-year outcome and mother–infant interactions at 2 months was no longer significant. Further investigation suggested, however, that the longer-term impact of interactions in infancy was principally confined to those infants whose interactive environment had been particularly impaired. In these cases, not only was the infants' cognitive outcome at 18 months relatively poor, but the developmental trajectory from 18 months to 5 years was considerably constrained by their earlier functioning.

The findings outlined previously, suggesting the importance of environmental factors, may appear at variance with a body of evidence emphasizing the role of intrinsic infant characteristics in the course of cognitive development. In particular, as noted earlier, infant cognitive functioning is well predicted by assessments of infant attention and habituation independent of interactions with the mother (Slater, 1995). Yet in the study described previously, no association was found between infant behavior in the standard interaction with the researcher at 2 months and cognitive outcome at either 18 months or 5 years. The apparent discrepancy here may be accounted for by a genuine progression in infant psychological functioning with parallels in brain growth and organization. Thus, there is accumulating evidence that experiential factors influence the course of infant brain development (Cicchetti & Tucker, 1994; Rothbart, Posner, & Rosicky, 1994; Trevarthen & Aitken, 1994). This is extremely rapid in the first weeks and months, with prodigious production of synapses, followed by extensive synaptic pruning, in which only functional connections are retained. Thus, when parents repeatedly respond sensitively to recruit the infant's engagement and then modulate their behavior in response to infant arousal and interest to sustain the infant's attention, it is likely that they directly influence the process of brain differentiation and organization. Our own and others' research (Pelaez-Nogueras, Cigales, Gonzalez, & Clasky, 1996) suggests that at 2 months postpartum there is still considerable flexibility in the infant's repertoire with, at best, a relatively modest generalization of infant behavior from interactions with the principal caretaker to those with others. Gradually, however, the form of the infant's adaptations in the interactions with the mother gain coherence and stability and, as the study of Field et al. (1988) suggests, the infant's consistent experience of particular patterns of interaction may eventually become incorporated in the infant's wider cognitive operations. Thus the mother's success in sustaining the infant's attention and involvement in face-to-face interactions, repeated over a period of some months, may, by 4 to 5 months, have influenced the infant's capacity to attend and process information in the wider social and the nonsocial environment. This age is precisely when researchers have found infant habituation and attention in nonsocial tasks to be predictive of later IQ. These infant characteristics might, therefore, have been shaped by specific features of their interpersonal experience.

Summary

The findings from our research concerning the outcome of the children of postnatally depressed and well mothers at 18 months and 5 years suggest that infant characteristics, as assessed in the neonatal period and at 2 months postpartum in a standard interaction with the researcher, do not reliably predict the course of development. By contrast, the quality of the early maternal environment does appear to be of predictive significance. Thus, the presence of behavioral difficulties in late infancy was found to be strongly associated with maternal mental state in the postpartum period, although the mechanisms mediating this association remain to be identified. With regard to cognitive development, analyses of face-to-face interactions reveal a significant role of maternal difficulties in sensitively engaging with the infant to sustain the infant's attention and involvement in play.

ACKNOWLEDGMENTS

The Cambridge research summarized in this chapter was supported by the Medical Research Council of Great Britain, the Winnicott Trust, and the Tedworth Charitable Trust.

REFERENCES

Appleby, L., Gregoire, A., Platz, C., Martin, P. L., & Kumar, R. (1994). Screening women for high risk of postnatal depression. *Journal of Psychosomatic Research, 38,* 539–545.

Bell, R. Q. (1968). A reinterpretation of the direction of effects in studies of socialization. *Psychological Review, 72,* 81–95.

Bernal, J. F. (1974). Attachment: Some problems and possibilities. In M. P. M. Richards (Ed.), *The integration of a child into a social world.* Cambridge, England: Cambridge University Press.

Bradley, S. B., & Trevarthen, C. B. (1978). Baby talk as an adaptation to the infant's communication. In N. Waterson & C. Snow (Eds.), *The development of communication.* New York: Wiley.

Brazelton, T. B. (1961). Psychophysiologic reactions in the neonate. I. The value of observations of the neonate. *Journal of Paediatrics, 58,* 508–512.

Brazelton, T. B. (1984). *Neonatal Behavioral Assessment Scale* (2nd ed.) (Clinics in Developmental Medicine, No. 88). London: S. I. M. P.

Brazelton, T. B., Koslowski, B., & Main, M. (1974). The origins of reciprocity: The early mother–infant interaction. In M. Lewis & L. A. Rosenblum (Eds.), *The effects of the infant on its caregiver.* New York: Wiley.

Brazelton, T. B., Tronick, E. Z., Adamson, L., Als, H., & Wise, S. (1975). Early mother–infant reciprocity. In M. Hofer (Ed.), *Parent–infant interaction.* Amsterdam: Elsevier.

Brown, G. W., & Harris, T. (1978). *Social origins of depression: A study of psychiatric disorder in women.* London: Tavistock.

Bushnell, I. W. R., Sai, F., & Mullin, J. T. (1989). Neonatal recognition of the mother's face. *British Journal of Developmental Psychology, 7,* 3–15.

Cernoch, J. M., & Porter, R. H. (1985). Recognition of maternal axillary odors by infants. *Child Development, 56,* 1593–1598.

Cicchetti, D., & Tucker, D. (1994). Development and self-regulatory structures of the mind. *Development and Psychopathology, 6,* 533–549.

Cogill, S., Caplan, H., Alexandra, H., Robson, K., & Kumar, R. (1986). Impact of postnatal depression on cognitive development in young children. *British Medical Journal, 292,* 1165–1167.

Cohn, J. F., Matias, R., Tronick, E. Z., Connell, D., & Lyons-Ruth, D. (1986). Face-to-face interactions of depressed mothers and their infants. In E. Z. Tronick & T. Field (Eds.), *Maternal depression and infant disturbance* (New Directions for Child Development, No. 34). San Francisco: Jossey-Bass.

Cohn, J. F., & Tronick, E. Z. (1983). Three-month-old infants' reaction to simulated maternal depression. *Child Development, 54,* 185–193.

Cooper, P. J., Murray, L., Hooper, R., & West, A. (1996). The development and validation of a predictive index for postpartum depression. *Psychological Medicine, 26,* 627–634.

Cox, J., Holden, J., & Sagovsky, R. (1987). Detection of postnatal depression: Development of the Edinburgh Postnatal Depression Scale. *British Journal of Psychiatry, 163,* 27–31.

Crockenberg, S. B. (1981). Infant irritability, mother responsiveness, and social support influences on the security of infant–mother attachment. *Child Development, 52,* 857–865.

Crockenberg, S. B. (1986). Are temperamental differences in babies associated with predictable differences in care giving? In J. V. & R. M. Lerner (Eds.), *Temperament and social interaction during infancy and childhood* (New Directions for Child Development, No. 31). San Francisco: Jossey-Bass.

Cutrona, C. E., & Troutman, B. R. (1986). Social support, infant temperament, and parenting self-efficacy: A mediational model of postpartum depression. *Child Development, 57,* 1507–1518.

De Casper, A. J., & Fifer, W. P. (1980). Of human bonding: Newborns prefer their mothers' voices. *Science, 208,* 1174–1176.

Eisenberg, R. B. (1975). *Auditory competence in early life. The roots of communicative behaviour.* Baltimore: University Park Press.

Fagen, J. W., Ohr, P. S., Fleckenstein, L. K., & Ribner, D. R. (1985). The effect of crying on long-term memory in infancy. *Child Development, 56,* 1584–1592.

Fantz, R. L. (1963). Pattern vision in newborn infants. *Science, 140,* 296–297.

Field, T. M. (1984). Early interactions between infants and their postpartum depressed mothers. *Infant Behavior and Development, 7,* 517–522.

Field, T. M. (1985). Neonatal perception of people: motivational and individual differences. In T. M. Field & N. A. Fox (Eds.), *Social perception in infants.* Norwood, NJ: Ablex.

Field, T. M., Healy, B., Goldstein, S., & Guthertz, M. (1990). Behavior-state matching and synchrony in mother–infant interactions in nondepressed versus depressed dyads. *Developmental Psychology, 26,* 7–14.

Field, T. M., Healy, B., Goldstein, S., Perry, S., Bendell, D., Schanberg, S., Zimmerman, E. A., & Kuhn, C. (1988). Infants of depressed mothers show "depressed" behavior even with nondepressed adults. *Child Development, 59,* 1569–1579.

Field, T. M., Sandberg, D., Garcia, R., Vega-Lahr, N., Goldstein, S., & Guy, L. (1985). Pregnancy problems, postpartum depression and early mother–infant interactions. *Developmental Psychology, 21,* 1152–1156.

Friedlander, B. (1970). Receptive language development in infancy. *Merrill–Palmer Quarterly, 16,* 7–51.

Goldberg, D. P., Cooper, B., Eastwood, M. R., Kedward, H. B., & Shepherd, M. A. (1970). A standardised psychiatric interview for use in community surveys. *British Journal of Preventative and Social Medicine, 25,* 91–109.

Goren, C. G., Sarty, M., & Wu, P. Y. K. (1975). Visual following and pattern discrimination of face-life stimuli by newborn infants. *Paediatrics, 56,* 544–549.

Hepper, P. G., Scott, D., & Shahidullah, S. (1993). Newborn and fetal response to maternal voice. *Journal of Reproductive and Infant Psychology, 11*(3), 147–153.

Hinchcliffe, M. K., Lancashire, M., & Roberts, F. J. (1971). A study of eye-contact changes in depressed and recovered psychiatric patients. *British Journal of Psychiatry, 119,* 213–215.

Kennerly, H., & Gath, D. (1989). "Maternity Blues": Detection and measurement by questionnaire. *British Journal of Psychiatry, 155,* 356–373.

Kugiumutzakis, G. (1985). *The origin, development and function of the early infant imitation.* Doctoral dissertation, Department of Psychology, University of Uppsala.

Kugiumutzakis, G. (1993). Intersubjective vocal imitation in early mother–infant interaction. In J. Nadel & L. Camaioni (Eds.), *New perspectives in early communicative development* (pp. 23–47). London: Routledge.

Leslie, A. M. (1984). Infant perception of a manual pick-up event. *British Journal of Developmental Psychology, 2,* 19–32.

Lester, B. M., Als, H., & Brazelton, B. (1982). Regional obstetric anesthesia and newborn behavior. A reanalysis towards synergistic effects. *Child Development, 56,* 15–27.

Levy, D. M. (1958). *Behavioural analysis.* New York: Thomas.

Lewinsohn, P. M., Weinstein, M. S., & Alper, T. (1970). A behavioral approach to the group treatment of depressed persons: Methodological contribution. *Journal of Child Psychology, 26,* 525–532.

Libert, J., & Lewinsohn, P. M. (1973). The concept of social skill with special reference to the behavior of depressed persons. *Journal of Consulting and Clinical Psychology, 40,* 304–312.

Maratos, O. (1973). *The origin and development of imitation in the first six months of life.* Doctoral dissertation, Department of Psychology, Geneva University.

Maratos, O. (1982). Trends in the development of imitation in early infancy. In T. G. Bever (Ed.), *Regressions in mental development: Basic phenomena and theories.* Hillsdale, NJ: Erlbaum.

McFarlane, J. (1975). Olfaction in the development of social preferences in the human neonate. In M. Hofer (Ed.), *Parent–infant interaction.* Amsterdam: Elsevier.

Meltzoff, A. N., & Moore, M. K. (1977). Imitation of facial and manual gestures by human neonates. *Science, 198,* 73–75.

Meltzoff, A. N., & Moore, M. K. (1983). Newborn infants imitate adult facial gestures. *Child Development, 54,* 702–709.

Murray, L. (1992). The impact of postnatal depression on infant development. *Journal of Child Psychology and Psychiatry, 33,* 543–561.

Murray, L., Fiori-Cowley, A., Hooper, R., & Cooper, P. J. (1996). The impact of postnatal depression and associated adversity on early mother infant interactions and later infant outcome. *Child Development, 67,* 2512–2526.

Murray, L., Hipwell, A., Hooper, R., Stein, A., & Cooper, P. J. (1996). The cognitive development of five year old children of postnatally depressed mothers. *Journal of Child Psychology and Psychiatry, 37,* 927–936.

Murray, L., Kempton, C., Woolgar, M., & Hooper, R. (1993). Depressed mothers' speech to their infants and its relation to infant gender and cognitive development. *Journal of Child Psychology and Psychiatry, 34,* 1083–1101.

Murray, L., Stanley, C., Hooper, R., King, F., & Fiori-Cowley, A. (1996). The role of infant factors in postnatal depression and mother–infant interactions. *Developmental Medicine and Child Neurology, 38,* 109–119.

Murray, L., & Trevarthen, C. B. (1985). Emotional regulation of interactions between two month olds and their mother's. In T. M. Field & N. A. Fox (Eds.), *Social perception in infants.* Norwood, NJ: Ablex.

Murray, L., & Trevarthen, C. (1986). The infant's role in mother–infant communication. *Journal of Child Language, 13,* 15–29.

Nugent, J. K., & Brazelton, T. B. (1989). Preventive intervention with infants and families: The NBAS model. *Infant Mental Health Journal, 10,* 84–99.

Papoušek, H., & Papoušek, M. (1975). Cognitive aspects of preverbal social interaction between human infants and adults. In. M. Hofer (Ed.), *Parent–infant interaction.* Amsterdam: Elsevier.

Pelaez-Nogueras, M., Cigales, M., Gonzalez, A., & Clasky, S. (1996). *Some myths about infant "depression": Infants of depressed mothers do not develop a "depressed mood style" of interaction.* Paper presented at the International Conference on Infant Studies, Providence, Rhode Island.

Richards, M. P. M. (1974). First steps in becoming social. In M. P. M. Richards (Ed.), *The integration of a child into a social world.* Cambridge, England: Cambridge University Press.

Richman, N., & Graham, P. (1971). A behavioural screening questionnaire for use with three-year-old children: Preliminary findings. *Journal of Child Psychology and Psychiatry, 12,* 5–33.

Rothbart, M. K., Posner, M. I., & Rosicky, J. (1994). Orienting in normal and pathological development. *Development and Psychopathology, 6,* 635–652.

St. James Roberts, I., & Wolke, D. (1988). Convergences and discrepancies among mothers' and professionals' assessments of difficult neonatal behaviour. *Journal of Child Psychology and Psychiatry, 29,* 21–42.

Schaffer, H. R., & Emerson, P. E. (1964). The development of social attachments in infancy. *Monographs of the Society for Research in Child Development, 29* (94).

Seligman, M. E. P. (1975). *Helplessness: On depression, development, and death.* San Francisco: Freeman.

Sharp, D., Hay, D., Pawlby, S., Schmucher, G., Allen, H., & Kumar, R. (1995). The impact of postnatal depression on boys' intellectual development. *Journal of Child Psychology and Psychiatry, 36,* 1315–1337.

Slater, A. (1995). Individual differences in infancy and later IQ. *Journal of Child Psychology and Psychiatry, 36,* 69–112.

Spitzer, R. L., Endicott, J., & Robins, E. (1978). Research diagnostic criteria: Rationale and reliability. *Archives of General Psychiatry, 35,* 773–782.

Spitzer, R. L., Williams, J. B. W., Gibbon, M., & First, M. B. (1989). *Structured Clinical Interview for DSM-III-R—Patient edition (with psychotic screen).* New York: Biometrics Research Department, New York State Psychiatric Institute.

Stern, D. N. (1974). The goal and structure of mother–infant play. *Journal of the American Academy of Child Psychiatry, 13,* 402–421.

Teasdale, J. D., Fogarty, S. J., & Williams, J. M. G. (1980). Speech rate as a measure of short-term variation in depression. *British Journal of Social and Clinical Psychology, 19,* 271–278.

Trevarthen, C. B. (1979). Communication and cooperation in early infancy: A description of primary intersubjectivity. In M. Bullowa (Ed.), *Before speech.* Cambridge, England: Cambridge University Press.

Trevarthen, C., & Aitken, K. J. (1994). Brain development, infant communication, and empathy disorders: Intrinsic factors in child mental health. *Development and Psychopathology, 6,* 597–633.

Trevarthen, C., & Hubley, P. (1978). Secondary intersubjectivity: Confidence, confiding and acts of meaning in the first year. In A. Lock (Ed.), *Action, gesture and symbol.* London: Academic Press.

Tronick, E. Z., Als, H., & Adamson, L. (1979). Structure of early face-to-face communicative interactions. In M. Bullowa (Ed.), *Before speech.* Cambridge, England: Cambridge University Press.

Tronick, E. Z., Als, H., Adamson, L., Wise, S., & Brazelton, T. B. (1978). The infants' response to entrapment between contradictory messages in face-to-face interaction. *Journal of the American Academy of Child Psychiatry, 17,* 1–13.

van Beek, Y., Hopkins, B., Hoeksma, J. B., & Samsom, J. F. (1994). Prematurity, posture and the development of looking behaviour during early communication. *Journal of Child Psychology and Psychiatry, 35,* 1093–1107.

van de Rijt-Plooij, H. H. C., & Plooij, F. X. (1992). Infantile regressions: Disorganization and the onset of transition periods. *Journal of Reproductive and Infant Psychology, 10,* 129–149.

van Wulfften Palthe, T., & Hopkins, B. (1993). A longitudinal study of neural maturation and early mother–infant interaction: A research note. *Journal of Child Psychology and Psychiatry, 34,* 1031–1041.

Whiffen, V. E., & Gotlib, I. H. (1989). Infants of postpartum depressed mothers: Temperament and cognitive status. *Journal of Abnormal Psychology, 98,* 274–279.

Yarrow, L. J. (1963). Research in dimensions of early maternal care. *Merrill–Palmer Quarterly, 9,* 101–114.

6

~

Maternal Cognitions
as Mediators of Child Outcomes
in the Context
of Postpartum Depression

Douglas M. Teti
University of Maryland, Baltimore County

Donna M. Gelfand
University of Utah

This chapter examines the role of maternal cognitions as mediators of relations between clinical depression during the postpartum period, depressed parents' behavior with their children, and children's developmental outcomes in the infancy and preschool periods. As such, this chapter addresses putative mechanisms central to a theory of intergenerational transmission of psychopathology from depressed parent to child. That clinical maternal depression places children of all ages at high risk for psychopathology is well documented in a number of comprehensive reviews (Cummings & Davies, 1994; Downey & Coyne, 1990; Gelfand & Teti, 1990; Goodman, 1992; Field, 1992; Rutter, 1990). During the infant and preschool periods, children of depressed mothers have more difficulty in emotion regulation (Zahn-Waxler, Cummings, Iannotti, & Radke-Yarrow, 1984; Zahn-Waxler, McKnew, Cummings, Davenport, &

Radke-Yarrow, 1984); are less responsive, more gaze avoidant, and distressed during interactions with mothers (Field, 1984; Field, Morrow, & Adelstein, 1993); show delays in cognitive and language development (Cox, Puckering, Pound, & Mills, 1987; Murray, 1992); and are more likely to establish insecure and insecure-disorganized attachments to their mothers (Murray, 1992; Radke-Yarrow, Cummings, Kuczynski, & Chapman, 1985; Teti, Gelfand, Messinger, & Isabella, 1995) in comparison to children of nondepressed controls. The degree of risk to children appears to relate in a straightforward manner to the severity and duration of mothers' depression following the child's birth (Campbell, Cohn, Meyers, Ross, & Flanagan, 1993; Teti et al., 1995).

The behavioral problems of children of depressed mothers appear to be directly linked to parenting deficits commonly associated with depressed women. Clinically depressed mothers have been variously characterized as incompetent, apathetic and uninvolved, ineffective, emotionally flat, insensitive, disengaged, and intrusive in interactions with their children (Cummings & Davies, 1994; Gelfand & Teti, 1990; Goodman, 1992). Regardless of maternal adjustment status, insensitive, incompetent mothering is identified as a central predictor of insecure attachments in early childhood (Ainsworth, Blehar, Waters, & Wall, 1978; Bretherton, 1985; Teti & Nakagawa, 1990); thus, it is not surprising that children of depressed mothers show increased rates of insecure attachments. Although not invariably predictive of later psychopathology, insecure attachment has been associated with psychiatric symptomatology in later childhood when accompanied by additional environmental risk factors such as high life stress (Bates & Bayles, 1988; Erickson, Sroufe, & Egeland, 1985; Fagot & Kavanagh, 1990; Lewis, Feiring, McGuffog, & Jaskir, 1984). Insecure children of depressed parents may be especially vulnerable because of the high levels of interpersonal stress and marital discord that so frequently co-occur with depression (Emery, Weintraub, & Neale, 1982; Gelfand, Teti, & Fox, 1992; Hammen, 1991).

In this chapter, we explore the organizational influences of depressed parental cognitions on depressed women's behavior with their infants and also the degree to which these cognitions can be shaped by depressed women's experiences with their babies. First, we discuss the general negative and distorted cognitions identified as central features of depression in theoretical formulations, and how such cognitions predispose the depressed individual to behave maladaptively in interpersonal contexts. We then address the impact of depression on mothers' perceptions of their children and of themselves as parents and discuss theoretical and empirical relations between parents' cognitive–affective schemas and parental behavior. Of particular importance is the mother's self-percept of parenting self-efficacy, its theoretical and empirical relation to maternal behavior, and how this percept might be influenced by factors in the caregiving environment other than maternal depression per se.

Finally, we conclude with a discussion of how the systematic study of cognition in depressed mothers can contribute to a more comprehensive understanding of the nature of individual differences in depressed mothers' parenting competence and, in turn, children's developmental outcomes.

DEPRESSION AND COGNITION

Although clinical depression is characterized primarily as a mood disorder (American Psychiatric Association, 1994), the lion's share of theoretical attention over the past three decades has focused on the role of cognition in the etiology, maintenance, and treatment of depression. Among the various theoretical perspectives giving cognition special status, Beck's cognitive theory (Beck, 1963, 1976, 1987) and Seligman's learned helplessness theory of depression (Overmeier & Seligman, 1967; Abramson, Seligman, & Teasdale, 1978) stand apart as the two most influential simply in terms of the sheer volume of research studies stimulated by them.

Beck's (1963, 1976) cognitive theory gives primacy to negative cognitions as symptoms of depression from which we can understand affective and motivational symptoms. Depressed individuals' negative thoughts are viewed as conforming to a "cognitive triad" in that subjective evaluations and appraisals about themselves, current environmental circumstances, and the future are uniformly negative despite the availability of contradictory evidence. These thoughts are viewed as automatic (i.e., unintentional and largely uncontrollable) and are believed to be governed by dysfunctional cognitive schemas or beliefs about the self that originally are latent but become activated by environmental events subjectively appraised by the individual as negative and stressful. In a review and critique of research on self-schemas as related to depression, Segal (1988) defines self-schemas as consisting of "organized elements of past reactions and experience that form a relatively cohesive and persistent body of knowledge capable of guiding subsequent perception and appraisals" (p. 147). When activated, dysfunctional self-schemas are assigned a causal role in the etiology of depression. Following Haaga, Dyck, and Ernst's (1991) analysis, if someone possessed the dysfunctional self-schema that failure at a subjectively valued task made him or her a "nobody," and then subsequently failed at that task, this schema would be activated and in turn predispose that individual to negative cognitions and sad affect. Once activated, dysfunctional cognitive schemas have a major impact on the processing of information by creating a "negative bias," which can lead to overselecting negative and filtering out positive information about oneself and others, selective recall of negative memories, and potential distortions of reality (Beck, 1976, 1987). Beck's theory has enjoyed considerable empirical support (for reviews, see Haaga et al., 1991; Kwon & Oei, 1994), although several investigators have emphasized the need to view the relation between cognition and depression as reciprocal rather than unidirectional, from cognition to depressed behavior, as Beck hypothesized (Bower, 1981; Clark & Teasdale, 1982; Isen, 1984; Teasdale & Fogarty, 1979). Teasdale and Fogarty (1979), for example, found that experimentally, depressed moods increase unpleasant thoughts and memories, which in turn fosters even more sad affect. Understanding the relation between depressed cognitions and depressed mood as bidirectional helps to explain why depression tends to persist even when more positive interpretations of environmental events are available to the depressed person.

Seligman's (Overmeier & Seligman, 1967) original formulation of the learned helplessness theory of depression viewed depression as an affective consequence of perceptions of helplessness derived from repeated exposure to highly stressful and inescapable events. When it was proved inadequate when applied to humans, the learned helplessness theory was reformulated (Abramson et al., 1978) to incorporate attributional processes as mediators of relations between noncontingent environmental events and expectations about future success. Both the original and the reformulated models propose that depression results directly from perceived lack of control. The reformulated model, however, posits that people who attribute the causes of negative, uncontrollable events to trait-like and generalized characteristics of themselves (i.e., internal, global, and stable characteristics) are more likely to become depressed than are people who attribute the causes of such events to specific and transient conditions. Seligman, Abramson, Semmel, and von Baeyer (1979) further proposed that individuals prone to depression should attribute good outcomes to external, specific, and unstable factors, for which they found partial empirical support. Thus, attributing uncontrollable negative outcomes to internal, global, and stable factors fosters an expectancy that future negative outcomes are beyond control and, therefore, unpreventable. This defeatist attribution leads to the affective and motivational deficits that characterize depression. Reformulated learned helplessness theory has some empirical support, although design limitations in many studies purporting to test the theory preclude an enthusiastic endorsement (for an extensive review, see Brewin, 1985).

The cognitive and learned helplessness theories of depression differ in emphasis and terminology but can be viewed as complementary. Whereas Beck's cognitive theory gives more attention to the role of prior cognitive organizations in guiding the processing of new information, learned helplessness theory addresses how individuals employ attributions to interpret the meaning of environmental outcomes and the consequences of these attributions for affective, cognitive, and behavioral functioning. The theories converge, however, in assigning a central role to depressogenic cognitive processes in the etiology of depressive states.

COGNITIONS OF DEPRESSED MOTHERS

Evidence is widespread that depressed mothers hold decidedly negative cognitions about their children and themselves. In comparison to nondepressed counterparts, depressed mothers have been found to hold more negative perceptions of themselves with regard to their enjoyment of and adequacy in the parenting role (Fleming, Ruble, Flett, & Shaul, 1988; Whiffen & Gotlib, 1989). Perceived parental adequacy is conceptually analogous to the construct of maternal self-efficacy, or mothers' feelings of competence and effectiveness in the parental role, and several studies have reported that depressed mothers feel less effective as parents relative to nondepressed mothers (Fox & Gelfand, 1994; Teti & Gelfand, 1991). Depressed mothers also have more negative perceptions of their children's social competence and psychiatric adjustment (Fox & Gelfand, 1994; Fergusson, Horwood, Gretten, & Shannon, 1985; Forehand, Lautenschlager, Faust, & Graziano, 1986; Friedlander, Weiss, & Traylor, 1986; Griest, Wells, & Forehand, 1979; Panaccione & Wahler, 1986; Rickard, Forehand, Wells, Griest, & McMahon, 1981; Rogers & Forehand, 1983; Schaughency & Lahey, 1985; Webster-Stratton & Hammond, 1988). Depression may lead mothers to overestimate the extent and seriousness of their children's problems.

Rickard et al. (1981) found that depressed mothers appeared more predisposed to perceive their children's behavior as more negative than objectively warranted, leading in turn to clinic referral for evaluation. However, it is unclear whether depressed mothers' negative perceptions of their children represent reality distortions or whether depressed mothers are reporting accurately that their children are maladjusted. In a thoughtful critique, Richters (1992) noted that the majority of studies purporting to find distortions in depressed mothers' perceptions of their children failed to compare depressed mothers' views with perceptions derived from other, more objective sources, such as professional observers of child behavior or other family members or teachers.

Brody and Forehand (1986), for example, found that depressed mothers' reports of child maladjustment coincided with independent home observations of high levels of child noncompliance. Conrad and Hammen (1989) actually found that depressed mothers were better able to distinguish highly deviant children from less symptomatic children on a child symptom checklist than were nondepressed mothers. Further, unlike nondepressed mothers, depressed mothers directed high levels of negative utterances only to children with more severe symptoms. This latter finding supports Brody and Forehand's (1986) finding that depressed mothers' reports of child maladjustment accurately reflected high levels of child noncompliance. Richters and Pellegrini (1989) found that depressed mothers' reports of children's behavior problems correlated strongly with teachers' reports, and Lovejoy (1991) found that depressed mothers' recollections of child misbehavior during an observational session correlated with independent observer reports of child transgressions. The preceding studies support a "depressive realism" hypothesis that depressed mothers' views of their children are largely accurate.

At least two recent studies, however, provide support for the depression–distortion hypothesis. Fergusson, Lynskey, and Horwood (1993) found small to moderate relations between mothers' depression and their tendencies to inflate reports of their children's maladjustment. In addition, in a very clever study, Field et al. (1993) had both mothers and trained, independent observers code infants' behavior during videotaped interactions with their mothers. Their results indicated that both observers and mothers coded the behavior of infants of depressed mothers as more distressed or sad than the behavior of infants of nondepressed mothers. However, depressed mothers coded their infants significantly more negatively than did the independent observers. Thus, the distortion and depressive realism hypotheses both have some empirical support. Indeed, it is unnecessary to view the negative realism and depression–distortion models as mutually exclusive. It is likely that depressed women's negative perceptions of their children are driven in part by the reality that children of depressed parents are indeed more symptomatic. Nevertheless, depressed women also tend to exaggerate problems of all types, including their children's behavioral problems. The degree to which parents overestimate their children's undesirable traits is likely correlated with the severity of their depression. Ironically, the mothers' severity of mood disorder is also likely to be correlated with the severity of her child's adjustment problems.

RELATIONS OF PARENTAL COGNITIONS TO PARENTING BEHAVIOR

Despite the "cognitive revolution" that has swept many fields in psychology over the last three decades, the study of parenting has been affected only recently (Maccoby & Martin, 1983; Main, Kaplan, & Cassidy, 1985; Miller, 1988; Sigel, 1985). Traditionally, parenting practices and family interaction patterns have been explained more in terms of learning and personality processes. It is widely assumed that cognition, emotion, and behavior are intimately intertwined, although considerable debate exists over the primacy of each (Goodnow, 1988).

Consistent with a transactional perspective on development (Bandura, 1986; Goodnow, 1988; Sameroff, 1975), there is evidence of complex interactive linkages between multiple systems. For example, in some circumstances, cognition is thought to drive behavior (Bandura, 1986; Teti & Gelfand, 1991). In others, cognitions are viewed as arising from individual experiences with the environment (Bandura, 1986; Goodnow, 1988).

Finally, cognitive appraisals of environmental events are seen as intimately tied to action tendencies, which in turn predispose emotion and behavior (Frijda, Kuipers, & ter Schure, 1989). Curiously, many social developmental theories have been somewhat more concerned with cognitive-behavioral relations in children rather than in parents. For example, attachment theorists (Ainsworth et al., 1978; Bowlby, 1973; Bretherton, 1985; Crittenden, 1992; Sroufe, 1983; Sroufe & Fleeson, 1986) propose that children develop a "working model" of their caregivers and themselves, conceptualized as a set of affectively laden cognitions or "rules" regarding interpersonal relationships, the content of which is shaped by the quality of care. These cognitive organizations are seen as (1) guiding the quality of ensuing behavior that young children exhibit toward caregivers and peers and (2) influencing the manner in which subsequent information from significant others is selected and interpreted (Main et al., 1985). From a somewhat different theoretical perspective of information processing, Dodge, Pettit, McClaskey, and Brown (1985) view the competence by which a child processes social information as crucial to the child's social competence with other children. They note that the enactment of a successful social response depends on the accuracy with which the child processes social information. Errors committed at any point in the sequence of encoding, interpretation, response search, response evaluation, and response enactment can lead to socially inept behavior. Similarly, other social–cognitive theorists view cognitive structures or schemas that develop in children as central influences on subsequent selective attention to and encoding of social–environmental inputs, and on children's behavior with others (Baldwin, 1992; Safran, 1990; Westen, 1991).

Interestingly, systematic attempts to examine cognitive-behavioral interfaces in parenting have emerged in earnest only in the last decade (e.g., Dix & Grusec, 1983; Sigel, 1985), despite some early attempts to identify cognitive mediators of parental functioning (e.g., Emmerich, 1969). Cognitions and emotions are now frequently placed at the heart of conceptualizations of parenting, with cognitive-affective organizations parents bring to the dyadic setting viewed as causal to parenting behavior and potentially open to modifiability as parent–child relationships proceed. Attachment theory and research, for example, have expanded to incorporate the effects of parental "working models" of relationships, believed to result at least in part from parents' early relationship histories, on parents' propensities to perceive children's cues without distortion and to respond to children sensitively and appropriately (Bakermans-Kranenburg & van IJzendoorn, 1993; Main et al., 1985; van IJzendoorn, 1992). Dix and his colleagues (Dix & Grusec, 1985; Dix & Lochman, 1990; Dix & Reinhold, 1991; Dix, Ruble, & Zambarino, 1989, Dix, Reinhold, & Zambarino, 1990; Dix, Ruble, Grusec, & Nixon, 1986) conceptualize parenting as a process mediated by parental attributions about such factors as the degree to which children are to be held responsible for their actions, children's intentions, and children's social competence, all of which are age- and gender-dependent.

In a further elaboration of this work, Dix (1991) has presented a model of parenting that places affective organizations at the center of the parenting process, conceptualized as a dynamic, reciprocal interplay between emotional activation, engagement, and regulation. Although this model places greater weight on the role of emotion, rather than on cognition in organizing parenting behavior, cognitions (e.g., appraisal processes) are viewed as central determinants of emotions, and both are thus closely intertwined. For example, a parent who is in a hurry to leave the house to make an appointment on time will likely appraise child behavior that is unresponsive to parental directives to "get ready to leave" as being in conflict with the parent's current concern. This in turn predisposes that parent to anger (emotion activation), which in turn leads to increased parental efforts to gain compliance from the child (engagement), which could take the form of raising one's voice and repeating the message to don the coat, some type of physical intervention such as detaining the child and putting the child's coat on for him, or perhaps both. As a final step, however, cognitions may further modulate the parent's irritation toward the child, before the parent acts, as the parent makes appraisals of situational factors that relate to the child's propensity to comply. A parent's irritation and ensuing response may be assuaged if he or she determines that the child was out of earshot when the parent made the request, lacked the skills to comply completely (e.g., too young to put on a coat without parental help), or was otherwise preoccupied (e.g., visiting the bathroom) so that immediate compliance was deemed impossible. On the other hand, parental anger at child noncompliance could be exacerbated, leading to a stronger and more forceful parental response, if the parent appraises the child's behavior as deliberately disobedient, if the parent expects disobedience because the child had a history of noncompliance, or if the parent's affective state (e.g., depression) renders the parent less tolerant of the child's misbehavior.

Whether it is cognition or emotion that immediately precedes parental responding at a given moment is a theoretical issue beyond the scope of this chapter and one that, we would argue, defies easy testing. In our view, cognition, emotion, and behavior are in constant reciprocal interplay, and attempts to establish primacy of any one over the others are fraught with difficulty. Our discussions of depressed parental cognitions as mediators of child outcomes operate from a level of analysis that views cognitive appraisal processes as both causal of and responsive to affective states and behavior.

Depressive Attributions about Child Behavior

Depressed mothers may be less tolerant of their children's misdeeds than are nondepressed mothers for similar transgressions (Conrad & Hammen, 1989), which may lead depressed mothers to attribute negative intentions and motives to their children's behavior more readily than would nondepressed mothers. In addition, depressed mothers may view themselves as suffering and in need of comforting, so perhaps they expect more social competence and responsibility from their children than would be developmentally warranted. Such unrealistic cognitive sets would be expected to provoke impatient, angry, even punitive behavior in response to children's inadvertant noncompliance. In addition, children's resistant, oppositional behavior can create negative maternal cognitive sets that influence disciplinary practices. Brunk and Henggeler (1984) convincingly demonstrated the impact of maternal cognitive sets on maternal behavior in a study in which two 10-year-old child confederates acted out internalizing ("anxious–withdrawn") and externalizing ("conduct-disordered") roles during interactions with normal-mood mothers. As predicted, mothers exhibited higher rates of commands and discipline in the conduct-disordered role play condition, and higher rates of nurturing behaviors in the anxious–withdrawn role play condition. However, sequential analyses revealed that mothers in the conduct-disordered condition were much more likely to display restricting, punitive behavior even when the child showed full compliance with mother's directives. By contrast, mothers in the anxious–withdrawn condition more frequently responded to child compliance with verbal rewards rather than discipline.

Depressed Mothers' Self-Perceptions of Caregiving Control

Depressed parents' perceptions of their own competence in the parental role would also be expected to affect parenting behavior. Presently, a small but growing number of studies are examining such self-appraisals as self-efficacy and judgments of control in the maternal role, and these studies highlight the important role of these constructs in the organization of parental behavior. In a compelling series of investigations, Bugental and her colleagues demonstrated that in comparison to mothers who saw caregiving outcomes as largely under their control, mothers who reported having little control showed more physiological reactivity to child unresponsivity (Bugental & Cortez, 1988) and were judged more negative and less affectively assertive during interactions with unresponsive children. The children, in turn, continued to be unresponsive to their mothers (Bugental & Shennum, 1984). Bugental, Blue, and Cruzcosa (1989) also found low levels of perceived control over caregiving failures to be more characteristic of mothers who had sought counseling from a child abuse agency and to be predictive of annoyance and irritation when mothers interacted with unrelated children designated to be at risk for abuse. Although these studies did not target depressed mothers per se, low levels of perceived control over caregiving outcomes are probably characteristic of depressed parents as well, given the evidence of depressed mothers' perceptions of themselves as less than adequate caregivers (Whiffen & Gotlib, 1989).

Depressed Mothers' Self-Efficacy Beliefs

An important line of research that links maternal depression, maternal self-appraisals of parenting effectiveness, and parenting behavior has been concerned with Bandura's (1982, 1986, 1989) concept of self-efficacy beliefs, or judgments about one's competency at a particular task or in a particular setting. Bandura's (1986) social–cognitive theory views self-efficacy as a central mediator of relations between knowledge and behavior. Self-efficacious individuals, who judge themselves as competent and effective in a given task, are expected to persist in their endeavors to achieve success even in the face of rather formidable obstacles, whereas self-inefficacious individuals are expected to lack such tenacity and give up prematurely, even though success is potentially achievable. Thus, Bandura (1982, 1986) conceptualizes self-efficacy beliefs as predictive of the degree of effort used to succeed at a given task. However, relations between self-efficacy beliefs and performance attainments are viewed as bidirectional in that how efficacious we feel at a given task is also related to our history of successes and failures at that task. Further, although self-efficacy is believed to be most strongly affected by performance attainments, it is also susceptible to other influences, such as affective state, vicarious experiences (e.g., modeling), and social persuasion from support figures.

Interestingly, researchers have only recently begun to examine maternal self-efficacy beliefs in relation to maternal behavior (e.g.,

Davis, 1990; Donovan & Leavitt, 1989; Gross & Conrad, 1992; Teti & Gelfand, 1991). This belated application of Bandura's formulations to parenting is in part because self-efficacy theory originally emerged from laboratory work that assessed self-efficacy change as a function of deliberate inductions of success or failure experience (Bandura & Wood, 1989), positive and negative moods (Kavanagh & Bower, 1985), or performance-contingent feedback (Newman & Goldfried, 1987). Not surprisingly, depressed mothers of young children report feeling less efficacious in the parenting role than do nondepressed mothers (Fox & Gelfand, 1994; Teti & Gelfand, 1991; Teti, Gelfand, & Pompa, 1990). Depressed mothers' self-inefficacy as parents may stem from several sources. Among the potential bases for low parenting self-efficacy in a depressed mother are the propensity of sad affect to foster negative, pessimistic, ruminative thought processes about ourselves and our environment (Clark & Teasdale, 1982; Isen, 1984; Teasdale & Fogarty, 1979); depressive mood's selective activation of memories of failure experiences (Bower, 1981); and perhaps a history of problematic caregiving with the infant. In turn, maternal self-efficacy should be closely linked to mothers' behavioral competence with their infants. Mothers who perceive themselves as efficacious in the parenting role should persist in attempting to establish harmonious relationships with their babies, flexibly using whatever external and internal resources are available to them. By contrast, inefficacious mothers' self-doubts should lead to relatively ineffective parenting marked by impatience, rigidity, and withdrawal.

Teti and Gelfand (1991) tested this hypothesis using 38 nondepressed and 48 clinically depressed, lower-middle to middle-class mothers and their first-year infants. In addition, Teti and Gelfand (1991) tested the hypothesis, based on Bandura's theory, that maternal self-efficacy mediated relations between maternal behavioral competence and severity of maternal depression, social–marital supports, and perceptions of infant temperament. All mothers were in therapy for their depression at recruitment and had received diagnoses according to the revised third edition of the *Diagnostic and Statistical Manual of Mental Disorders* (DSM-III-R; American Psychiatric Association, 1987) of either major depression, dysthymia, or adjustment disorder with depressed mood from their therapists. Nondepressed mothers were recruited from the same neighborhoods as the depressed mothers. Severity of depressive symptoms was assessed with the Beck Depression Inventory (BDI; Beck, Ward, Mendelson, Mock, & Erbaugh, 1961). Social–marital supports were measured with a standardized composite score derived from the marital harmony scales of Locke and Wallace (1959) and Spanier (1976) and social support subscales of the Interview Schedule for Social Interaction (Henderson, Byrne, & Duncan-Jones, 1981). The Fussy–Difficultness subscale of the Infant Characteristics Questionnaire (Bates, Freeland, & Lounsbury, 1979) obtained mothers' perceptions of infant temperamental difficulty. Maternal self-efficacy was examined with a scale developed by the authors that inquired about self-efficacy beliefs in nine domains of parenting specific to mothers of first-year infants (e.g., soothing, understanding baby's wishes, maintaining baby's attention), with a final question that inquired about the women's global sense of self-efficacy as parents. A single score for maternal self-efficacy was obtained by summing the individual scores of the 10 items (alpha = .86). Finally, maternal behavioral competence was derived from observations of mothers' behavior in contexts of feeding and free play. Individual dimensions of mothers' behavior rated by "blind" observers were adapted from scales developed by Zoll, Lyons-Ruth, and Connell (1984) and included sensitivity, warmth, flatness of affect, disengagement, and anger. These ratings were adjusted so that higher scores always reflected more competent behavior, and the 10 ratings (5 per context) were summed to create a composite maternal behavioral competence index. Interrater (Pearson $r = .87$ on 18 dyads) and internal reliability (alpha = .86) on this composite were adequate.

As expected, maternal self-efficacy beliefs correlated negatively with mothers depressive symptomatology and perceptions of infant temperament, indicating that mothers felt less efficacious as parents when their depression levels were high and when they perceived their infants as difficult. In addition, maternal self-efficacy beliefs correlated positively with mothers' social–marital supports and with independent observers' judgments of their behavioral competence with their infants. Subsequent multiple regression analyses indicated that maternal self-efficacy beliefs continued to predict maternal behavioral competence even after the other variables were statistically controlled (i.e., maternal depressive symptomatology, social–marital supports, and perceptions of infant temperament). In addition, relations of maternal depressive symptoms, social–marital supports, and perceptions of infant temperament to maternal behavioral competence were substantially reduced when maternal self-efficacy beliefs were statistically controlled. These findings emphasize the sensitivity of mothers' self-efficacy beliefs' to maternal affective states and mothers' perceptions of their social environments. In addition, this study gave support to the mediational role of maternal self-efficacy in the prediction of parenting behavior.

Parent Attentional Processes in Depression

In addition to fostering negative cognitions about children and about oneself, depressive affect may affect parental cognitive processes by narrowing parents' attentional field and undermining problem-solving ability, thus predisposing the individual to parenting deficits. Consistent with this view, depressed parents have been characterized as self-absorbed, ruminative, and preoccupied, leading to inattentiveness and insensitivity to children's health, safety, and psychological needs (Gelfand & Teti, 1990). Other work (Wahler & Dumas, 1989) cites the role of environmental stressors, so frequently found to be correlates of parental depression (Hammen et al., 1987), in producing deficiencies in parental attention, monitoring, and information-processing skills. Such deficiencies further undermine parental judgments and narrow the field of response options that parents perceive (e.g., Vasta, 1982). Indeed, it has been suggested that high levels of distress distract parents from attending properly to their children and make parents intolerant of children's misdeeds and more prone to inappropriate, indiscriminate, controlling, and/or punitive parenting styles (Dumas & Wahler, 1986; Fox & Gelfand, 1994; Lahey, Conger, Atkeson, & Treiber, 1984; Mash, Johnston, & Kovitz, 1983).

In their interbehavioral model of parenting, Wahler and Dumas (1989) propose that successful parenting depends on the parents' ability to judge and respond to their children's behavior despite stresses that have no immediate relevance to the parent–child relationship. Stated more concretely, sophisticated parents do not confuse work or marital stressors with problems with their children. The degree of success at "compartmentalizing" and cognitively isolating stressors external to caregiving should help reduce the impact of such stressors on parental functioning.

VARIATION IN DEPRESSED MOTHER–CHILD OUTCOMES: THE ROLE OF MATERNAL COGNITIONS

Children of depressed mothers have varied developmental outcomes (Conrad & Hammen, 1993; Radke-Yarrow & Brown, 1993; Teti et al.,

1990), and not all experience adjustment difficulties. Reasons for individual differences in the outcomes of children in high-risk environments,
however defined, are complex, but most formulations center around risk
factors that increase children's vulnerability to psychopathology (e.g.,
"constitutional" factors such as low intelligence) or resilience factors that
buffer children against the negative effects of inadequate caregiving environments (e.g., social competence with peers) (Cicchetti & Aber, 1986;
Conrad & Hammen, 1993; Garmezy, 1987; Rutter, 1987).

A full discussion of risk and resilience factors as they apply to the
development of children of depressed parents is beyond the scope of this
chapter. We emphasize, however, that along with such child factors as high
intelligence, academic success, and appealing physical appearance (Masten, Best, & Garmezy, 1990), variation in outcomes of children of depressed mothers should be a function of individual differences in mothers' behavioral competence with their children (Cohn, Matias, Tronick, et
al., 1986; Teti et al., 1990). Such differences, we propose, can be linked
directly to differences in maternal appraisals of themselves and their children, in keeping with a model of cognitive mediation. This view acknow-
ledges that depressed mothers' appraisals of their infants and themselves
need not be, and probably are not, driven solely by severity of depressive
symptomatology. In this final section, we explore some social–familial
factors that might be expected to influence the cognitions of depressed
mothers and, in turn, their behavior with their children.

Infant Temperament

Of the constitutional factors in infancy thought to influence maternal–infant relations, infant temperament has garnered the lion's share of attention. Although variously conceptualized, temperament in infancy is generally believed to be genetically based and can be operationally defined by
such dimensions as emotionality, activity, predictability of daily cycles
and rhythms, adaptability to novel environmental stimuli, and sociability
(Bates et al., 1979; Buss & Plomin, 1975; Carey & McDevitt, 1978; Goldsmith et al., 1987; Rothbart, 1981; Thomas & Chess, 1977). A fussy, active,
slow-to-adapt, unpredictable baby may be challenging for any mother,
who might then develop negative perceptions of the baby and of herself as
a parent.

Goldberg (1977) has argued that mothers' self-appraisals of effectiveness in the caregiving role (i.e., maternal feelings of efficacy) are fostered

by easy-to-manage, predictable infants. Conversely, self-appraisals of ineffectiveness would be expected if mothers are faced with chronically fussy, difficult-to-read, and unpredictable babies. Researchers have found infant fussiness to relate negatively to maternal self-efficacy (Cutrona & Troutman, 1986; Davis, 1990; Gross & Conrad, 1992; Teti & Gelfand, 1991), supporting Goldberg's (1977) formulations and those of Bandura (1982, 1986), who proposes that self-efficacy beliefs are based on performance attainments. Teti and Gelfand (1991) propose that maternal self-efficacy is crucial to an understanding of the construct of "goodness of fit" between parent and child characteristics (Thomas & Chess, 1977). Indeed, relations between infant temperamental difficulty and maternal responsivity are inconsistent, with some studies showing positive, negative, or even no effect of infant temperament on maternal behavior (Crockenberg, 1986). One explanation for these discrepancies is that difficult infant temperament may affect different mothers differently, depending on mothers' initial levels of self-efficacy. A woman with a difficult baby but high levels of maternal self-efficacy would be expected to try harder, to make better use of her personal and social resources to achieve a successful, harmonious relationship with her infant than would a woman with an equally difficult baby but low maternal self-efficacy. The first woman might view her baby as "feisty, vigorous, and full of life"; the second might view her baby as "noisy, tiresome, and difficult."

Depressed mothers report lower levels of self-efficacy than do nondepressed mothers (Fox & Gelfand, 1994; Gross & Rocissano, 1988; Teti & Gelfand, 1991), and thus depressed mothers as a group are more vulnerable to perceiving a temperamentally difficult baby negatively and to developing performance deficits in mothering. Further, the combination of maternal depression and infant difficulty makes it particularly problematic for mothers to develop feelings of competence in the parental role. Teti and Gelfand (1991), for example, found in multiple regression analyses that maternal BDI and perceptions of infant difficulty scores interacted in predicting mothers' feelings of efficacy. Maternal self-efficacy was highest (predicted mean = 29.38) among mothers whose depressive symptoms were relatively mild and who saw their infants as temperamentally easy. Intermediate self-efficacy scores were obtained from mothers who reported high levels of depressive symptoms but who perceived their infants as easy (predicted mean = 20.63) and from mothers who reported low levels of depressive symptoms but who saw their infants as difficult (predicted mean = 26.28). By contrast, maternal self-efficacy was lowest (predicted mean = 13.01), and lower than would have been expected from a purely additive model of relations among these variables, in mothers who reported high levels of depressive symptomatology and who perceived their infants to be difficult. Thus, the "double jeopardy" combination of moderate–severe depression and a perceived difficult baby may place mothers at substantially high risk for parenting disturbances with their babies than the presence of either risk factor alone.

Interestingly, recent evidence (Murray, Stanley, Hooper, King, & Fiori-Cowley, 1996) indicates that high infant irritability and poor motor tonus, based on Neonatal Behavioral Assessment Scores (Brazelton, 1984), predicted maternal depression at 8 weeks postpartum. These data are important for at least two reasons. First, they indicate that postpartum depression in mothers is in part a function of infant characteristics during the neonatal period, characteristics that very likely interact with mothers' hormonal milieu to influence their postpartum affective states. Second, this study represents an important methodological advance in that the predictive relations obtained cannot be explained by shared method variance attributable to having mothers as the sole source of data for all measures.

Social–Marital Supports

Another putative influence on mother–child relations in infancy and early childhood is the quality of instrumental and social supports provided by intimates. Mothers with low social support and unhappy marriages behave less optimally with their infants than do mothers with good support networks and happy marriages (Cox, Owen, Lewis, & Henderson, 1989; Crnic, Greenberg, Ragozin, Robinson, & Basham, 1983; Crockenberg & McCluskey, 1986; Goldberg & Easterbrooks, 1984). Like infant temperament, social–marital supports should affect maternal functioning via their impact on maternal percepts and feelings. Self-efficacy theory (Bandura, 1982, 1986) suggests that support from intimates directly affects mothers' self-efficacy via modeling influences (e.g., learning about successful child care routines by watching competent relatives and friends) and positive consequences in the form of encouragement and praise.

This position receives support from several studies that have reported positive relations between quality of social–marital supports and mothers' self-efficacy (Davis, 1990; Donovan & Leavitt, 1989; Teti & Gelfand, 1991). In addition, social–marital supports may influence mothers' perceptions of their infants' difficult temperament, as evidenced by a significant negative correlation (Pearson r (84) = - .38, p .01) found between the two (Teti & Gelfand, 1991). Finally, Crockenberg (1981) found that temperamentally difficult infants were significantly more likely to become securely attached to their mothers when their mothers' levels of social support were high. We would thus expect that mothers prone to depression but whose marriages and support networks were at least adequate would tend to have more positive perceptions of themselves and their infants and would be more behaviorally competent with their infants.

CONCLUSION

We have argued that maternal cognitions are central to an understanding of the effects of maternal depression on depressed mothers' behavior with their children. Similarly, cognitive factors help determine the goodness of fit between parents' and children's characteristics and can be influenced by the depressed mothers' social milieu. Research evidence that depressed mothers' perceptions of themselves and their children are not linked solely to affective states suggests several areas of inquiry that are worth pursuing.

The first potential research area involves more systematic examination of the role of infant temperament and mothers' social–marital supports in the development of depressed mothers' appraisals of their infants and of themselves in the caregiving role. Surprisingly little is known about how infant temperament, maternal depression, and mothers' social–marital supports interact to influence maternal cognitions and mothers' behavior with their children. A difficult baby of a depressed mother may be less at risk for maladjustment if the mother has access to positive, caring support figures who can help her perceive her baby "objectively" (i.e., that her baby's difficulty is not the product of her incompetence as a mother). On this note, the classic findings of the New York Longitudinal Study (Thomas & Chess, 1977; Thomas, Chess, & Birch, 1970) are pertinent: Among the babies identified in this sample as very temperamentally difficult (i.e., as "mother killers") (Thomas et al., 1970), 70% were later identified as showing behavioral problems with parents and peers, whereas the remaining 30% of the difficult babies had more positive outcomes. An examination of parental differences between these two groups indicated that parents of the difficult children with more positive outcomes responded to them with more consistency, firmness, and patience and also reported less anxiety and self-blame over their children's temperamental problems than did the parents of difficult infants with later behavioral problems. Thus, more positive child outcomes for difficult babies were fostered when mothers were able to maintain more positive and "objective" perceptions of their babies and of themselves. These mothers may well have been less depressed than those who were less competent and self-confident. Research examining the impact of infant temperament on depressed women's parental cognitions would benefit from ongoing assessments of infant temperament provided by independent, trained observers in addition to those based on maternal report. Such an approach would circumvent the confounds of maternal personality, social desirability, and mood that are inherent in studies of the effects of infant temperament on parenting.

The ability to maintain positive appraisals of oneself and one's baby should depend in part on the quality of support received from intimates. Parents with difficult babies who can work as a team and support each other's efforts in child care should be successful at viewing their baby's difficulties as independent of their behavior. The combination of maternal depression, marital harmony, and seamless child care may be somewhat rare, however, given the stress that a mother's depression creates for other family members. Coyne et al. (1987) found that spouses of depressed women reported being stressed by their wives' lack of interest in normal social activities, persistent fatigue, feelings of hopelessness, and chronic worrying, and many of them were found to be depressed themselves. Gelfand and Teti (1990) propose that the marital relationship is an important focus of therapeutic efforts with depressed mothers. The spouse of a depressed woman who is given an opportunity to develop a clearer understanding of his wife's affective disorder may be better equipped psychologically to respond to his wife's negative cognitions and ruminations with emotional support and instrumental assistance rather than irritation and withdrawal. This may be especially important in depressed families with a younger, and perhaps temperamentally difficult, infant.

A second avenue of research that has received scant attention to date is the degree to which maternal appraisals in caregiving contexts have roots in mothers' experiences prior to childbirth. Conceivably, mothers' perceptions of their adequacy as caregivers and of their children may be tied to specific experiences in caregiver-like roles, such as babysitting and caring for younger siblings. Presumably, the more practiced individuals are for a particular task, the more ready and capable those individuals perceive themselves to be to undertake that task. More broadly, specific cognitive–affective predispositions created by childhood experiences with her family of origin could color a woman's readiness for parenthood and her perceptions of her child and her maternal competence. Ambivalence or anxiety about impending parenthood, which might be defined as having doubts about having children or about how effective we will be in the parenting role, may have links to childhood trauma (e.g., physical, sexual, and/or emotional abuse) or perhaps to nonabusive but consistently negative attitudes toward children expressed by our parents. Such cognitive–affective states may dispose women to make negative self- and infant appraisals, especially in the face of a temperamentally difficult baby and a poor marriage. Teti and Gelfand (1991) propose that self-efficacious mothers will make every effort to establish harmonious relationships with their babies, even temperamentally difficult ones, in contrast to self-inefficacious mothers who are expected to withdraw in defeat from a challenging infant. This view suggests that cognitive appraisals about motherhood may predate the actual experience of motherhood and may later influence maternal percepts. This issue clearly is best studied prospectively, but retrospective approaches may still be of value in hypothesis generation.

Finally, we support direct intervention efforts to foster successful caregiving experiences for depressed mothers of infants, which should in turn foster more positive self- and infant appraisals in depressed mothers and, in turn, maternal behavior. We (Gelfand & Teti, 1989) conducted an early intervention study to aid depressed mothers and their infants. The intervention consisted of weekly visits to the homes of clinically depressed mothers participating in psychotherapy using trained public health nurses. The nurses attempted to improve mothers' recognition of and responsivity to infant social cues, to help mothers enjoy their infants more fully, and to function as important support figures in the mothers' lives. This program was successful in reducing depressed mothers' reports of depressive symptoms relative to a matched group of depressed mothers who were not given the intervention. The program was also successful in improving mothers' perceptions of their infants, reducing daily minor stressors, and decreasing the proportion of disorganized infant–mother attachment relationships (Gelfand & Teti, 1993). Although such efforts should prove most beneficial in tandem with psychotherapy and medication to treat depression, behavioral interventions should be important in their own right if they foster mothers' performance attainments in the caregiving role.

ACKNOWLEDGMENTS

Preparation of this chapter was supported in part by National Institute of Mental Health Grant No. MH 41474, awarded to the authors. We wish to thank Laureen Teti and the members of our research group for their insightful comments on earlier versions of this chapter.

REFERENCES

Abramson, L. Y., Seligman, M. E. P., & Teasdale, J. D. (1978). Learned helplessness in humans: Critique and reformulation. *Journal of Abnormal Psychology, 87,* 49–74.

Ainsworth, M. D. S., Blehar, M. C., Waters, E., & Wall, S. (1978). *Patterns of attachment: A psychological study of the strange situation.* Hillsdale, NJ: Erlbaum.

American Psychiatric Association. (1987). *Diagnostic and statistical manual of mental disorders* (3rd ed., rev.). Washington, DC: Author.

American Psychiatric Association. (1994). *Diagnostic and statistical manual of mental disorders* (4th ed.). Washington, DC: Author.

Bakermans-Kranenburg, M. J., & van IJzendoorn, M. H. (1993). A psychometric study of the Adult Attachment Interview: Reliability and discriminant validity. *Developmental Psychology, 29,* 870–879.

Baldwin, M. W. (1992). Relational schemas and the processing of social information. *Psychological Bulletin, 112,* 461–484.

Bandura, A. (1982). Self-efficacy mechanisms in human agency. *American Psychologist, 84,* 191–215.

Bandura, A. (1986). *Social foundations of thought and action: A social–cognitive theory.* Englewood Cliffs, NJ: Prentice Hall.

Bandura, A. (1989). Regulation of cognitive processes through perceived self-efficacy. *Developmental Psychology, 25,* 729–735.

Bandura, A., & Wood, R. (1989). Effect of perceived controllability and performance standards on self-regulation of complex decision making. *Journal of Personality and Social Psychology, 56,* 805–814.

Bates, J. E., & Bayles, K. (1988). Attachment and the development of behavior problems. In J. Belsky & T. Nezworski (Eds.), *Clinical implications of attachment* (pp. 253–299). Hillsdale, NJ: Erlbaum.

Bates, J. E., Freeland, C. A., & Lounsbury, M. L. (1979). Measurement of infant difficultness. *Child Development, 50,* 794–803.

Beck, A. (1976). *Cognitive therapy and the emotional disorders.* New York: International Universities Press.

Beck, A. T. (1963). Thinking and depression: I. Idiosyncratic content and cognitive distortions. *Archives of General Psychiatry, 9,* 324–333.

Beck, A. T. (1987). Cognitive models of depression. *Journal of Cognitive Psychotherapy: An International Quarterly, 1,* 5–37.

Beck, A. T., Ward, C. H., Mendelson, M., Mock, J., & Erbaugh, J. (1961). An inventory for measuring depression. *Archives of General Psychiatry, 4,* 561–571.

Bower, G. H. (1981). Mood and memory. *American Psychologist, 2,* 129–148.

Bowlby, J. (1973). *Attachment and loss: Vol. 2. Separation.* New York: Basic Books.

Brazelton, T. B. (1984). *Neonatal Behavioral Assessment Scale* (2nd ed.). London: Spastics International Medical Publications.

Bretherton, I. (1985). Attachment theory: Retrospect and prospect. In I. Bretherton & E. Waters (Eds.), Growing points of attachment theory and research. *Monographs of the Society for Research in Child Development, 50*(1–2, Serial No. 209), 167–193.

Brewin, C. R. (1985). Depression and causal attributions: What is their relation? *Psychological Bulletin, 98,* 297–309.

Brody, G. H., & Forehand, R. (1986). Maternal perceptions of child maladjustment as a function of the combined influence of child behavior and maternal depression. *Journal of Consulting and Clinical Psychology, 54,* 237–240.

Brunk, M. A., & Henggeler, S. W. (1984). Child influences on adult controls: An experimental investigation. *Developmental Psychology, 20,* 1074–1081.

Bugental, D. G., Blue, B., & Cruzcosa, M. (1989). Perceived control over caregiving outcomes: Implications for child abuse. *Developmental Psychology, 25,* 532–539.

Bugental, D. B., & Cortez, V. (1988). Physiological reactivity to responsive and unresponsive children—As modified by perceived control. *Child Development, 59,* 686–693.

Bugental, D. B., & Shennum, W. A. (1984). "Difficult" children as elicitors and targets of adult communication patterns: An attributional–behavioral analysis. *Monographs of the Society for Research in Child Development, 49*(1, Serial No. 205), 1–81.

Buss, A. H., & Plomin, R. (1975). *A temperament theory of personality.* New York: Wiley.

Campbell, S. B., Cohn, J. F., Meyers, T. A., Ross, S., & Flanagan, C. (1993, March). Chronicity of maternal depression and mother–infant interaction. In D. Teti (Chair), *Depressed mothers and their children: Individual differences in mother–child outcome.* Symposium conducted at the meeting of the Society for Research in Child Development, New Orleans.

Carey, P. H., & McDevitt, S. C. (1978). Revision of the Infant Temperament Questionnaire. *Pediatrics, 61,* 735–739.

Cicchetti, D., & Aber, L. (1986). Early precursors of later depression: An organizational perspective. In L. Lipsitt & C. Rovee-Collier (Eds.), *Advances in infancy* (Vol. 4, pp. 87–137). Norwood, NJ: Ablex.

Clark, D. M., & Teasdale, J. D. (1982). Diurnal variation in clinical depression and accessibility of memories of positive and negative experiences. *Journal of Abnormal Psychology, 91*, 87–95.

Cohn, J. F., Matias, R., Tronick, E. Z., Connell, D., & Lyons-Ruth, K. (1986). Face-to-face interactions of depressed mothers and their infants. In E. Z. Tronick & T. Field (Eds.), *Maternal depression and infant disturbance: New directions for child development* (pp. 31–45). San Francisco: Jossey-Bass.

Conrad, M., & Hammen, C. (1989). Role of maternal depression in perceptions of child maladjustment. *Journal of Consulting and Clinical Psychology, 57*, 663–667.

Conrad, M., & Hammen, C. (1993). Protective and resource factors in high- and low-risk children: A comparison of children with unipolar, bipolar, medically ill, and normal mothers. *Development and Psychopathology, 5*, 593–608.

Cox, A. D., Puckering, C., Pound, A., & Mills, M. (1987). The impact of maternal depression in young children. *Journal of Child Psychology and Psychiatry, 28*, 917–928.

Cox, M. J., Owen, M. T., Lewis, J. M., & Henderson, V. K. (1989). Marriages, adult adjustment, and early parenting. *Child Development, 60*, 1015–1024.

Coyne, J. C., Kessler, R. C., Tal, M., Turnbull, J., Wortman, C. B., & Greden, J. F. (1987). Living with a depressed person. *Journal of Consulting and Clinical Psychology, 55*, 347–352.

Crittenden, P. (1992). Attachment in the preschool years. *Development and Psychopathology, 4*, 209–241.

Crnic, K. A., Greenberg, M. T., Ragozin, A. S., Robinson, N. M., & Basham, R. (1983). Effects of stress and social support on mothers and premature and full-term infants. *Child Development, 54*, 209–217.

Crockenberg, S., & McCluskey, K. (1986). Changes in maternal behavior during the baby's first year of life. *Child Development, 57*, 746–753.

Crockenberg, S. B. (1981). Infant irritability, mother responsiveness, and social support influences on the security of infant–mother attachment. *Child Development, 52*, 857–865.

Crockenberg, S. B. (1986). Are temperamental differences in babies associated with predictable differences in caregiving? In J. V. Lerner & R. H. Lerner (Eds.), *Temperament and social interaction in infants and children* (pp. 53–73). San Francisco: Jossey-Bass.

Cummings, E. M., & Davies, P. T. (1994). Maternal depression and child development. *Journal of Child Psychology and Psychiatry, 35*, 73–112.

Cutrona, C. E., & Troutman, B. R. (1986). Social support, infant temperament, and parenting self-efficacy: A mediational model of postpartum depression. *Child Development, 57*, 1507–1518.

Davis, A. L. (1990, April). *Clarifying the role of maternal self-confidence in maternal interactional competence.* Paper presented at the 7th International Conference on Infant Studies, Montreal.

Dix, T. (1991). The affective organization of parenting: Adaptive and maladaptive processes. *Psychological Bulletin, 110*, 3–25.

Dix, T., & Grusec, J. (1983). Parental influence techniques: An attributional analysis. *Child Development, 54,* 645–652.

Dix, T., & Lochman, J. (1990). Social cognition and negative reactions to children: A comparison of mothers of aggressive and nonaggressive boys. *Journal of Social and Clinical Psychology, 9,* 418–438.

Dix, T., & Reinhold, D. P. (1991). Chronic and temporary influences on mothers' attributions for disobedience. *Merrill–Palmer Quarterly, 37,* 251–271.

Dix, T., Reinhold, D. P., & Zambarino, R. J. (1990). Mothers' judgment in moments of anger. *Merrill–Palmer Quarterly, 36,* 465–486.

Dix, T., Ruble, D. N., Grusec, J. E., & Nixon, S. (1986). Social cognition in parents: Inferential and affective reactions to children of three age levels. *Child Development, 57,* 879–894.

Dix, T., Ruble, D. N., & Zambarano, R. J. (1989). Mothers' implicit theories of discipline: Child effects, parent effects, and the attribution process. *Child Development, 60,* 1373–1391.

Dodge, K. A., Pettit, G. S., McClaskey, C. L., & Brown, M. L. (1985). Social competence in children. *Monographs of the Society for Research in Child Development,* (2, Serial No. 213).

Donovan, W. L., & Leavitt, L. A. (1989). Maternal self-efficacy and infant attachment: Integrating physiology, perceptions, and behavior. *Child Development, 60,* 460–472.

Downey, G., & Coyne, J. C. (1990). Children of depressed parents: An integrative review. *Psychological Bulletin, 108,* 50–76.

Dumas, J. E., & Wahler, R. G. (1986). Indiscriminant mothering as a contextual factor in aggressive–oppositional child behavior. *Journal of Abnormal Child Psychology, 13,* 1–17.

Emery, R., Weintraub, S., & Neale, J. M. (1982). Effects of marital discord on the school behavior of children of schizophrenic, affectively disordered, and normal parents. *Journal of Abnormal Child Psychology, 10,* 215–228.

Emmerich, W. (1969). The parental role: A functional–cognitive approach. *Monographs of the Society for Research in Child Development, 34*(No. 8, Serial No. 132), 1–71.

Erickson, M. F., Sroufe, L. A., & Egeland, B. (1985). The relationship between quality of attachment and behavior problems in preschool in a high-risk sample. In I. Bretherton & E. Waters (Eds.), Growing points of attachment theory and research. *Monographs of the Society for Research in Child Development, 50*(1–2, Serial No. 209), 147–166.

Fagot, B. I., & Kavanagh, K. (1990). The prediction of antisocial behavior from avoidant attachment classifications. *Child Development, 61,* 864–873.

Fergusson, D. M., Horwood, L. J., Gretten, M. E., & Shannon, F. T. (1985). Family life events, maternal depression, and maternal and teacher descriptions of child behavior. *Pediatrics, 75,* 30–35.

Fergusson, D. M., Lynskey, M. T., & Horwood, L. J. (1993). The effect of maternal depression on maternal ratings of child behavior. *Journal of Abnormal Child Psychology, 21,* 245–269.

Field, T. M. (1984). Early interactions between infants and their postpartum depressed mothers. *Infant Behavior and Development, 7,* 517–522.

Field, T. M. (1992). Infants of depressed mothers. *Development and Psychopathology, 4,* 49–66.

Field, T., Morrow, C., & Adelstein, D. (1993). Depressed mothers' perceptions of infant behavior. *Infant Behavior and Development, 16,* 99–108.

Fleming, A. S., Ruble, D. N., Flett, G. L., & Shaul, D. L. (1988). Postpartum adjustment in first-time mothers: Relations between mood, maternal attitudes, and mother–infant interactions. *Developmental Psychology, 24,* 71–81.

Forehand, R., Lautenschlager, G. J., Faust, J., & Graziano, W. G. (1986). Parent perceptions and parent–child interactions in clinic-referred children: A preliminary investigation of the effects of maternal depressive moods. *Behaviour Research and Therapy, 24,* 73–75.

Fox, C. R., & Gelfand, D. M. (1994). Maternal depressed mood and stress as related to vigilance, self-efficacy, and mother–child interactions. *Early Development and Parenting, 3,* 233–243.

Friedlander, S., Weiss, D. S., & Traylor, J. (1986). Assessing the influence of maternal depression on the validity of the Child Behavior Checklist. *Journal of Abnormal Child Psychology, 14,* 123–133.

Frijda, N. H., Kuipers, P., & ter Schure, E. (1989). Relations among emotion, appraisal, and emotional action readiness. *Journal of Personality and Social Psychology, 57,* 212–228.

Garmezy, N. (1987). Stress, competence, and development: Continuities in the study of schizophrenic adults, children vulnerable to psychopathology, and the search for stress-resistant children. *American Journal of Orthopsychiatry, 57,* 159–174.

Gelfand, D. M., & Teti, D. M. (1989, August). *Intervention to aid infants of depressed mothers: First results.* Paper presented at the 97th Annual Convention of the American Psychological Association, New Orleans.

Gelfand, D. M., & Teti, D. M. (1990). The effects of maternal depression on children. *Clinical Psychology Review, 10,* 329–353.

Gelfand, D. M., Teti, D. M., & Fox, C. E. R. (1992). Sources of parenting stress for depressed and nondepressed mothers of infants. *Journal of Clinical Child Psychology, 21,* 262–272.

Goldberg, S. (1977). Social competence in infancy: A model of parent–infant interaction. *Merrill–Palmer Quarterly, 23,* 163–177.

Goldberg, W., & Easterbrooks, M. A. (1984). Role of marital quality in toddler development. *Developmental Psychology, 10,* 504–514.

Goldsmith, H. H., Buss, A. H., Plomin, R., Rothbart, M. K., Thomas, A., Chess, S., Hinde, R. A., & McCall, R. B. (1987). Roundtable: What is temperament? Four approaches. *Child Development, 58,* 505–529.

Goodman, S. H. (1992). Understanding the effects of depressed mothers on their children. In E. F. Walker, R. H. Dworkin, & B. A. Cornblatt (Eds.), *Progress in experimental personality and psychopathology research* (pp. 47–109). New York: Springer.

Goodnow, J. J. (1988). Parents' ideas, actions, and feelings: Models and methods from developmental and social psychology. *Child Development, 59,* 286–320.

Griest, D. L., Wells, K. C., & Forehand, R. (1979). An examination of predictors of maternal perceptions of maladjustment in clinic-referred children. *Journal of Abnormal Psychology, 88,* 277–281.

Gross, D., & Conrad, B. (1992, May). *A longitudinal model of maternal confidence and maternal mental health during toddlerhood.* Paper presented at the 8th International Conference on Infant Studies, Miami, FL.

Gross, D., & Rocissano, L. (1988). Maternal confidence in toddlerhood: Its measurement for clinical practice and research. *Nurse Practitioner, 13,* 19–29.

Haaga, D. A. F., Dyck, M. J., & Ernst, D. (1991). Empirical status of cognitive theory of depression. *Psychological Bulletin, 110,* 215–236.

Hammen, C. (1991). Generation of stress in the course of unipolar depression. *Journal of Abnormal Psychology, 100,* 555–561.

Hammen, C., Adrian, C., Gordon, D., Burge, D., Jaenicke, C., & Hiroto, D. (1987). Children of depressed mothers: Maternal strain and symptom predictors of dysfunction. *Journal of Abnormal Psychology, 96,* 190–198.

Henderson, S., Byrne, D. G., & Duncan-Jones, P. (1981). *Neurosis and the social environment.* Sydney: Academic Press Australia.

Isen, A. M. (1984). Toward understanding the role of affect in cognition. In R. Wyer & T. Srull (Eds.), *Handbook of social cognition* (pp. 179–236). Hillsdale, NJ: Erlbaum.

Kavanagh, D. J., & Bower, G. H. (1985). Mood and self-efficacy: Impact of joy and sadness on perceived capabilities. *Cognitive Therapy and Research, 9,* 507–525.

Kwon, S-M., & Oei, T. P. A. (1994). The roles of two levels of cognitions in the development, maintenance, and treatment of depression. *Clinical Psychology Review, 14,* 331–358.

Lahey, B. B., Conger, R. D., Atkeson, B. M., & Treiber, F. A. (1984). Parenting behavior and emotional status of physically abusive mothers. *Journal of Consulting and Clinical Psychology, 52,* 1062–1071.

Lewis, M., Feiring, C., McGuffog, C., & Jaskir, J. (1984). Predicting psychopathology in six-year-olds from early social relations. *Child Development, 55,* 1232–1236.

Locke, H., & Wallace, K. (1959). Short marital-adjustment and prediction tests: Their reliability and validity. *Marriage and Family Living, 21,* 251–255.

Lovejoy, M. C. (1991). Maternal depression: Effects on social cognition and behavior in parent–child interactions. *Journal of Abnormal Child Psychology, 19,* 693–706.

Maccoby, E. E., & Martin, J. P. (1983). Socialization in the context of the family: Parent–child interaction. In E. M. Hetherington (Ed.) & P. H. Mussen (Series Ed.), *Handbook of child psychology: Vol 4. Socialization, personality, and social development* (pp. 1–101). New York: Wiley.

Main, M., Kaplan, N., & Cassidy, J. C. (1985). Security in infancy, childhood and adulthood: A move to the level of representation. In I. Bretherton & E. Waters (Eds.), Growing points of attachment theory and research. *Mono-*

graphs of the Society for Research in Child Development, 50(1–2, Serial No. 209), 66–104.

Masten, A. S., Best, K. M., & Garmezy, N. (1990). Resilience and development: Contributions from the study of children who overcome adversity. Development and Psychopathology, 2, 425–444.

Mash, E. J., Johnston, C., & Kovitz, K. (1983). A comparison of the mother–child interactions of physically abused and nonabused children during play and task situations. Journal of Clinical Child Psychology, 12, 337–346.

Miller, S. A. (1988). Parents' beliefs about children's cognitive development. Child Development, 59, 259–285.

Murray, L. (1992). The impact of postnatal depression on infant development. Journal of Child Psychology and Psychiatry, 33, 543–561.

Murray, L., Stanley, C., Hooper, R., King, F., & Fiori-Cowley, A. (1996). The role of infant factors in postnatal depression and mother–infant interactions. Developmental Medicine and Child Neurology, 38, 109–119.

Newman, C., & Goldfried, M. R. (1987). Disabusing, negative self-efficacy expectations via experiences, feedback, and discrediting. Cognitive Therapy and Research, 11, 401–417.

Overmeier, J. B., & Seligman, M. E. P. (1967). Effects of inescapable shock upon subsequent escape and avoidance learning. Journal of Comparative and Physiological Psychology, 63, 28–33.

Panaccione, V. F., & Wahler, R. G. (1986). Child behavior, maternal depression, and social coercion as factors in the quality of child care. Journal of Abnormal Child Psychology, 14, 263–278.

Radke-Yarrow, M., & Brown, E. (1993). Resilience and vulnerability in children of multiple-risk families. Development and Psychopathology, 5, 581–592.

Radke-Yarrow, M., Cummings, E. M., Kuczynski, L., & Chapman, M. (1985). Patterns of attachment in two- and three-year-olds in normal families and families with parental depression. Child Development, 56, 884–893.

Richters, J. E. (1992). Depressed mothers as informants about their children: A critical review of the evidence of distortion. Psychological Bulletin, 112, 485–499.

Richters, J. E., & Pellegrini, D. (1989). Depressed mothers' judgments about their children: An examination of the depression–distortion hypothesis. Child Development, 50, 1068–1075.

Rickard, K. M., Forehand, R., Wells, K. C., Griest, D. L., & McMahon, R. J. (1981). Factors in the referral of children for behavioral treatment: A comparison of mothers of clinic-referred deviant, clinic-referred non-deviant and non-clinic children. Behaviour Research and Therapy, 19, 201–205.

Rogers, T. R., & Forehand, R. (1983). The role of parent depression in interactions between mothers and their clinic-referred children. Cognitive Therapy and Research, 7, 315–324.

Rothbart, M. K. (1981). Measurement of temperament in infancy. Child Development, 52, 569–578.

Rutter, M. (1987). Psychosocial resilience and protective mechanisms. American Journal of Orthopsychiatry, 57, 316–331.

Rutter, M. (1990). Commentary: Some focus and process considerations regarding effects of parental depression on children. *Developmental Psychology, 26,* 60–67.

Safran, J. D. (1990). Towards a refinement of cognitive therapy in light of interpersonal theory: I. Theory. *Clinical Psychology Review, 10,* 87–105.

Sameroff, A. J. (1975). Early influences on development: Fact or fancy? *Merrill-Palmer Quarterly, 21,* 3–33.

Schaughency, E. A., & Lahey, B. B. (1985). Mothers' and fathers' perceptions of child deviance: Roles of child behavior, parental depression, and marital satisfaction. *Journal of Consulting and Clinical Psychology, 53,* 718–723.

Segal, Z. V. (1988). Appraisal of the self-schema construct in cognitive models of depression. *Psychological Bulletin, 103,* 147–162.

Seligman, M. E. P., Abramson, L. Y., Semmel, A., & von Baeyer, C. (1979). Depressive attributional style. *Journal of Abnormal Psychology, 88,* 242–247.

Sigel, I. E. (Ed.). (1985). *Parental belief systems.* Hillsdale, NJ: Erlbaum.

Spanier, G. B. (1976). Measuring dyadic adjustment: New scales for assessing the quality of marriage and similar dyads. *Journal of Marriage and the Family, 38,* 15–28.

Sroufe, L. A. (1983). Infant–caregiver attachment and patterns of adaptation in preschool: The roots of maladaptation and competence. In M. Perlmutter (Ed.), *Minnesota symposium on child psychology* (Vol. 16, pp. 41–81). Hillsdale, NJ: Erlbaum.

Sroufe, L. A., & Fleeson, J. (1986). Attachment and the construction of relationships. In W. Hartup & Z. Rubin (Eds.), *The nature and development of relationships* (pp. 51–71). Hillsdale, NJ: Erlbaum.

Teasdale, J. D., & Fogarty, S. J. (1979). Differential effects of induced mood on retrieval of pleasant and unpleasant events from episodic memory. *Journal of Abnormal Psychology, 88,* 248–257.

Teti, D. M., & Gelfand, D. M. (1991). Behavioral competence among mothers of infants in the first year: The mediational role of maternal self-efficacy. *Child Development, 62,* 918–929.

Teti, D. M., Gelfand, D. M., Messinger, D. S., & Isabella, R. (1995). Maternal depression and the quality of early attachment: An examination of infants, preschoolers, and their mothers. *Developmental Psychology, 31,* 364–376.

Teti, D. M., Gelfand, D. M., & Pompa, J. (1990). Depressed mothers' behavioral competence with their infants: Demographic and psychosocial correlates. *Development and Psychopathology, 2,* 259–270.

Teti, D. M., & Nakagawa, M. (1990). Assessing attachment in infancy: The Strange Situation and alternate systems. In E. D. Gibbs & D. M. Teti (Eds.), *Interdisciplinary assessment of infants: A guide for early intervention professionals* (pp. 191–214). Baltimore: Paul H. Brookes.

Thomas, A., & Chess, S. (1977). *Temperament and development.* New York: Brunner/Mazel.

Thomas, A., Chess, S., & Birch, H. (1970). The origin of personality. *Scientific American, 223,* 102–109.

van IJzendoorn, M. H. (1992). Intergenerational transmission of parenting: A review of studies in nonclinical populations. *Developmental Review, 12,* 76–99.

Vasta, R. (1982). Physical child abuse: A dual-component analysis. *Developmental Review, 2,* 125–149.

Wahler, R. G., & Dumas, J. E. (1989). Attentional problems in dysfunctional mother–child interactions: An interbehavioral model. *Psychological Bulletin, 105,* 116–130.

Webster-Stratton, C., & Hammond, M. (1988). Maternal depression and its relationship to life stress, perceptions of child behavior problems, parenting behaviors, and child conduct problems. *Journal of Abnormal Child Psychology, 16,* 299–315.

Whiffen, V. E., & Gotlib, I. H. (1989). Infants of postpartum depressed mothers: Temperament and cognitive status. *Journal of Abnormal Psychology, 98,* 274–279.

Zahn-Waxler, C., Cummings, E. M., Ianotti, R. J., & Radke-Yarrow, M. (1984). Altruism, aggression, and social interactions in young children with a manic–depressive parent. *Child Development, 55,* 112–122.

Zahn-Waxler, C., McKnew, D. H., Cummings, E. M., Davenport, Y., & Radke-Yarrow, M. (1984). Problem behavior and peer interactions of young children with a manic–depressive parent. *American Journal of Psychiatry, 141,* 236–240.

Zoll, D. A., Lyons-Ruth, K., & Connell, D. (1984, August). *Infants at psychiatric risk: Maternal behavior, depression, and family history.* Paper presented at the 92nd Annual Convention of the American Psychological Association, Toronto.

7

The Timing and Chronicity
of Postpartum Depression:
Implications for Infant Development

Susan B. Campbell
Jeffrey F. Cohn
University of Pittsburgh

A growing body of research has focused on the characteristics of women experiencing a postpartum depression on the assumption that this may be a unique disorder (e.g., Hopkins, Marcus, & Campbell, 1984; Pitt, 1968). However, recent studies suggest that postpartum depression occurs at similar rates (Campbell & Cohn, 1991; Cooper, Campbell, Day, Kennerly, & Bond, 1988), has similar antecedents and correlates (O'Hara, Zekoski, Philipps, & Wright, 1990; Whiffen & Gotlib, 1993), and follows a similar course (Cooper et al., 1988; Whiffen & Gotlib, 1993) to depressions at other times in women's lives (see O'Hara, Chapter 1, this volume). Despite these similarities, the occurrence of postpartum depression raises unique issues about the adaptation to parenthood, the mother–infant relationship (Campbell, Cohn, Flanagan, Popper, & Meyers, 1992), and the potential impact of the depression on the infant at a time of particular vulnerability and dependency (Beardslee, Bemporad, Keller, & Klerman, 1983), underscoring the importance of studying postpartum depression in its own right.

Depression in the postpartum period may have a particularly delete-rious effect on the developing mother–infant relationship insofar as the symptoms of depression interfere with the mothering role (Radke-Yarrow, Cummings, Kuczynski, & Chapman, 1985). Mothers of younger infants, especially when it is their first child, must adjust to their baby and learn to understand their infant's communications and needs. This task is more difficult if the mothers are feeling despondent, fatigued, and over-whelmed by the responsibilities attendant upon the transition to parent-hood (e.g., Belsky, Rovine, & Fish, 1989; Campbell et al., 1992). Thus, researchers hypothesize that the sadness, irritability, and social with-drawal that characterize depressed women compromise their ability to provide a responsive, sensitive, nurturing environment for their younger babies (e.g., Cohn & Campbell, 1992; Cohn, Campbell, Matias, & Hop-kins, 1990; Field, 1992; Radke-Yarrow et al., 1985; Tronick, 1989). Theo-retically, the symptoms of depression should be reflected in mothers' less-ened ability to support the infant in regulating affect, in less positive and synchronized affect expression, and in lower levels of maternal stimula-tion and responsiveness (Cohn & Campbell, 1992; deMulder & Radke-Yarrow, 1991; Field, 1992; Field, Healy, Goldstein, & Guthertz, 1990). A result of these early and less optimal patterns of maternal behavior should be a more irritable, less self-regulated, and more withdrawn infant who develops an insecure attachment relationship with his or her relatively unresponsive and disengaged mother.

This formulation seems plausible, even likely, from a theoretical per-spective, and it points to several important issues. In particular, it suggests that one of the major mechanisms through which maternal depression influences infant outcome is parenting behavior (Cummings & Davies, 1994; Radke-Yarrow et al., 1985). This perspective has gained growing acceptance, despite the recognition that genetic mechanisms are also in-volved (Kendler, Neale, Kessler, Heath, & Eaves, 1992). Thus, although a genetic diathesis may render some offspring of depressed women more vulnerable to the impact of insensitive or inconsistent maternal care, it seems important to examine early indices of relationship quality if we are to identify proximal and modifiable processes in the mother–infant rela-tionship that lead to negative outcomes.

Despite the logic of this argument, a number of issues cloud the interpretation of extant findings. These issues include the heterogeneity of depression, the timing and course of the depression relative to infant age and developmental needs, the way depression has been defined in various studies, and the inevitable confounding of depression with other risk factors such as marital distress and other indicators of family adversity.

Many of the studies that document differences between depressed and nondepressed mother–infant dyads have focused on high-risk groups selected on the basis of elevated scores on symptom checklists. Thus, for example, Field et al. (1990) delineated differences in patterns of early interaction and maternal synchrony in depressed inner-city women; Lyons-Ruth, Connell, Grunebaum, and Botein (1990) reported differences in the rates of disorganized attachment and maternal hostility and intrusiveness in a small sample of depressed women identified as experiencing parenting problems and receiving community services.

Both these investigators studied multiproblem, single mothers living in poverty, so the elevated symptom ratings may reflect anxiety and stress as well as feelings of demoralization, rather than a diagnosable depression (Garrison & Earls, 1986). Furthermore, in these high-risk groups, depression may interact with other risk factors to lead to more dysfunctional patterns of caregiving and poorer infant outcome (Rutter, 1990).

When carefully diagnosed samples of women with depression in the postpartum period are studied, the results point to a less consistent pattern of differences between depressed and nondepressed mothers and their babies, especially in social behavior and quality of interaction. This appears to be true whether one studies high-risk women with a history of psychiatric treatment (e.g., Sameroff, Seifer, & Zax, 1982), women currently in treatment for depression (Teti & Gelfand, 1991), or low-risk women from the community experiencing a depression after the birth of their first baby (Campbell et al., 1992; Campbell, Cohn, & Meyers, 1995). Thus, Sameroff et al. (1982) reported relatively few group differences when mothers with a history of depression, those with a history of other disorders, and control mothers with no disorder were observed extensively in the home with their babies at 4 months. Even though mothers with a history of depression were less spontaneous and vocalized to their infants less, the behavior of their infants did not differ from that of other infants. Moreover, these once depressed mothers were neither less responsive nor more negative, nor did they spend less time than comparison mothers in face-to-face interaction. Chronicity and severity of psychiatric disorder, social status indicators, and parity all were more important predictors of mother–infant interaction, infant functioning, and child outcome in the preschool period than was maternal diagnosis. Teti and Gelfand (1991) found that although there were differences between depressed and control mothers in their competence during caretaking and play, these differences were accounted for by feelings of self-efficacy in the maternal role rather than depression per se in a group of postpartum women in treatment. Thus, these studies suggest that depression in and of itself may be less relevant to understanding parenting difficulties than other psychosocial factors that accompany the depression. This possibility has been raised in several recent reviews of maternal depression (Cummings & Davies, 1994; Downey & Coyne, 1990).

One issue that has been largely overlooked in studies of maternal depression and its effects on offspring is the timing and chronicity of the depression and whether it is present at the time of assessment. One might argue that any occurrence of depression during a woman's lifetime suggests an underlying personality characteristic that may compromise her parenting skills. Factors that make her vulnerable to depression may also lead to relationship difficulties, even in the absence of full-blown symptoms of depression (Billings & Moos, 1983; Coyne, Downey, & Boergers, 1992; Murray, 1992; Stein et al., 1991; Weissman & Paykel, 1974; Whiffen & Gotlib, 1993). For these reasons, many studies of mother–child interaction and maternal depression are based on the assumption that a history of depression will be associated with less optimal parenting. However, in a study formally addressing this question, no differences were identified between a control group and one in which the mother had a history of severe depression but no depression during the child's lifetime. No differences were found in the quality of mother–infant interaction at 2 months or infant outcome at 18 months (Murray, 1992; Murray, Kempton, Woolgar, & Hooper, 1993).

An alternative view is that the mother–child dyad is more likely to appear dysfunctional when the depression is current and more longstanding effects will be observed only when the depression persists over a significant portion of a child's life. The timing and chronicity of the depression may be especially important in infancy, given the dependency of the infant on the emotional and social responsiveness of the primary caregiver, usually the mother (Beardslee et al., 1983). Thus, in the postpartum period, chronic depressions may make infants particularly vulnerable to negative outcomes, whereas short-lived depressions may have fewer consequences for infant development or for the quality of the mother–infant relationship. Although Hammen, Adrian, Gordon, Burge, and Jaenicke (1987) reported that current symptom levels were more important than a positive history of depression in predicting psychopathology in school-age offspring of depressed mothers, few studies have actually addressed this complicated issue in infants.

Finally, the occurrence of short-lived depressions in the first few months postpartum raises the question of sensitive periods (see Hay, Chapter 4, and Murray & Cooper, Chapter 5, this volume). Hay and Murray and Cooper argue that maternal withdrawal and variability in contingent responding, especially in the early months, may compromise infant regulation of attention and affect, with implications for cognitive and socioemotional development.

Although the data supporting this argument are equivocal at best, there is some suggestion that postpartum depression potentiates the effects of other risk factors, especially as they relate to poorer cognitive functioning in boys. Although our data are not consistent with this position (Campbell et al., 1995), our sample consists of low-risk women and their infants in whom the protective effects of higher maternal education and the availability of emotional and instrumental support for both mother and baby may offset any potentially longer-term effects on the infant of early maternal depression. Clearly, this hypothesis merits further research with larger samples, stratified by risk status and depression chronicity. However, findings such as those reviewed by Hay and Murray and Cooper may indicate a sensitive period in the infant for the consolidation of particular interactive skills and cognitive processes, or they may indicate that the postpartum depression is associated with continued differences in maternal responsiveness that last beyond the depression itself.

In one study examining the question of the timing and chronicity of depression, Stein et al. (1991) found that a history of depression in the postpartum period had an impact on the quality of mother–infant interaction and infant outcome at 19 months, even when the depression was no longer current. In this study, mothers and their toddlers were observed at home during a structured play interaction. Mothers who were depressed in the first postpartum year were less likely to facilitate child exploration, their children engaged in less affective sharing, and the dyad interacted less overall than demographically matched comparison dyads without a history of depression. It is interesting, however, that the groups did not differ in maternal warmth. When the subgroup of formerly depressed women who were no longer depressed at 9 months was compared with controls, differences were still observed in maternal facilitation and toddlers' affective sharing. These findings, then, suggest that although women in the midst of an episode may be more unresponsive than women whose depressions have remitted, women who have experienced a severe depression during their infants' early months may continue to engage in lower rates of affective communication and sharing with their toddlers. Thus, depression effects or personality factors associated with depression may last beyond the period of the depression itself, suggesting that the presence of depression is enough to disrupt aspects of the mother–infant relationship. The paucity of research directly addressing this question, however, makes it difficult to draw conclusions.

One important consideration regarding the impact of maternal depression on the infant is that its timing and chronicity may be more important for certain outcomes than for others. Among the most salient outcomes for the infant is the quality of attachment. Attachment theory posits that early mother–infant interaction, especially maternal sensitivity and responsiveness during the 6- to 12-month period when the attachment relationship is consolidating, will be a particularly important determinant of the quality of attachment that develops (Bowlby, 1969). Thus, infants who experience a prolonged period of maternal unavailability, withdrawal, or inconsistency will be more likely to show avoidant, resistant, or disorganized patterns of attachment in toddlerhood, whereas those whose mothers are more appropriately responsive will be more likely to be secure (Ainsworth, Blehar, Waters, & Wall, 1978; Bates, Maslin, & Frankel, 1985; Belsky, Rovine, & Taylor, 1984). If we assume that the symptoms of depression compromise maternal responsiveness and sensitivity to infant communications, it seems logical to argue that chronicity of depression is a more robust predictor of attachment quality than the mere presence of a brief depressive episode at some time during the first year. Thus, short-lived postpartum depressions with an onset in the first postpartum weeks that resolve themselves by 4 or 5 months should have less of an impact on the quality of attachment than depressions that last through 6 months and beyond.

For these reasons, the course and timing of the depression may be important for understanding the associations among maternal depression, less optimal early caretaking, and later deleterious effects on the infant and toddler attachment to the mother. However, data relating attachment security to maternal depression have been surprisingly sparse and equivocal. Although the findings of Radke-Yarrow et al. (1985) linking depression to insecure attachment in toddlers have been widely cited, a later report on the National Institute of Mental Health sample indicated that higher rates of insecure attachment were accounted for *only* by the bipolar group (deMulder & Radke-Yarrow, 1991; see also Cohn & Campbell, 1992). Similarly, in the landmark study of the offspring of psychiatrically ill women, Sameroff et al. (1982) found no differences in attachment security as a function of either diagnosis, severity, or chronicity of psychiatric illness.

On the other hand, two studies of depressed women and their offspring demonstrated higher rates of insecurity in the depressed mother–infant dyads, consistent with theoretical predictions. Teti and Gelfand (1993) found higher rates of insecure and disorganized attachments in the toddler offspring of depressed than comparison women. Murray (1992) likewise found higher rates of insecurity in the offspring of depressed than comparison women at 18 months. Furthermore, neither duration nor severity of depression was related to attachment status in Murray's study, suggesting, as in the study of Stein et al. (1991), that women experiencing depression in the early postpartum period may continue to have difficulties in their relationship with their infant, despite the remission of symptoms.

It is difficult to make sense of these conflicting findings because in all four of these studies women met diagnostic criteria for depression. The differences cannot be accounted for by treatment utilization. The women who took part in the Radke-Yarrow and Murray studies were recruited from the community, and the women in the Sameroff and Teti studies had sought treatment. However, the timing of the depression in the woman's life relative to infant functioning may be relevant to understanding these apparently discrepant findings. In the Teti study, women were in treatment at the time of recruitment and many had chronic depressions; in most instances the current episode was not their first. Thus, it is reasonable to assume that their depressions lasted through a significant portion of the infant's first year, and especially the period preceding the assessment of attachment. Moreover, it is unclear from the data presented whether the attachment insecurity in this sample was associated with other risk factors that often co-occur with depression.

Although Murray (1992) also reported more insecurity in the offspring of her depressed women, and only 10 women were depressed at the 18-month assessment of attachment, she also found that adversity associated with attachment issues mediated the insecurity (Murray, Fiori-Cowley, Hooper, & Cooper, 1996).

The findings of Sameroff et al. (1982) and deMulder and Radke-Yarrow (1991) are especially counterintuitive because diagnosed major depression was not associated with elevated rates of insecurity relative to controls.

However, in the Sameroff et al. study, data on chronicity and severity of illness reflected lifetime history, and it is impossible to determine how many women were depressed during their infants' early months or concurrent with the assessment of attachment. The Radke-Yarrow data are relevant to this discussion as well. First, data from Radke-Yarrow et al. (1985) indicate that co-occurring risk factors and factors related to the depression were associated with greater rates of insecure attachment, but only with mixed avoidant and resistant (A/C) attachment, the classification similar to the disorganized attachment described by Main and Solomon (1990). Thus, depressed women living without partners were more likely to have insecure babies; women whose depressions were more severe, who were more likely to have been in treatment, and who had been depressed for a greater proportion of their child's lifetime were also more likely to have insecure toddlers. However, interpretation of these findings is complicated further because women with major depression and bipolar disorder were combined into one category of severe depression. Women experiencing unipolar and bipolar disorders are likely to provide quite different social and emotional environments for their infants and toddlers (deMulder & Radke-Yarrow, 1991; Hipwell & Kumar, Chapter 11, this volume). Therefore, studies that examine depression as a single entity rather than a complex process oversimplify the issues as they relate to parenting.

In further analysis of the data set of Radke-Yarrow and colleagues, it became clear that attachment security per se was unrelated to a diagnosis of unipolar major depression (deMulder & Radke-Yarrow, 1991). However, maternal mood and affect observed in a naturalistic environment within several weeks of the attachment assessment predicted attachment security, but only within the depressed group of mothers and toddlers. Depressed and bipolar mothers who demonstrated the highest rates of sad mood and anger/irritability when observed in an apartment-like setting with their child were more likely to have toddlers who were insecure, and this was especially the case for depressed mothers and their daughters. Within the control group, concurrent observations of negative mood were unrelated to attachment security, presumably because the negative mood was not part of a long-term pattern of negative affective exchange.

These data underscore the importance of current symptoms but also highlight the heterogeneity of depression. Thus, despite diagnoses of depression, many mothers exhibited neither sad mood nor anger/irritability when observed with their toddlers, and their toddlers were likely to be securely attached. On the other hand, some mothers with a depression diagnosis were quite negative and sad, and their toddlers were less likely to seek them out for comfort and support when distressed. These data indicate that insecurity may be specific to dyads in which the mothers' depression is either prolonged and chronic or occurs in the context of a dysphoric personality style that persists between episodes. Less severe and chronic depressions may have fewer consequences for the quality of mother–toddler relationships.

Studies of postpartum depression have tended to focus on the initial diagnosis, with rather limited data available on course. However, it appears that many depressions in the immediate postpartum period are quite brief. This means that studies of postpartum women often combine women with short-lived, though intense, negative reactions to the stresses of childbirth and child care (e.g., Hopkins, Campbell, & Marcus, 1987; O'Hara, Neunaber, & Zekoski, 1984; O'Hara, Chapter 1, this volume) with women experiencing more serious depressions. Thus, differences in course and severity, as well as the specific manifestations of the depression vis-à-vis the baby, must enter into a discussion of the impact of depression on the infant and the infant–mother relationship.

In this chapter, we report data on the course of depression in first-time mothers over the first 24 months postpartum and its relation to early mother–child interaction, as well as attachment security at 12 and 18 months. We examine satisfaction with marital support over this same period because this appears to be an important concomitant of postpartum adjustment (e.g., Campbell et al., 1992; O'Hara et al., 1990; Whiffen & Gotlib, 1993). We also illustrate different patterns of depression course with prototypical case studies. Our sample represents a low-risk community sample of married, middle-class women. They were selected specifically to minimize the impact of such co-occurring risk factors as poverty, single parenthood, low social support, and closely spaced multiparity, all of which have been associated with self-reported depression as well as with less optimal parenting (e.g., Brown & Harris, 1978; Field et al., 1990; Lyons-Ruth et al., 1990; McLoyd, 1990; Sameroff et al., 1982).

METHOD

Overview of Study Procedure

Women were screened for depression during a telephone interview at 6 to 8 weeks postpartum. Women who met screening criteria for depression (see the next section) and a comparable group of nondepressed women were recruited for a longitudinal study of postpartum adaptation and infant development. Women who agreed to participate were interviewed at home at 2, 4, and 6 months postpartum. They were assessed for depression and asked more generally about the baby and their postpartum adaptation. At the 2-month visit, lifetime history and family history of psychiatric disorder also were assessed. Women completed questionnaires and were observed interacting with their infants at 2, 4, and 6 months (see Campbell et al., 1995).

Depression assessments were repeated at 9, 12, 18, and 24 months postpartum. At 9 and 24 months, interviews were conducted on the telephone. At 12 and 18 months, they were conducted in the infant development laboratory in the context of additional assessments of infant attachment security. Women who could not come into the laboratory for an appointment were interviewed on the telephone.

Recruitment and Depression Screening

A sample of 2,760 women who delivered babies at Magee–Women's Hospital between July 1986 and August 1991 were contacted shortly after birth and asked for permission to be interviewed on the telephone at about 6 weeks postpartum. Only primiparous women delivering full-term, healthy, singleton infants without major complications were included in the screening sample. To be eligible for the study, women also had to be Caucasian, married, and between 18 and 35 years of age and had to have at least a high school education. Women with adoptive or stepchildren in the home full-time were excluded.

Between 6 and 8 weeks after delivery, women were telephoned and asked if they were willing to answer some questions about how they had been feeling since the birth of the baby: 69% of potentially eligible women were reached; of these, 79% agreed. Women were then interviewed to confirm that they met demographic inclusion criteria (8% were excluded) and to determine whether they met approximate Research Diagnostic Criteria (RDC; Spitzer, Endicott, & Robins, 1978) for depression, on a version of the Schedule for Affective Disorders and Schizophrenia (SADS; Endicott & Spitzer, 1978), as modified by O'Hara et al. (1984) for postpartum samples. A total of 1,439 women who met inclusion criteria completed the telephone interview.

Women who reported 2 weeks of depressed mood and at least three other symptoms were considered to have met screening criteria for depression. Women who met screening criteria were asked if they were willing to participate in the full study; a comparable group of women who did not meet depression screening criteria were also invited to participate (for more details on the screening interview, see Campbell & Cohn, 1991). Of the 126 women (8.8%) who met screening criteria for depression, 74 (59%) agreed to participate in the longitudinal study and 70 comparison women agreed (53% of those contacted). Another three depressed women in treatment were also added to the depressed group.

Main Study Sample

These women were then visited at home and additional interviewing was carried out to determine whether they actually met the RDC for minor depression (definite) or major depression (probable or definite) (for details see Campbell et al., 1992). Five women from the depressed group were dropped at this stage because they did not meet criteria; data from another two depressed women were not included in the analyses because they became psychotic. Five control women were dropped after the initial home visit because they reported some clinically significant depressive symptoms. Data from another two control women were not included in the analyses because of other reported problems. The final sample consisted of 70 depressed women and 63 nondepressed women; groups were well matched on demographic variables. They did not differ in age (M's = 28.9 and 29.7), educational level (M's = 5.5 and 5.7), or occupational level (M's = 6.1 and 5.9) as scored on the Hollingshead (1975) scale; 87% of the sample had at least some post-high school education and 51% had graduated from college. Women were primarily in secretarial, administrative, and professional occupations. The distribution of infant gender was comparable across groups (68 boys, 65 girls). Groups also were comparable in work status (working full-time, part-time, or not at all) and number of hours working across the period of the study.

At 2 months, 70% of the women in the sample were still at home full-time, but by 12 months, 62% of the sample had returned to work at least part-time.

Assessment of Depression

Women were interviewed at home at 2 months postpartum and followed up at regular intervals when the SADS was readministered. Women were considered to be in remission if they had a period of 8 weeks during which they did not report depressed mood or clinically significant symptoms (Coryell, Endicott, & Keller, 1990). However, women who were receiving psychotropic medication to treat their depression but did not endorse enough symptoms to meet the RDC were still considered to be in a continuing episode (see Shea et al., 1992). Women with two continuing symptoms and clinically significant depressed mood or with depressed mood and more than three subclinical symptoms also were considered to be in a continuing episode. Women who reported a period of 8 weeks without symptoms that met criteria but who endorsed either sad mood and two subclinical symptoms or sad mood and one symptom at a clinically significant level were not given a diagnosis of depression but were considered to be showing ongoing subclinical depression (Wells, Burnam, Rogers, Hays, & Camp, 1992). Finally, women with a clear period of at least 8 weeks without symptoms who then experienced a new period of depressed mood and at least three additional symptoms for at least 2 weeks were considered to have relapsed (Coryell et al., 1990).

The reliability of diagnoses at 2 months was determined on 39 cases selected at random, but with a distribution of two depressed women for every control. All interviews were audiotaped and a second independent trained interviewer listened to the audiotape, made ratings on mood and symptoms, and gave a diagnosis. Agreement on diagnosis (depressed vs. not depressed) was 97%. The mean interrater reliability on symptom scores was $r = .84$, with reliability on most symptoms above $r = .90$. The interrater reliability on the summed symptom score at 2 months was $r = .97$. Diagnostic agreement at 6 months, determined on 12 cases, was 100% (depressed, subclinical, or not depressed), and the mean interrater reliability on mood and symptom ratings was $r = .76$. Interrater reliability on the summed symptom severity score was $r = .95$. At 12 months, six cases were selected at random and agreement was 83%; the mean reliability on symptom ratings was $r = .80$ and the reliability on total symptom severity score was $r = .78$.

At the 2-month interview, when the lifetime version of the SADS, the SADS-L, was administered, interviewers asked questions about previous history of affective disorder. The number of prior episodes of depression was coded as none, one, two, or three or more. Questions about treatment utilization, including medication and psychotherapy, were asked at each assessment. Questions about family history were included in the initial interview.

Postpartum Spousal Support

At each interview, mothers were asked specifically about how much help they were receiving from their husbands and responses were coded on a 3-point scale. In addition, women were asked how much emotional support they received from their spouse and whether their relationship with their spouse had changed since the prior assessment. Ratings on these questions were summed to form a composite marital support score because at each age they showed moderate internal consistency (alphas from .49 to .70). Higher scores indicated more satisfaction with spousal support.

Observations of Mother–Infant Interaction

Interviewers observed mothers and infants in several contexts during home visits at 2, 4, and 6 months. At each age, they asked mothers to play with their infants in the face-to-face position for 3 minutes and the interactions were videotaped for later scoring by observers blind to group designation (depressed or control). Mother–infant face-to-face interaction was coded on a second-by-second basis and scores for maternal positive engagement and maternal negative engagement were derived. Feeding interactions were also observed and rated from videotapes at 2 and 4 months; a composite feeding rating was obtained reflecting more harmonious interactions. At 4 months, mothers and infants were also observed interacting during play with an age-appropriate toy. Behavior was rated by different sets of blind observers and composite maternal positive affect and sensitivity scores were derived. Details of coding, data reduction and coding reliability may be found in Campbell et al. (1995). Finally, at the completion of the home visit, interviewers (who were not blind to depressed vs. control status) rated the overall quality of maternal positive and negative engagement (for details, see Campbell et al., 1992).

Attachment Security

At 12 and 18 months, mothers and infants came to our laboratory for an assessment that included the Ainsworth Strange Situation (Ainsworth et al., 1978). We followed the usual sequence of separations and reunions with and without the female stranger present and all strange situations were videotaped for later scoring. Both 12- and 18-month strange situation tapes were coded by Douglas Teti and his assistants; coders were blind to diagnosis and different coders rated the 12- and 18-month tapes. Reliability on classification was above .90 at both ages.

RESULTS

Subject Attrition

Four depressed women and one control woman dropped out of the study between the 2-month interview and the 6-month follow-up. Between 9 and 24 months another 13 depressed and 3 control women were lost or dropped out. Thus, there is a clear pattern of higher attrition in the depressed group (6% vs. 24%). Several of the depressed women who dropped out reported that talking about their mood and symptoms made them feel worse. However, depressed women who dropped out of the study by 24 months did not differ from those who remained in age, education, or occupational level or in initial depression severity. These rates of attrition are comparable to rates reported in other studies of depression (e.g., Wells et al., 1992).

Course of Postpartum Depression

Of the 70 women who met depression criteria at 2 months postpartum, 39 women (56%) met the RDC for a definite major depression (depressed mood and at least five symptoms); 23 women (33%) met criteria for a probable major depression (depressed mood and four symptoms); the remaining 8 women (11%) met the RDC for a minor depression (depressed mood and three symptoms).

Figure 7.1 displays data on the course of depression through 24 months postpartum. Following Shea et al. (1992), women who were on psychotropic medication were considered to be in a continuing episode even if they no longer reported enough clinically significant symptoms to meet the RDC. At the 4-month follow-up, 48% of women continued to meet depression criteria; 24% continued to report low-level symptoms; the remaining 28% reported being free of symptoms since the previous interview. By 6 months, only 30% of the depressed women were still in the postpartum episode; 41% continued to report subclinical symptoms, although they did not report enough symptoms to meet the RDC. At the 9-month assessment, 25% of the depressed women met depression crite-

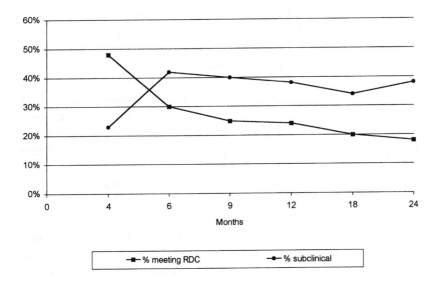

FIGURE 7.1. Cross-sectional data on the percentage of women meeting the RDC and reporting subclinical symptoms at each follow-up assessment.

ria and 38% reported low-level symptoms; at 12 months, 24% were depressed; at 18 months, 18% were depressed; at 24 months, 13% of the women in the original depressed group met criteria for depression. However, a relatively large proportion of women continued to report subclinical symptoms even if they no longer met the RDC: 36% at 12 months, 31% at 18 months, and 35% at 24 months.

Only eight women reported using psychotropic medication; of these, five women remained on medication from 6 through 12 months. Only one woman remained on medication continuously through the 24-month follow-up. In addition to the women on medication, several women were in psychotherapy only: one at 4 months, one at both 4 and 6 months, one at 12 months, one at 18 months, and three at 24 months. Overall, only 15 women in the depressed sample sought treatment at any time during the 24-month follow-up interval. These data underscore the limited treatment utilization in this community sample of depressed women with young babies (see also Cooper & Murray, Chapter 8, this volume).

The data reported so far reflect cross-sectional assessments of whether or not women met depression criteria, reported low-level but clinically significant symptoms, or were on medication at each assessment. However, data also indicate that a number of women had depressions that showed a chronic course, and this pattern is underestimated when cross-sectional data are examined.

Chronicity was defined in terms of either a continuing diagnosis of major depression, an intermittent diagnosis punctuated by periods of subclinical depression, or continued treatment with psychotropic medication; 17 women (30% of the depressed women with complete data through 24 months) showed a chronic course. The pattern of continuing low-level symptoms punctuated with clear episodes of depression may be akin to the "double depression" described by Keller, Lavori, Endicott, Coryell, and Klerman (1983). Another 10 women (18%) showed an episodic course. To be considered episodic, women had to report a period of at least 8 weeks without clinically significant sad mood or symptoms, followed by the recurrence of clinically significant symptoms. These 27 women (17 chronic, 10 episodic) were grouped together under "chronic" for purposes of data analyses on the assumption that their depressions reflected a more severe underlying depressive process. Two of the chronically depressed women on medication were hospitalized during the course of the follow-up interval.

Symptoms and Risk Factors as a Function of Depression Chronicity

As noted previously, women in the depressed group were classified into three subgroups based on the course of their depression. Data were then examined for these subgroups of depressed women: chronic ($n = 27$), subclinical ($n = 13$), and remitted ($n = 15$).

Two risk factors for depression were examined first: family history of depression and a personal history of prior episodes. Both these risk factors differentiated depressed from control groups at initial assessment (Campbell et al., 1992). However, women in the chronic group were no more likely to report a family history of depression (57%) than were women in the subclinical (46%) or remitted (47%) groups. Surprisingly, chronic depression was also unrelated to a history of depression prior to this postpartum episode: 39% of those in the chronic group, 46% of those considered subclinical, and 53% of the remitted group reported experiencing at least one prior episode of depression.

Patterns of symptoms over time were examined next. The sum of symptom ratings on the SADS was examined using a repeated-measures analysis of variance (ANOVA) with time (2, 4, 6, 9, 12, 18, 24 months) as the within-subjects factor and group as the between-subjects factor (control, remitted, subclinical, chronic). Not surprisingly, both group and time main effects were significant ($p < .001$), and they were qualified by a significant group by time interaction, $F(18,276) = 6.01$, $p < .001$. This is depicted graphically in Figure 7.2, which indicates that the three depressed subgroups were equally symptomatic at 2 months, differing significantly from controls but not from each other on total symptom ratings. By 4 months, although the three depressed subgroups showed a significant and substantial decrease in symptoms relative to their initial high levels, only the remitted subgroup had dropped to the level of the control group on overall symptom ratings; by 6 months, only the chronic subgroup continued to show statistically elevated symptom ratings and they remain elevated throughout the follow-up interval, despite some variability in symptom severity from one assessment to the next. Although these patterns are partly an artifact of how we defined subgroups, it is noteworthy that the group that no longer met criteria by 4 months

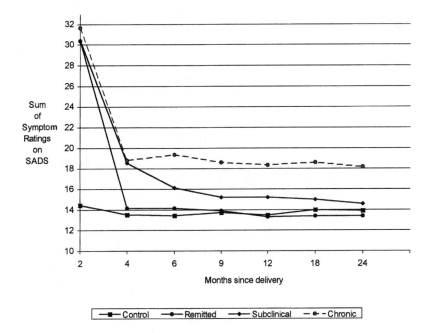

FIGURE 7.2. Sum of symptom ratings over time by depression subgroup.

and stayed remitted throughout the follow-up period was already back to the level of the normal controls by 4 months, underscoring the intense but brief depressions experienced by some women. In addition, women who remain depressed showed a relatively persistent level of moderate symptoms after the initial postpartum period.

Spousal Support

At each follow-up interview (4–24 months), women were asked about their spouse's emotional support, his help with child care, and the quality of the current relationship. Ratings on these questions were combined into one composite marital support score, with higher scores reflecting greater satisfaction with support. A group by time-repeated-measures ANOVA revealed only a group main effect, $F(3,84) = 5.38, p < .002$, but no significant effect of time or group by time interaction. Follow-up one-way ANOVAs indicated that women in the chronically depressed group reported significantly less satisfaction with spousal support than did control women at each assessment period; women with subclinical and remitted depressions fell in between. Women whose depressions had remitted early were significantly more satisfied with spousal support at the 4-, 18-, and 24-month assessments than were women whose depressions were chronic; women in the subclinical group were less satisfied with spousal support than control women at the 6- and 9-month assessments. These data are presented graphically in Figure 7.3.

Case Descriptions

Despite the variability in outcome that is reflected in the data on course, there were some clear themes that emerged from our rich interview data with these postpartum women, and they have implications for understanding both the course of the depression and the difficulties that confront new mothers adapting to the birth of a baby. These themes include concerns about being a good mother, problems with breast feeding and subsequent guilt about changing to bottle feeding, ambivalence and guilt about working, concerns about spousal support, and difficulties adjusting to the marked change in lifestyle (see also Cramer, Chapter 10, this volume). What is striking in these cases is the similarity of themes and worries as well as prior history of depression, despite very different adaptational patterns.

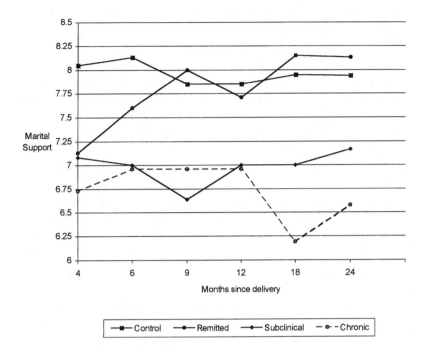

FIGURE 7.3. Marital support scores over time by depression subgroup.

Early Remission

Mrs. X, a 26-year-old, college-educated nurse was depressed for the first 2 months postpartum. On the initial SADS interview she endorsed eight symptoms at clinically significant levels, including an extreme level of depressed mood, a moderate decrease in appetite, sleep problems including insomnia, marked fatigue, lack of interest in formerly pleasurable activities, feelings of guilt that were focused on her dislike of breast feeding, difficulties with concentration, agitation, and fleeting suicidal thoughts. Overall, her sum of symptom ratings at 2 months was 40.

Mrs. X described a difficult pregnancy with much nausea and other health concerns, although she also reported that her relationship with her husband improved during the pregnancy. Although the delivery was uneventful, her daughter had some minor medical problems shortly after birth that quickly resolved. Overall, Mrs. X felt overwhelmed by the responsibilities of caring for a new baby. She missed working and felt that her husband did not provide enough help with child care. Mrs. X described her baby as difficult, with irregular sleep patterns and frequent crying; she also reported feeding difficulties. Observations of face-to-face interaction during play revealed that Mrs. X was very tense with her baby. She was noted to grimace and grit her teeth as well as pinch and poke at the baby who was drowsy and not interested in play. This was seen as an atypical and dysfunctional pattern of interaction, similar to the anger–poke pattern described by Cohn, Matias, Tronick, Connell, and Lyons-Ruth (1986).

On the SADS-L, Mrs. X reported one prior episode of depression about 3 years earlier. At that time she also reported suicidal ideation and five additional symptoms. Her physician suggested medication, but she decided against taking antidepressant medication. The depression lifted after about 1 month. She reported no other mental health problems.

When followed up at 4 months, Mrs. X no longer reported clinically significant sad mood or other symptoms, with the exception of low levels of guilt focused primarily on not providing enough attention to the baby. Mrs. X had stopped breast feeding by the 4-month visit and had returned to work part-time. She attributed her improved sense of well-being to these changes, although she still saw her husband as providing inadequate help with child care and not giving her enough emotional support. Over the course of the follow-up period, Mrs. X continued to report low levels of guilt around the baby. She no longer acknowledged dissatisfaction with spousal support and at 12 months reported that her marriage was improving. At the 18-month visit, Mrs. X was again pregnant. She delivered a second child, a boy, when her daughter was 27 months old, and although she was somewhat "blue" during the third postpartum week, she did not develop a full-blown episode of depression after the birth of her second child.

Mrs. X is typical of many of the women in the remitted subgroup who reported quite severe symptoms initially, symptoms as severe as those of the women with more prolonged depressions, but bounced back to their normal levels of functioning quite quickly. In many instances, a return to work or other normal activities and a decrease in initial infant fussiness were associated with symptom remission.

Ongoing Subclinical Symptoms

Mrs. Y, a 29-year-old health professional, reported feeling "blue," sad, and overwhelmed and crying off and on during the first 6 weeks after delivery. She had a decrease in appetite, quite severe sleep problems that included both difficulty falling asleep and waking in the middle of the night, concentration problems, especially forgetfulness, and feelings of guilt. Mrs. Y had returned to work half-time at 2 months and her guilt focused on her return to work and consequent concerns about being a bad mother.

Mrs. Y's son was born without complications, although the pregnancy was extremely difficult, with nausea, toxemia, and other complications. This fueled Mrs. Y's worry about the baby, worry that was partly ascribed to a history of birth complications in her family of origin. Mrs. Y found her husband initially helpful and supportive.

Mrs. Y had a history of at least four prior episodes of depression. She had been in psychotherapy in the past and on anti-anxiety medication. She also reported a family history of other problems including maternal depression and paternal alcohol abuse. Even at the 2-month visit, the interviewer's impression was that Mrs. Y might be dysthymic, which is consistent with her continuing history of low-level symptoms.

At the 4-month interview, Mrs. Y still met criteria for depression. She noted some improvement in her mood when the baby started sleeping though the night, but she also still reported feeling depressed several days each week. Other symptoms were still present, and she described her infant as somewhat fussy and irritable. Mrs. Y was concerned that she did not have enough energy or time for her spouse; she considered marriage counseling but also reported that her husband was helpful. She was offered the names of several mental health facilities, but she did not actually seek treatment. At the 6-month interview, Mrs. Y's continuing guilt and concern about her marital relationship were evident. She noted that her relationship with her husband would never be the same and that they had been much closer before the birth of the baby. Now the demands of work and child care meant that they had little time to spend together, and she was concerned about the impact of these circumstances on her marriage. Despite these concerns, Mrs. Y continued to report that her husband was helpful and supportive, and she blamed herself for any change in the relationship. At the 6-, 9-, and 12-month interviews, Mrs. Y reported continued low levels of fatigue, guilt, and sad mood, but she did not meet the RDC. At 18 months, Mrs. Y acknowledged concerns about her husband's lack of support. She was again pregnant and experiencing nausea. She delivered a daughter by cesarean-section close to the 24-month interview. Her low-level symptoms continued, but she did not have another full-blown episode of depression after the birth of her second child.

Chronic Depression

By contrast, Mrs. Z, a 29-year-old executive with a college degree, presented a picture of chronic depression that continued through the 18-month follow-up. Moreover, her symptoms worsened over time. Mrs. Z initially described herself as feeling blue and anxious and as crying a good deal during the second and third postpartum weeks. She was particularly anxious about being alone with the baby and afraid that she would not know what to do. She described herself as feeling lonely and desperate during the day. At the initial assessment, Mrs. Z reported sleep problems, profound loss of interest, including lack of interest in the baby, and difficulty concentrating and making decisions. She experienced difficulties breast feeding and gave up after a week; although she felt guilty about this, she also did not have the energy or motivation to continue. Mrs. Z noted that she was "not the same person I used to be."

Mrs. Z's pregnancy was planned and uneventful; both parents were pleased with the pregnancy, which had a positive effect on their marriage. Mr. Z was involved with his daughter after the birth; marital problems were not reported and spousal support, including involvement in child care, was reported to be satisfactory throughout. Mrs. Z did not describe her baby as difficult. However, Mrs. Z had had a prior episode of depression 11 months before becoming pregnant. There is no other family history of depression reported.

At the 4-month visit, Mrs. Z had returned to work full-time and she reported some improvement in her mood and symptoms. However, her depression had worsened by the 6-month visit and continued to be quite severe throughout the 18-month assessment.

Mrs. Z reported feeling drained, washed out, and wanting to escape; her sleep was severely impaired. Overall, sad mood, sleep problems, fatigue, loss of interest, and guilt continued at clinically significant levels through the 18-month interview, although Mrs. Z noted that she did get some pleasure from her work, something that fueled her guilt about not being a good mother. In addition, Mrs. Z felt continuously anxious and, although she never sought treatment, she did self-medicate to some degree with alcohol to alleviate feelings of anxiety. At the 24-month interview, Mrs. Z reported residual guilt and fatigue, but she noted that she had "finally adjusted" to her toddler and was getting some pleasure from her.

These case vignettes suggest that despite the variability in the course of depression, these women were grappling with similar initial concerns about competence in the maternal role. In addition, despite some improvement in mood and well-being after returning to work, this transition was complicated by feelings of guilt about the baby. The consistent focus of these women on difficult issues of adaptation and the data reported next underscore the complexity of issues that surround depression in the postpartum period.

Early Mother–Infant Interaction

Details of these analyses are reported in Campbell et al. (1995). Women meeting the RDC for depression at 2 months postpartum did not differ from nondepressed controls in maternal negative or positive affect expression or maternal sensitivity observed during a playful face-to-face interaction at 2, 4, or 6 months postpartum, during a toy play episode at 4 months, or during a feeding interaction at either 2 or 4 months. In addition, negative maternal behavior during face-to-face interaction was exceedingly rare in either group of mothers. However, women who were depressed at 2 months were less likely to be breast feeding (25%) than were comparison women (66%), a significant difference, $\chi^2(1) = 10.62, p < .01$.

Although there were few differences between the controls and the depressed group considered as a whole, when our data were examined for chronicity effects, a number of differences emerged.

Women whose depressions were chronic through 6 months postpartum were less positive with their infants during face-to-face interaction at 2, 4, and 6 months; their feeding interactions were less optimal at 2 and 4 months; and they showed less positive affect during toy play at 4 months than women whose depressions had remitted by 6 months. In addition, their infants were less positive during face-to-face interaction. Ratings by observers at the completion of each home visit also indicated that women who ultimately were classified as chronically depressed were less positive with their babies at 4 and 6 months than women whose depressions were less prolonged. These findings, then, highlight the importance of examining the course of depression in new mothers as one important factor that may influence the impact of maternal depression on offspring adjustment and may have particular ramifications for understanding attachment security.

Attachment

Attachment security, therefore, was examined in terms of depression chronicity. Infants whose attachments were classified as disorganized or were considered unclassifiable were grouped with the resistant and avoidant insecure infants. Depressions that were chronic through 6 months were unrelated to attachment security at 12 months, although there was a trend for remitted depressions to be associated with a higher rate of security at 18 months $X^2(2) = 5.35, p = .07$; given the generally null findings (see later), however, this is best viewed as a chance result (although see Cooper & Murray, Chapter 8, this volume).

When chronicity was defined in terms of the pattern of depression over the entire follow-up period, depression chronicity was unrelated to attachment security, $X^2(3) < 1$, at either 12 or 18 months (see Table 7.1). Surprisingly, at both 12 and 18 months, half the control infants were classified as insecure.

In view of the arguments about the timing of the depression in relation to the assessment, attachment security was also examined in relation to current depression. Infants whose mothers met depression criteria at 12 months were not more likely to be insecure than were offspring of other depressed women; the same held true for attachment security at 18-months in relation to 18 month diagnosis.

Thus, it seems crucial to ask what factors might be buffering secure infants of chronically depressed mothers. One possibility is that support from spouse around child care as well as care from others while mother works may provide sufficient stimulation and responsiveness from other attachment figures to buffer the effects of mother's chronic depression. However, within the chronically depressed group, marital satisfaction and work status did not vary with attachment security. But chronically depressed women with insecure infants reported more severe symptoms at 12 months, $t(24) = 2.10, p = .046$, M's = 21.75 and 16.67, suggesting that concurrent mood may be more important than diagnosis in predicting insecurity, consistent with the findings of deMulder and Radke-Yarrow (1991).

TABLE 7.1. Attachment Classifications by Chronicity of Depression

	Control		Remitted		Subclinical		Chronic	
	n	%	n	%	n	%	n	%
12 months								
Avoidant	18	(33)	1	(8)	2	(18)	5	(19)
Secure	26	(47)	9	(69)	9	(82)	18	(69)
C, D, U	11	(20)	3	(23)	0	(0)	3	(12)
	55		13		11		26	
18 months								
Avoidant	19	(37)	2	(14)	3	(30)	9	(41)
Secure	24	(46)	9	(64)	6	(60)	13	(59)
C, D, U	9	(17)	3	(21)	1	(10)	0	(0)
	52		14		10		22	
Stability								
Stable secure	11	(22)	4	(33)	5	(50)	10	(45)
Stable insecure	11	(22)	1	(8)	1	(10)	4	(18)
Secure–insecure	14	(23)	4	(29)	3	(33)	5	(30)
Insecure–secure	13	(14)	3	(27)	1	(25)	3	(10)
	49		12		10		22	

There were also subtle indications of more problems early on. At the initial interview, mothers who ultimately were chronically depressed and whose infants were insecure were more likely to note that their pregnancy was unplanned; of the eight chronically depressed women with insecure infants, five (63%) reported that their pregnancies were unplanned; only 28% of the chronically depressed women with secure infants reported at the initial visit that the pregnancy was unplanned (Fisher's exact test, p = .11). Global ratings of mother–infant interaction in the home at 2, 4, and 6 months made at completion of each home visit suggested that chronically depressed mothers of infants who eventually became insecure at 12 months were more negative at 2 months ($t(22)$ = 2.04, p = .053) and less positive at 4 ($t(23)$ = 1.78, p = .089) and 6 months ($t(23)$ = 2.11, p = .046). These differences were found only on the global ratings of the entire home visit and not for the videotaped observations of feeding and play. These data, therefore, must be interpreted with caution because they were obtained on a small sample and are inconsistent across measures. However, they may suggest that home visitors were picking up something about the quality of maternal behavior that was missing from the more structured interactions and that these qualitative features of the more prolonged interactions in the chronically depressed women have implications for security of attachment at 12 months. Insecurity at 18 months was not systematically related to earlier measures of mother–infant interaction within the chronically depressed subgroup. However, there was a trend for chronically depressed women with insecure infants to be at home full-time (63%); chronically depressed women with infants who were secure at 18 months were more likely to be working, at least part-time (85%) (Fisher's exact test = .055, two-tailed).

It was also possible to examine stability of attachment (see Table 7.1). Of the 93 subjects who were assessed at both 12 and 18 months, 49 controls and 44 depressed mother–infant pairs, only 41 (44%) retained the same classification, and this figure did not vary by depression status (39% of controls and 50% of the depressed group showed stable attachments). Within the depressed group, stability of attachment was unrelated to chronicity: 45% of infants with chronically depressed mothers were stably secure in comparison to 41% of the offspring of the remaining depressed women; among the chronic group, 14% of those who were insecure at 12 months became secure at 18 months; the comparable figure for the remaining depressed women was 18%.

DISCUSSION

These data underscore the heterogeneity of depression in the postpartum period and the variable relations between the course of depression and the mother–infant relationship. First, the course of depression was quite variable, with many women showing only short-lived depressions with little effect on the quality of early mother–infant interactions. Other women showed continuing low-level symptoms that were not associated with less involved or positive interactions with their infants. Subgroups of women whose depressions remitted quickly or who showed only low-level symptoms beyond the 4-month visit did not differ from comparison women in their interactions with their infants. Thus, despite the early concerns and symptoms reported by these women, they were able to provide sufficiently responsive and positive environments for their infants. Only women with more chronic depressions appeared to show less positive and sensitive behavior with their babies during the first 6 months postpartum. These findings would appear to run counter to the "sensitive period" hypothesis put forth by Hay (Chapter 4, this volume), at least in regard to the socioemotional development of the infants of mothers with short-lived postpartum depression. These findings are also inconsistent with those of Stein et al. (1991) in that dysfunctional patterns of mother–infant interaction were not in evidence once the depression remitted (see also Campbell et al., 1995), even in women who experienced continuing low-level symptoms.

In addition, and contrary to expectation, neither chronicity of depression nor depression concurrent with attachment assessments predicted higher rates of insecurity. Although these findings are counterintuitive and inconsistent with attachment theory, they suggest that even most of these more chronically depressed women provided a "good enough" environment for their babies. However, within the chronically depressed group, insecurity was associated with an unplanned pregnancy, as well as subtle signs of early relationship difficulties reflected in more negative interaction at 2 months and less positive interaction, as rated by home visitors at 4 and 6 months. Moreover, although diagnosis per se at 12 months was unrelated to attachment security, within the chronically depressed group, insecurity was associated with more severe symptoms. This may indicate that the combination of an unplanned pregnancy and a more severe and prolonged depression have the potential to compromise the quality of the early mother–infant relationship, suggesting one pathway to insecurity at 12 months. However, in view of the instability of attachment in this sample, even these relationships appear to be transient.

These data suggest quite clearly, then, that depression in the postpartum period is not inevitably a risk factor for either early or later problems in the mother–infant relationship. Given the heterogeneity of depression and the variability in outcome, most mother–infant dyads appeared to function adequately. This is an important finding because roughly 1 in 10 women become depressed after the birth of an infant. Thus it becomes important to delineate which mothers and infants are at risk to target prevention efforts wisely. In a depressed group of otherwise low-risk married, middle-class women without serious delivery complications and with healthy newborns, it appears that most will function at least adequately in the maternal role. Those women with more prolonged depressions, especially those for whom the pregnancy was unplanned, may be among the more vulnerable for difficulties as caregivers. It may be these women and their husbands who would benefit most from interventions aimed at dealing with adaptation to the pregnancy and the attendant life transitions and role changes that will occur, the depression itself, and the needs of young infants.

These data also indicate that despite the long-held view that infants of depressed mothers are at risk for attachment difficulties, this need not be the case in low-risk samples. This finding may be partly consistent with arguments of Sameroff and others (e.g., Cummings & Davies, 1994; Hammen, 1992; Sameroff, Seifer, Baldwin, & Baldwin, 1993) that maternal depression must be viewed from the context of multiple risk. Focus on depression in and of itself may be inadequate to explain variations in patterns of caretaking or mother–infant interaction. Some depressed women, despite feeling sad and drained, were responsive and nurturant with their infants. In addition, the focus on infants raises questions about the role of alternative caregivers. In the current study, we focused on stable, two-parent families; in addition, in many instances extended family members were nearby. Thus, fathers and other family members may have provided enough support to mothers early on to help circumvent potential interactional problems with the infant, or alternative caregivers may have buffered the infant directly from stressful interactions with a depressed mother. Other studies have found that father presence and level of functioning are important in understanding the consequences of maternal depression for children (e.g., Goodman, Brogan, Lynch, & Fielding, 1993; Hammen, 1992; Radke-Yarrow et al., 1985). Although chronically depressed women in this study reported less satisfaction with spousal support, these fathers were in the home and they were involved with their children, at least to some extent. Further, data on satisfaction with spousal support may be as much a reflection of the depression itself as a comment on paternal involvement in the family system.

The role of maternal employment is also worthy of further study. Data from the 18-month assessment of attachment suggest that maternal employment may serve as a protective factor for infants of chronically depressed women. Women who return to work and feel fulfilled outside the home despite their depressive symptoms may have more energy for their infants than do women at home full-time. Alternatively, other caregivers may play a buffering role. Prior analyses of portions of this data set at 2 months also suggested that maternal employment might serve as a buffering factor for depressed women and their infants (Cohn et al., 1990).

One caveat must be kept in mind when reviewing these data. First, roughly 40% of the women who met depression screening criteria were unwilling to participate in the longitudinal portion of the study. Although this refusal rate was not different from the refusal rate from control women and women who refused did not report more severe initial symptoms on the screening interview (Campbell et al., 1992), it is possible that other biases exist in the sample. In addition, the depressed group had more attrition, and more depressed than control women missed the laboratory visits in which attachment was assessed. Attrition is common in studies of depression. However, it may compromise the findings to some degree. For example, depressed women who are concerned about their relationship with their baby may be less willing to participate in an observation of mother–infant interaction than other depressed women.

CONCLUSION

In summary, then, it is important to consider the heterogeneity, timing, and course of depression, as well as co-occurring risk and protective factors, when making predictions about whether offspring of depressed women are at risk. Interactional processes, especially interactional processes that occur over time and reflect more severe symptomatology and more dysfunctional patterns of caregiving, may be important, whereas relatively brief periods of maternal unresponsiveness, especially in the very early months, may be less salient. This may be the case especially when other caregivers are available to meet the infant's needs.

ACKNOWLEDGMENTS

This research was supported by National Institute Of Mental Health Grant No. 5R01 40867 to Drs. Campbell and Cohn. Appreciation is expressed to Teri Meyers, Clare Flanagan, and Ginger Moore for help with data coding and analysis.

REFERENCES

Ainsworth, M. D., Blehar, M. C, Waters, E., & Wall, S. (1978). *Patterns of attachment: A psychological study of the strange situation.* Hillside, NJ: Erlbaum.

Bates, J. E., Maslin, C. A., & Frankel, K. A. (1985). Attachment security, mother–child interaction, and temperament as predictors of behavior problem ratings at age three years. In I. Bretherton & E. Waters (Eds.), Growing points of attachment theory and research. *Monographs of the Society for Research in Child Development*(1–2, Serial No. 209), *50*, 167–193.

Beardslee, W. R., Bemporad, J., Keller, M. B., & Klerman, G. L. (1983). Children of parents with major depressive disorder: A review. *American Journal of Psychiatry, 54,* 1254–1268.

Belsky, J., Rovine, M., & Fish, M. (1989). The developing family system. In M. Gunnar (Ed.), *Minnesota Symposia on Child Psychology: Vol. 22. Systems and development* (pp. 119–166). Hillsdale, NJ: Erlbaum.

Belsky, J., Rovine, M., & Taylor, D. (1984). The Pennsylvania infant and family development project: III. The origins of individual differences in infant–mother attachment. *Child Development, 55,* 718–728.

Billings, A. G., & Moos, R. H. (1983). Comparison of children of depressed and nondepressed parents: A social environmental perspective. *Journal of Abnormal Child Psychology, 11,* 483–496.

Bowlby, J. (1969). *Attachment and loss: Vol. 1. Attachment.* New York: Basic Books.

Brown, G. W., & Harris, T. (1978). *Social origins of depression.* London: Tavistock.

Campbell, S. B., & Cohn, J. F. (1991). Prevalence and correlates of postpartum depression in first-time mothers. *Journal of Abnormal Psychology, 100,* 594–599.

Campbell, S. B., Cohn, J. F., Flanagan, C., Popper, S., & Meyers, T. (1992). Course and correlates of postpartum depression during the transition to parenthood. *Development and Psychopathology, 4,* 29–47.

Campbell, S. B., Cohn, J. F., & Meyers, T. (1995). Depression in first-time mothers: Mother–infant interaction and depression chronicity. *Developmental Psychology, 31,* 349–357.

Cohn, J. F., & Campbell, S. B. (1992). Influence of maternal depression on infant affect regulation. In D. Cicchetti & S. Toth (Eds.), *Rochester Symposium on Developmental Psychopathology: Vol. 4. A developmental approach to affective disorders* (pp. 103–130). Rochester, NY: University of Rochester Press.

Cohn, J. F., Campbell, S. B., Matias, R., & Hopkins, J. (1990). Face-to-face interactions of postpartum depressed and nondepressed mother–infant pairs at 2 months. *Developmental Psychology, 26,* 15–23.

Cohn, J. F., Matias, R., Tronick, E. Z., Connell, D., & Lyons-Ruth, K. (1986). Face-to-face interactions of depressed mothers and their infants. In T. Field & E. Z. Tronick (Eds.), *Maternal depression and child disturbance* (New Directions for Child Development, No. 34, pp. 31–46). San Francisco: Jossey-Bass.

Cooper, P. J., Campbell, E. A., Day, A., Kennerly, H., & Bond, A. (1988). Non-psychotic psychiatric disorder after childbirth: A prospective study of prevalence, incidence, course and nature. *British Journal of Psychiatry, 152,* 799–806.

Coryell, W., Endicott, J., & Keller, M. (1990). Outcome of patients with chronic affective disorder: A five year follow-up. *American Journal of Psychiatry, 147,* 1627–1633.

Coyne, J. C., Downey, G., & Boergers, J. (1992). Depression in families: A systems perspective. In D. Cicchetti & S. Toth (Eds.), *Rochester Symposium on Developmental Psychopathology: Vol. 4. A developmental approach to affective disorders* (pp. 211–250). Rochester, NY: University of Rochester Press.

Cummings, E. M., & Davies, P. T. (1994). Maternal depression and child development. *Journal of Child Psychology and Psychiatry, 35,* 73–112.

DeMulder, E. K., & Radke-Yarrow, M. (1991). Attachment with affectively ill and
well mothers: Concurrent behavioral correlates. *Development and Psychopathology, 3,* 227–242.

Downey, G., & Coyne, J. C. (1990). Children of depressed parents: An integrative
review. *Psychological Bulletin, 108,* 50–76.

Endicott, J., & Spitzer, R. L. (1978). A diagnostic interview: The Schedule for
Affective Disorders and Schizophrenia. *Archives of General Psychiatry, 35,*
837–844.

Field, T. M. (1992). Infants of depressed mothers. *Development and Psychopathology, 4,* 49–66.

Field, T. M., Healy, B., Goldstein, S., & Guthertz, M. (1990). Behavior state matching and synchrony in mother–infant interactions of nondepressed vs. depressed dyads. *Developmental Psychology, 26,* 7–14.

Garrison, W. T., & Earls, F. J. (1986). Epidemiological perspectives on maternal
depression and the young child. In T. M. Field & E. Z. Tronick (Eds.), *Maternal depression and child disturbance* (New Directions for Child Development, No. 34., pp. 13–30). San Francisco: Jossey-Bass.

Goodman, S. H., Brogan, D., Lynch, M. E., & Fielding, B. (1993). Social and
emotional competence in children of depressed mothers. *Child Development, 64,* 513–531

Hammen, C. (1992). Cognitive, life stress, and interpersonal approaches to a
developmental psychopathology model of depression. *Development and
Psychopathology, 4,* 189–206.

Hammen, C., Adrian, C., Gordon, G., Burge, D., & Jaenicke, C. (1987). Children of
depressed mothers: Maternal strain and symptom predictors of dysfunction. *Journal of Abnormal Psychology, 96,* 190–198.

Hollingshead, A. G. (1975). *Four factor index of social status.* New Haven: Yale
University, Department of Sociology.

Hopkins, J., Campbell, S. B., & Marcus, M. D. (1987). The role of infant-related
stressors in postpartum depression. *Journal of Abnormal Psychology, 96,*
237–241.

Hopkins, J., Marcus, M. D., & Campbell, S. B. (1984). Postpartum depression: A
critical review. *Psychological Bulletin, 95,* 498–515.

Keller, M. B., Lavori, P. W., Endicott, J., Coryell, W., & Klerman, G. (1983). "Double
depression": Two-year follow-up. *American Journal of Psychiatry, 140,* 689–
694.

Kendler, K. S., Neale, M. C., Kessler, R. C., Heath, A. C., & Eaves, J. (1992). A
population-based twin study of major depression in women. *Archives of
General Psychiatry, 49,* 257–266.

Kochanska, B., Kuczynski, L., Radke-Yarrow, M., & Welsh, J. D. (1987). Resolution
of control episodes between well and affectively ill mothers and their young
children. *Journal of Abnormal Child Psychology, 15,* 441–456.

Lyons-Ruth, K., Connell, D. B., Grunebaum, H. U., & Botein, S. (1990). Infants at
social risk: Maternal depression and family support services as mediators of

infant development and security of attachment. *Child Development, 61,* 85–98.

Main, M., & Solomon, J. (1990). Procedures for identifying infants as disorganized–disoriented during the Ainsworth Strange Situation. In M. T. Greenberg, D. Cicchetti, & E. M. Cummings (Eds.), *Attachment in the preschool years: Theory, research, and intervention* (pp. 121–160). Chicago: University of Chicago Press.

McLoyd, V. C. (1990). The impact of economic hardship on black families and children: Psychological distress, parenting, and socioemotional development. *Child Development, 61,* 311–346.

Murray, L. (1992). The impact of postnatal depression on infant development. *Journal of Child Psychology and Psychiatry, 33,* 543–561.

Murray, L., Fiori-Cowley, A., Hooper, R., & Cooper, P. (1996). The impact of postnatal depression and associated adversity on early mother infant interactions and later infant outcome. *Child Development, 67,* 2512–2526.

Murray, L., Kempton, C., Woolgar, M., & Hooper, R. (1993). Depressed mothers' speech to their infants and its relation to infant gender and cognitive development. *Journal of Child Psychology and Psychiatry, 31,* 1083–1101.

O'Hara, M. W., Neunaber, D. J., & Zekoski, E. M. (1984). Prospective study of postpartum depression: Prevalence, course, and predictive factors. *Journal of Abnormal Psychology, 93,* 158–171.

O'Hara, M. W., Zekoski, E. M., Philipps, L. H., & Wright, E. J. (1990). A controlled, prospective study of postpartum mood disorders: Comparison of childbearing and non-childbearing women. *Journal of Abnormal Psychology, 99,* 3–15.

Pitt, B. (1968). "Atypical" depression following childbirth. *British Journal of Psychiatry, 114,* 1325–1335.

Radke-Yarrow, M., Cummings, M., Kuczynski, L., & Chapman, M. (1985). Patterns of attachment in two- and three-year-olds in normal families and in families with parental depression. *Child Development, 56,* 884–893.

Rutter, M. (1990). Some focus and process considerations regarding effects of parental depression on children. *Developmental Psychology, 26,* 60–67.

Sameroff, A. J., Seifer, R., Baldwin, A., & Baldwin, C. (1993). Stability of intelligence from preschool to adolescence: The influence of social and family risk factors. *Child Development, 64,* 80–97.

Sameroff, A. J., Seifer, R., & Zax, M. (1982). Early development of children at risk for emotional disorder. *Monographs of the Society for Research in Child Development, 47*(7, Serial No. 199).

Shea, M. T., Elkin, I., Imber, S. D., Sotsky, S. M., Watkins, J. T., Collins, J. F., Pilkonis, P. A., Beckham, E., Glass, D. R., Dolan, R. T., & Parloff, M. B. (1992). Course of depressive symptoms over follow-up.—Findings from the National Institute of Mental Health Treatment of Depression Collaborative Research Program. *Archives of General Psychiatry, 49,* 782–787.

Spitzer, R. L., Endicott, J., & Robins, E. (1978). Research Diagnostic Criteria: Rationale and reliability. *Archives of General Psychiatry, 36,* 773–782.

Stein, A., Gath, D. H., Bucher, J., Bond, A., Day, A., & Cooper, P. J. (1991). The relationship between post-natal depression and mother–child interaction. *British Journal of Psychiatry, 158,* 46–52.

Teti, D. M., & Gelfand, D. M. (1991). Behavioral competence among mothers of infants in the first year: The mediational role of maternal self-efficacy. *Child Development, 62,* 918–929.

Teti, D. M., & Gelfand, D. M. (1993, March). Attachment security among infants of depressed mothers: Associations with mother-infant behavior and maternal functioning. In D. Teti (Chair), *Depressed mothers and their children: Individual differences in outcome.* Symposium presented at the Society for Research in Child Development, New Orleans.

Tronick, E. (1989). Emotions and emotional communication in infants. *American Psychologist, 44,* 112–119.

Weissman, M. M., & Paykel, E. D. (1974). *The depressed woman: A study of social relationships.* Chicago: University of Chicago Press.

Wells, K. B., Burnam, A., Rogers, W., Hays, R., & Camp, P. (1992). The course of depression in adult outpatients. Results from the Medical Outcomes Study. *Archives of General Psychiatry, 49,* 788–794.

Whiffen, V. E., & Gotlib, I. H. (1993). Comparison of postpartum and nonpostpartum depression: Clinical presentation, psychiatric history, and psychosocial functioning. *Journal of Consulting and Clinical Psychology, 61,* 485–495.

IV

THE TREATMENT OF POSTPARTUM DEPRESSION AND ASSOCIATED MOTHER–INFANT DISTURBANCES

8

The Impact of Psychological Treatments of Postpartum Depression on Maternal Mood and Infant Development

Peter J. Cooper
Lynne Murray
University of Reading

There is surprisingly little systematic information on the clinical management of nonpsychotic postpartum depression. There are a number of possible explanations for the paucity of research. First, postpartum depression commonly goes undetected by the primary health care team (Seeley, Murray, & Cooper, 1996), and despite the fact that there are solid epidemiological data attesting to its high prevalence in the general population (O'Hara, Chapter 1, this volume), it may well be regarded clinically as quite rare. Second, in psychiatric terms this disorder represents a relatively minor disturbance which tends, in any event, to remit spontaneously within a few months (Cooper, Campbell, Day, Kennerly, & Bond, 1988; Murray, 1992; Campbell & Cohn, Chapter 7, this volume) and, as such, postpartum depression could be regarded as not of great psychiatric significance. Finally, when physicians do detect depression in the early postpartum period, there may be a reluctance to prescribe an antidepressant, the standard medical treatment for depression occurring at any time, because of the difficulties of doing so in breast-feeding women.

There is one exception in the research literature to the reluctance to administer antidepressant medication in the immediate postpartum period. Appleby, Warner, Whitton, and Faragher (in press), in a factorial design involving the use of fluoxetine or placebo in combination with one or six counseling sessions, demonstrated an impressive antidepressant effect for both the active drug and the psychological treatment over a 3-month treatment period. However, there was no additive effect of the two treatments, and drug treatment was not superior to the psychological treatment. Given that of the 188 women with depression invited to take part in the study less than half agreed, and that the main reason for refusal was "reluctance to take medication," the role of fluoxetine in the treatment of postpartum depression, or indeed that of any other antidepressant medication, must be questioned.

In another placebo-controlled trial of a pharmacological agent (Henderson, Gregoire, Kumar, & Studd, 1991), treatment with estradiol skin patches for 2 months was found to produce a greater elevation in mood than placebo, but because the patients in this study were all medical referrals they are likely to have been a sample selected for a greater severity of depression than is typical of the population of depressed postpartum women, and the extent to which the findings from this study can be generalized must, therefore, be questioned.

Given the strong evidence for the importance of psychological and social factors in the etiology of postpartum depression (Cooper, Murray, & Stein, 1991), the case for a psychological intervention is a strong one. However, the literature on the use of such treatments is surprisingly sparse. The only trial of the efficacy of a psychological treatment delivered to depressed postpartum women identified by a screen of the community involved the use of counseling delivered by British health visitors (community nurses). Holden, Sagovsky, and Cox (1989) found considerable improvement in maternal mood in women treated over eight weekly sessions by health visitors trained in nondirective counseling, with no improvement evident in the control group that received routine primary care.

Therefore, it is clear that postpartum depression can be effectively treated in the short term by antidepressant medication, but the majority of women are likely to refuse this form of management. It is also clear that nondirective counseling, which is highly acceptable to women, is also an effective short-term treatment. However, it is unfortunate that, given the considerable body of evidence implicating postpartum mood disorder in impairments in parenting and in a raised incidence of infant behavioral problems, insecure attachment, and compromised cognitive development (Murray & Cooper, 1997), there is no information on the impact of treatment on these crucial dimensions of outcome in women with postpartum affective disorder. This issue is of both clinical and theoretical importance. The clinical significance is straightforward: If postpartum depression is associated with impairments in infant cognitive and emotional development, it is important to develop and evaluate treatments that prevent these adverse infant outcomes. The theoretical issues are more complex. Although postpartum depression is associated with adverse infant outcomes, the precise mechanisms whereby such outcomes arise are far from clear. Certainly, the evidence from the Cambridge longitudinal study (Murray, 1992; Murray, Kempton, Woolgar, & Hooper, 1993; Murray, Hipwell, Hooper, Stein, & Cooper, 1996) indicates that the impairments in parenting associated with postpartum depression, rather than some other factor, are the major causal force (at least in relation to cognitive outcome). However, this association affords two quite variant causal accounts. On the one hand, it has been widely assumed that the maternal depression is primary and the parenting deficits are a secondary phenomenon. From this assumption it can be predicted that a treatment that elevates maternal mood, in the absence of any attention to the mother–infant relationship, would be of incidental benefit to the mother–infant relationship and, as a consequence, would improve infant outcome. There is an alternative view of the causal chain, namely, that difficulties in the mother–infant relationship are primary and the maternal mood disorder arises as a consequence of these interpersonal difficulties (Brockington & Brierley, 1984; Cramer, Chapter 10, this volume). This account is consistent with particular neonatal characteristics raising the risk of postpartum depression (see Murray & Cooper, Chapter 5, this volume), as well as with the finding that for some women the risk of depression is significantly raised in the postpartum period (Cooper & Murray, 1995). If this view were correct, it could be predicted that it might not be possible to effect an enduring improvement on maternal mood without focusing directly on the mother–infant relationship. As a corollary to this prediction, it would follow that if maternal mood could be elevated independently of the mother–infant relationship (say, using fluoxetine), the quality of mother–infant engagement would not be significantly improved and infant outcome would remain compromised. A third account must be considered; namely, both the maternal mood disorder and the impaired parenting are causally related to some other factor, such as general social adversity. If this were the case, it might well be that no form of treatment that does not address the wider social circumstances which obtain (or whatever third factor variable is critical) would have a significant and enduring impact on either maternal mood or the associated impairments in the mother–infant relationship.

There is a considerable literature on interventions designed to improve the quality of mother–infant interactions. For example, Field (Chapter 9, this volume) describes a variety of techniques that have been shown to enhance mothers' sensitivity to infant cues and to improve both maternal and infant affective state. Thus, Field and her colleagues have shown that with overstimulating intrusive mothers, instructing the mother to imitate the infant improves the quality of the mother–infant interaction; with withdrawn mothers, instructing them on how to attract and maintain their infant's attention has similar beneficial effects on the interaction (Malphurs et al., 1996).

Despite these encouraging short-term findings, little information is available on the impact of more comprehensive treatment approaches on the longer-term outcome of depressed mothers and their infants. Two distinct theoretical lines have been advanced, both of which have produced promising clinical results. First is the "brief mother–baby psychotherapy" described by Cramer and colleagues (Cramer & Stern, 1988; Cramer et al., 1990; Cramer, Chapter 10, this volume). The focus of this psychodynamic treatment is the mother's representation of her infant and of her relationship with that infant in terms of the projections made which relate to unresolved conflicts dating from the mother's own childhood. Cramer makes the argument that there are core conflictual themes which are activated and enacted in the relationship with the mother's own infant. Interpretation linking the past to the present and the mother's representations to the current interactions is considered the cardinal force for change. Evidence for the efficacy of this form of treatment comes from a comparative trial carried out in Geneva of a sample of children aged 6 months to 2½ years referred for treatment of "psychofunctional problems," such as sleeping difficulties, feeding problems, and disturbances in attachment (Cramer et al., 1990). The treatment, which was delivered to a group selected on the basis of a judgment of their suitability for this form of clinical management, was associated with marked improvements in the mother's representations of herself, her infant, and their relationship; in the quality of the mother–infant interactions; and in the symptoms for which the child was referred. Clearly, this model of treatment, with its emphasis on issues of attachments, provides one possible therapeutic approach to the treatment of women with postpartum depression.

The second approach to the treatment of disturbances in the mother–infant relationship focuses directly on the mother–infant interaction, for example, the "interaction guidance" treatment described by McDonnough (1993). This treatment aims, in the context of a strong therapeutic alliance, to improve the quality of the mother–infant relationship by using support, practical advice, and education together with strong reinforcement of good parenting practice. The therapist focuses the therapeutic intervention on the interactive behaviors taking place within the therapy session. In a comparison of this form of treatment with the dynamic psychotherapy described earlier, equivalent degrees of improvement were found on all maternal, infant, and interactive outcome measures (Cramer et al., 1990). Although this form of treatment was developed to provide help to severely disadvantaged groups where there were marked disturbances in the mother–infant relationship, it provides a model that, with some modification, could be useful in the treatment of postpartum depression.

The treatment literature reviewed briefly above raises a number of questions of both clinical and theoretical importance concerning the treatment of postpartum depression and the associated disturbances in the mother–infant relationship. Principal among these are the following:

1. Would a treatment of postpartum depression directed solely at the elevation of maternal mood, in the absence of any specific attention to the mother–infant relationship, indirectly improve the quality of mother–infant engagement and of infant outcome? This question could be investigated by studying the impact of either a pharmacological treatment or a nondirective counseling therapy on mood, the mother–infant relationship, and infant cognitive and emotional outcome. Because counseling is an acceptable treatment to women and antidepressant medication is, to a significant proportion, not, it seems sensible to address this question by studying the impact of the psychological form of intervention.

2. Would a treatment directed explicitly at the immediate quality of the mother–infant relationship, independent of the mother's own per-

sonal history, be an effective antidepressant, improve the quality of mother–infant engagement, and enhance infant development? This question could be investigated by studying the efficacy of a treatment such as that described by McDonnough (1993), which essentially uses cognitive-behavioral strategies to improve the mother's parenting capacities and enhance her perception of her efficacy as a mother.

3. Would a treatment that explored with the mother the quality of her current relationship with her infant in terms of her own early history be an effective antidepressant, improve the quality of mother–infant engagement, and enhance child development? This question could be investigated by studying the efficacy of a psychodynamic attachment treatment, as described by Cramer and Stern (1988).

THE CAMBRIDGE TREATMENT TRIAL

Atreatment trial designed to address the questions enumerated previously has recently been completed in Cambridge. It was a study in which a large consecutive series of primiparous women (i.e., 3,222) were screened for mood disturbance in the early postpartum period, those with suspected postpartum depression were systematically assessed, and then those found to be suffering from postpartum depression were invited to take part in a study in which "different forms of help to mothers" were being compared. In all, a total of 207 women were identified who fulfilled DSM-III-R (American Psychiatric Association, 1987) criteria for current major depressive disorder. Of these, only 13 refused to take part in the study. The remaining 194 women were randomly assigned to one of four conditions as follows:

1. Routine primary care, involving the normal care provided by the primary health care team with no additional input (apart from assessment) from the research team;

2. Nondirective counseling, replicating the treatment provided in the Edinburgh study by Holden et al. (1989), in which women were provided with the opportunity of airing their feelings about any current concerns, such as marital problems or financial difficulties, as well as concerns they might raise about their infant.

3. Cognitive-behavioral therapy (CBT), in which the full range of CBT techniques (Hawton, Salkovskis, Kirk, & Clark, 1989) was used in the

context of an appropriately modified form of the interaction guidance treatment described by McDonnough (1993). The treatment was directed not at the maternal depression itself but at problems identified by the mother in the management of her infant (e.g., concerning feeding or sleeping), as well as at observed problems in the quality of the mother–infant interaction. In the context of a supportive therapeutic relationship, the mother was provided with advice about managing particular infant problems, was helped to solve such problems in a systematic way, was encouraged to examine her patterns of thinking about her infant and herself as a mother, and was helped through modeling and reinforcement to alter aspects of her interactional style.

4. Dynamic psychotherapy, using the treatment techniques described by Cramer and Stern (Stern, 1995), in which an understanding of the mother's representation of her infant and her relationship with her infant was promoted by exploring aspects of the mother's own early attachment history.

In addition to the scientific objectives of the study outlined previously, there was also a pragmatic consideration. Clearly, it would be of considerable clinical significance to demonstrate that a treatment of postpartum depression could materially influence the course of the mother–infant relationship and improve infant outcome. For this reason, the three active treatments were explicitly designed to be deliverable within the British National Health Service: they were, therefore, brief treatments that could be provided by health visitors who had received some specific training.

Fifty-two women were assigned to the control condition (i.e., routine primary care), but 4 moved away and were lost to follow-up. One hundred thirty-nine women were assigned to one of the three research treatments: 49 to the counseling condition (of whom 7 dropped out of treatment early), 42 to the CBT (of whom 1 dropped out early), and 48 to the psychodynamic treatment (of whom 8 dropped out early). Data are reported here on the 171 who completed treatment.

Therapy was conducted in the women's own homes on a weekly basis from 8 weeks to 18 weeks postpartum. There were six study therapists. They included a specialist in each of the three research treatments and three generalists (including two National Health Service health visitors) who were each trained in two of the treatments. This allowed for both therapist effects and expertise effects to be investigated. Assessments of maternal mental state, the quality of the mother–infant relationship, and infant behavioral problems were made before treatment, immediately after treatment, and at 9 and 18 months postpartum; infant cognitive development was assessed at 9 and 18 months postpartum; and infant attachment was assessed at 18 months postpartum. The first three waves of assessments were made in the women's' own homes and the fourth assessment was carried out in the research unit. All assessments were made by assessors unaware of the treatment group to which the women had been assigned.

There were no therapist or expertise effects with respect to any of the maternal or infant outcome measures.

Maternal Mood

Maternal mood was assessed using a self-report measure, the Edinburgh Postnatal Depression Scale (EPDS; Cox, Holden, & Sagovsky, 1987), as well as by interview, using the depression section of the Structured Clinical Interview for DSM-III-R (SCID; Spitzer, Williams, Gibbon, & First, 1989). There was no difference between the four groups in terms of the mean EPDS score before treatment.

Figure 8. 1 shows the percentage reduction in EPDS score for the four groups. It is apparent that (1) the control group which received routine primary care experienced minimal change in terms of mood over the 10-week period, (2) all three treatment groups experienced a substantial benefit from treatment, and (3) there was no difference in terms of their antidepressant effects between the three forms of treatment. These conclusions were no different when the data were examined in terms of remission rates: By the end of the treatment phase, 40% of the control group no longer satisfied DSM-III-R criteria for major depressive disorder, as compared with 52% of those who received counseling, 59% of those who received CBT, and 75% of those who received the psychodynamic treatment.

The degree of mood change effected by the treatments was substantial. It compares favorably with that reported in other controlled psychological treatment trials, such as the National Institute of Mental Health comparison of cognitive therapy and interpersonal psychotherapy (Elkin et al., 1987).

It is apparent from Figure 8.1 that the improvements in mood achieved by treatment were well maintained: Although it appears that maintenance of change was best for the CBT group, the differences be-

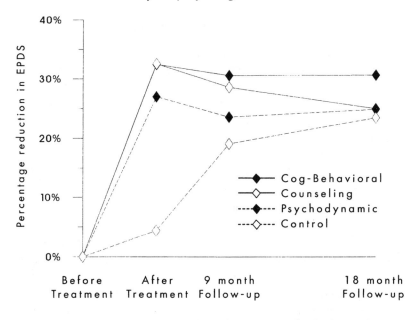

FIGURE 8.1. Improvement in maternal mood: Percentage reduction in EPDS score.

tween the treatment groups at 9 and 18 months postpartum were not significant. Indeed, by 9 months postpartum there was no difference in terms of improvement in mood between all four groups: There had been substantial spontaneous recovery for those in the control group, as has been previously found in prospective epidemiological studies (Cooper et al., 1988; Murray, 1992), and statistical analysis revealed no significant effect of treatment by 9 months postpartum.

The findings from the counseling group replicate those of Holden et al. (1989). It is clear that a brief intervention in which nondirective support is provided is of considerable benefit to women with postpartum depression. It is also apparent from this study that other forms of psychological intervention have an equivalent antidepressant effect. Both the cognitive-behavioral treatment and the psychodynamic treatment effected substantial change in maternal mood. Indeed, all three treatments served to speed up the natural remission rate of postpartum depression to a significant degree.

Mother–Infant Interactions

Videotapes of the mother and infant interacting in a play session at the 8- and 18-week postpartum assessments (i.e., before treatment and at the end of treatment) were rated by an independent assessor using the global rating scales devised by Murray and colleagues (Murray, Fiori-Cowley, Hooper, & Cooper, 1996). This rating system, in common with others used to assess the quality of engagement between depressed mothers and their infants (e.g., Field, Healy, Goldstein, & Guthertz, 1990; Cohn, Matias, Tronick, Connell, & Lyons-Ruth, 1986), includes microanalytic assessments of maternal sensitivity to infant cues and the quality of maternal responsiveness. Ratings are made of the mother's tendency to override infant expressions and initiatives (i.e., maternal intrusiveness) and to fail to respond to infant communicative cues (i.e., maternal withdrawal). In the current study, although there was some improvement across the two assessments, it was not substantial. Furthermore, improvement in the quality of the mother–infant interactions was not associated with either receiving treatment or early remission from depression. This is illustrated in Figure 8.2. This figure provides two scatterplots in a two-dimensional space (a "sensitive–insensitive" axis and an "intrusive–withdrawn" axis), one comparing those who had received treatment with those who had not and one comparing those whose depression had remitted and those

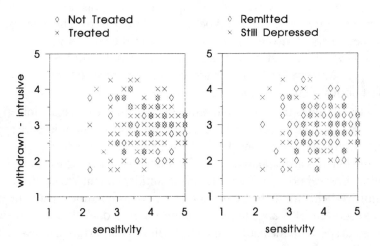

FIGURE 8.2. Mother–infant face-to-face engagement: The impact of treatment and of remission.

whose depression persisted. There was no difference between the three forms of intervention in terms of their impact on the quality of mother–infant engagement.

The fact that the counseling treatment did effect a substantial improvement in maternal mood but that this was not associated with a corresponding improvement in the mother–infant relationship provides an answer to part of the first question this study set out to address, namely, "Would a treatment of postpartum depression directed solely at the elevation of maternal mood, in the absence of any specific attention to the mother–infant relationship, indirectly improve the quality of mother–infant engagement and of infant outcome?" Clearly, no such indirect effect was apparent. Because no discernible benefit in terms of the quality of mother–infant engagement was apparent from the cognitive-behavioral or the psychodynamic treatment, a negative answer to the second and third questions posed was also provided: These two forms of treatment, explicitly designed to address difficulties in the mother–infant relationship, failed to effect any significant change in the quality of face-to-face engagement.

It is clearly important to speculate on the reasons for the failure of the two treatments designed to improve the quality of the mother–infant relationship to effect an improvement in face-to-face interactions. One plausible explanation is that there was a ceiling effect: That is, as the disturbances in interactions found in British community samples of depressed women are subtle in nature (Murray, Fiori-Cowley, et al., 1996; Murray, Hipwell, et al., 1996), there was relatively little room for improvement. The population of depressed mothers recruited for the Cambridge treatment study does not resemble the severely impaired clinical samples described, for example, by Field et al. (1990) but is much more like the community sample described by Campbell and Cohn (Cohn, Campbell, Matias, & Hopkins, 1990; Campbell, Cohn, & Myers, 1995) in which only minor degrees of interactional disturbance were detected. It is, therefore, unreasonable to expect that either treatment or early remission from depression could have a major impact on maternal sensitivity and the general quality of the mother–infant engagement.

A second explanation for the failure of the treatments to improve the quality of the mother–infant interactions, which must be given serious consideration, is the possibility that the relationship disturbances found in the context of maternal depression arise because of factors other than the maternal affective disorder. For example, it may well be that intrinsic infant factors drive the disturbed interactions. However, as Murray and Cooper have argued (Chapter 5, this volume), although infant factors clearly do play a part in determining the onset of maternal mood disorder and do influence the quality of the infant's behavior with the mother, they are not a major determining factor in the quality of the mother–infant relationship. It might also be the case that maternal factors other than the mood disorder determine the interaction difficulties. There is some evidence to support this idea, because Murray, Fiori-Cowley, et al. (1996) found social adversity in nondepressed women to be associated with the same degree of impairment in the mother–infant relationship as was found in the context of maternal depression. In the current sample, inspection of the data did reveal an association between social adversity and suboptimal mother–infant engagement, and although maternal mood improved with treatment, the social disadvantage (and, presumably, its influence on maternal sensitivity) was left unchanged.

A third explanation for the failure of any of the treatments to have a significant impact on the quality of mother–infant engagement, which merits consideration, is that the interventions were initiated rather late in the process of the development of the mother–infant relationship. Several studies have shown that infants learn the features of their interpersonal environment and their regularities at a very early stage, and a certain pattern of interactions between mother and infant may well have become established by 8 weeks postpartum. It therefore seems plausible that this pattern may be difficult to shift with therapeutic sessions held only weekly for 8 weeks. It further suggests that if it is important to later infant outcome that these features of their early interpersonal environment are changed, treatments should either be carried out for a longer period or should be initiated at an early stage in the process. This latter suggestion raises an important question, namely, would the prevention of postpartum depression in vulnerable women also prevent the disturbances in the mother–infant relationship found to obtain in the context of postpartum affective disorder? The answer to this question would considerably elucidate the processes whereby the disturbed mother–infant relationships arise.

Infant Cognitive and Emotional Development

Cognitive Development

Infant cognitive development was assessed at 9 months using Stage IV of Piaget's Object Concept task, and at 18 months using Stage V of the

Piagetian task as well as the Bayley Scales of Infant Development (Bayley, 1969). No impact on any of these measures of outcome of either treatment or early remission from maternal depression was found, and no one treatment had a better outcome in terms of any of these measures than any other. Thus, at 18 months postpartum the pass rate on Stage V of the Object Concept task was 42% for the control group and 47% for those in the three treatments groups. Similarly, the mean score on the Mental Development Index of the Bayley Scales at 18 months postpartum was 114.6 for the untreated controls and 114.1 for those in the three treatment groups.

Infant emotional development was investigated in a number of ways.

Early Infant Behavioral and Relationship Problems

A checklist was devised specifically for this project covering infant behavioral problems (feeding, sleeping, crying) and relationship problems (infant demands on attention, separation problems, playing difficulties, and general difficulties in relating to the infant). The mothers rated these on a 4-point severity scale (from "not at all" to "a great deal") before treatment and immediately after treatment. The presence of any behavioral problem in moderate or marked degree was reported by 53% of the women before treatment, and the presence of any relationship problem of similar severity was reported by 65% before treatment. These rates are substantially higher than those found in samples of nondepressed postpartum women (Seeley, Murray, & Cooper, 1996). Figure 8.3 shows the change in the frequency of such problems with treatment for each of the four conditions. For the behavioral problems it is apparent from the control condition that there was a considerable natural improvement with time. Thus, although those who received treatment improved substantially on this measure, they did not improve any more than those in the control group. Furthermore, there was no association between improvement and the early remission from depression. The absence of an effect of treatment or of early remission from maternal depression is clearly a function of the marked improvement in the control condition. There are three possible explanations for this latter finding. First, there is a natural improvement in infant problems (crying, sleeping, feeding) with infant maturation and the improvement shown by the control group could simply reflect this maturation. Second, with the experience of a further 8 weeks of motherhood, those in the control condition might have become more competent (or felt more confident) at managing infant behavioral problems. Finally, the improvement evident in the control condition might reflect the input

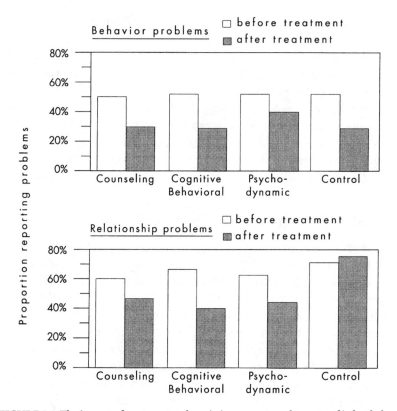

FIGURE 8.3. The impact of treatment and remission on maternal reports of infant behavioral and relationship problems.

received from the health visitors who routinely focus on providing mothers with help in managing just these infant behavioral problems.

It is apparent from Figure 8.3 that the situation was very different for relationship problems. In this case there was no natural improvement over time: Those in the control group showed no improvement across the two assessments on this measure. In contrast, those who received treatment improved substantially in terms of the reporting of relationship problems. Indeed, both treatment and the early remission from depression were associated with significant improvement on this measure.

Although it might appear from Figure 8.3 that the CBT was especially successful at improving maternal reports of relationship problems, the difference between the three treatments was not a significant one. In view of this equivalence between the three treatment conditions, one might be tempted to interpret this finding as a simple antidepressant effect. However, this does not appear to be correct because an examination of the subgroup of treated women who did not recover from depression revealed a significant benefit of treatment. It would seem that the opportunity to think about and discuss aspects of the relationship with the infant, whatever the theoretical context in which this is provided, is beneficial to a mother's perception of that relationship.

Later Infant Behavioral Problems

At 18 months postpartum all the women were interviewed using the Behavioural Screening Questionnaire (Richman & Graham, 1971) modified for use with this age group (Murray, 1992). Again, although there was no difference between the three forms of treatment, those who had received treatment reported significantly fewer infant behavioral problems than those among the control group.

Infant Attachment

Infant attachment to the mother was assessed at 18 months in the research unit using the Ainsworth Strange Situation procedure (Ainsworth, Blehar, Waters, & Wall, 1978). Trained independent assessors rated attachment as secure or insecure (avoidant or resistant). Figure 8.4 shows the rates of

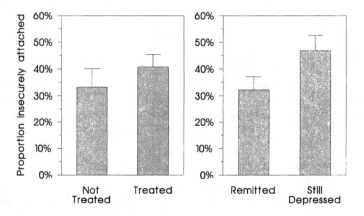

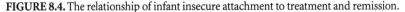

FIGURE 8.4. The relationship of infant insecure attachment to treatment and remission.

secure and insecure attachment for those infants whose mothers had received treatment compared to those infants whose mothers had not, and it shows the rates for those infants whose mothers' depression had remitted by 18 weeks postpartum compared to those infants whose mothers' depressions persisted. It is apparent that there was no effect of treatment: The rate of insecure attachment among those who had received treatment (i.e., 41%) was no different from the rate among those who had not received treatment (i.e., 33%). The rate of insecurity for the three treatments was very similar. Early remission from maternal depression was, on the other hand, associated with less insecurity of infant attachment: Among the group whose depression persisted beyond 18 weeks, the rate of infant insecurity was 47%, as compared with a rate of 32% among those where the maternal mood disorder had lifted by 18 weeks postpartum.

The fact that early remission from postpartum depression was associated with a better attachment outcome provides some support for the idea that postpartum depression is causally implicated in the insecure attachments found in these samples. However, the lack of a specificity of treatment effect suggests that no particular pathway to maternal recovery is preferable with respect to this index of infant outcome.

CONCLUSION

1. All three treatments were equally effective at speeding up the natural rate of remission from depression. There was little evidence of relapse within any of the treatment conditions. Indeed, there was evidence of a trend to a natural recovery and by 9 months postpartum, the spontaneous recovery rate within the control group had caught up with the rate achieved by treatment.

2. None of the treatments produced any more change in the quality of face-to-face engagements than that evident in the control group. A number of reasons for this negative finding were discussed earlier in this chapter. Paramount among them must be the fact that the degree of disturbance in the mother–infant relationship evident in this community sample of depressed women was small and there was, therefore, little room for change.

3. The rate of maternal reports of relationship problems was significantly reduced by treatment, but all three treatments were equally effective. This did not appear to be simply an incidental consequence of the elevation of the maternal mood disorder because there was an impact of

treatment independent of its antidepressant effect. A common feature of all three treatments was that they provided the women with the opportunity to discuss their problems with managing their infants, and it is conceivable that this opportunity enabled therapeutic change of this dimension.

4. No treatment had any impact on infant cognitive development. Because no association between cognitive impairment and maternal depression was evident in this sample, again there was little scope for a specific effect of treatment. In addition, because markedly disturbed early mother–infant interactions have been found to predict compromised cognitive development, and no such disturbance obtained in this sample, the absence of an impact of treatment or early remission on cognitive outcome was to be expected.

5. Although there was no significant impact of treatment on infant attachment status, early remission from maternal depression, itself significantly related to receiving treatment, was associated with a reduced rate of insecure attachments. However, there was no relationship between attachment status and the method by which that remission from depression was achieved. Although this confirms the fact that early maternal depression is associated with insecure infant attachment, it suggests that a rapid remission from that depression, however effected, is sufficient to shift whatever features of the early relationship are implicated in later attachment status.

The findings of this study suggest that if maternal depression could be prevented, the infant problems associated with such depression, in particular infant behavioral problems and insecure attachment, would themselves be prevented. The existence of a predictive index for postpartum depression affords the opportunity to address this question.

The findings of this study also suggest that infant development in the context of postpartum depression would benefit from a community-based intervention. This has recently been demonstrated in a study of British health visitors—that is, community-based nurses with special responsibility for the welfare of mothers and young children (Seeley, Murray, & Cooper, 1996). Training was provided to all the health visitors working in the Cambridge National Health Service sector. This training consisted of 6 weekly half-day sessions and involved training in basic counseling skills as well as basic cognitive-behavioral strategies. A cohort study was conducted with information collected (by maternal self-report) on the health visitors' clientele before their training and then the same information was collected for a posttraining period. The findings with respect to maternal mood and maternal reports of relationship problems were precisely the same as those that obtained for the Cambridge controlled trial reported earlier: Compared with the pretraining period, following training health visitors effected substantial improvements on both these dimensions of outcome.

ACKNOWLEDGMENTS

The research discussed in this chapter was supported by grants from Birthright and the Department of Health. We are grateful to Sian Coker, Jenny Corrigal, Bridget Halnan, Sheelah Seeley, and Claire Wilson for their help with carrying out the treatments; to Alison Hipwell, Fiona King, Agnese Fiori-Cowley, Charlie Stanley, and Anji West for their help with the assessments; and to Richard Hooper for help with the data analysis. We are indebted to all the women and their families who took part in this study.

REFERENCES

Ainsworth, M. D., Blehar, M. C., Waters, E., & Wall, S. (1978). *Patterns of attachment: A psychological study of the strange situation.* Hillsdale, NJ: Erlbaum.

American Psychiatric Association. (1970). *Diagnostic and statistical manual of mental disorders* (3rd ed., rev.). Washington DC: Author.

Appleby, L., Warner, R., Whitton, A., & Faragher, B. (in press). A controlled study of fluoxetine and cognitive-behavioural counseling in the treatment of postnatal depression. *British Medical Journal.*

Bayley, N. (1969). *Bayley Scales of Infant Development.* New York: Psychological Corporation.

Brockington, I. F., & Brierley, E. (1984). Rejection of a child by his mother successfully treated after three years. *British Journal of Psychiatry, 145,* 316–318.

Campbell, S. B., Cohn, J. F., & Meyers, T. (1995). Depression in first-time mothers: Mother–infant interaction and depression chronicity. *Developmental Psychology, 31,* 349–357.

Cohn, J. F., Campbell, S. B., Matias, R., & Hopkins, J. (1990). Face-to-face interaction of postpartum depressed and nondepressed mother–infant pairs at 2 months. *Developmental Psychology, 26*(1), 15–23.

Cohn, J. F., Matias, R., Tronick, E., Connell, D., & Lyons-Ruth, K. (1986). Face-to-face interactions of depressed mothers and their infants. In E. Z. Tronick & T. Field (Eds.), *Maternal depression and infant disturbance.* San Francisco: Jossey-Bass.

Cooper, P. J., Campbell, E. A., Day, A., Kennerly, H., & Bond, A. (1988). Non-psychotic psychiatric disorder after childbirth: A prospective study of prevalence, incidence, course and nature. *British Journal of Psychiatry, 152,* 799–806.

Cooper, P. J., & Murray, L. (1995). The course and recurrence of postnatal depression: Evidence for the specificity of the diagnostic concept. *British Journal of Psychiatry, 166,* 191–195.

Cooper, P. J., Murray, L., & Stein, A. (1991). Postnatal depression. In A. Seva (Ed.), *European handbook of psychiatry and mental health.* Zaragosa, Spain: Anthropos.

Cox, J. L., Holden, J. M., & Sagovsky, R. (1987). Detection of postnatal depression: Development of the Edinburgh Postnatal Depression Scale. *British Journal of Psychiatry, 150,* 782–786.

Cramer, B., & Stern, D. (1988). Evaluation of changes in mother–infant brief psychotherapy: A single case study. *Infant Mental Health Journal, 9,* 20–45.

Cramer, B., Robert-Tissot, C., Stern, D., Serpa-Rusconi, S., De Muralt, M., Besson, G., Palacio-Esoasa, F., Bachmann, J. -P., Knauer, D., Berney, C., & D'Arcis, U. (1990). Outcome evaluation in brief mother–infant psychotherapy: A preliminary report. *Infant Mental Health Journal, 11,* 278–300.

Elkin, I., Shea, M. T., Watkins, J. T., Imber, S. D., Sotsky, S. M., Collins, J. F., Glass, D. R., Pilkonis, P. A., Leber, W. R., Docherty, J. P., Fiester, S. J., & Parloff, M. B. (1989). NIMH treatment of depression collaborative research program: General effectiveness of treatments. *Archives of General Psychiatry, 46,* 971–983.

Field, T., Healy, B., Goldstein, S., & Guthertz, M. (1990). Behavior-state matching and synchrony in mother–infant interactions of nondepressed versus depressed dyads. *Developmental Psychology, 26,* 7–14.

Hawton, K., Salkovskis, P., Kirk, J., & Clark, D. M. (Eds.). (1989). *Cognitive-behavioural approaches to adult psychiatric disorders.* Oxford, England: Oxford University Press.

Henderson, A. F., Gregoire, A. J. P., Kumar, R., & Studd, J. W. W. (1991). Treatment of severe postnatal depression with oestrodiol skin patches. *Lancet, 338,* 816–817.

Holden, J., Sagovsky, R., & Cox, J. L. (1989). counseling in a general practice setting: A controlled study of health visitor intervention in the treatment of postnatal depression. *British Medical Journal, 298,* 223–226.

Malphurs, J., Larrain, C., Field, T., Pickens, J., Pelaez-Nogueras, M., Yando, R., & Bendell, D. (1996). Altering withdrawn and intrusive interaction behaviors of depressed mothers. *Infant Mental Health Journal, 17,* 152–160.

McDonnough, S. C. (1993). Interaction guidance: Understanding and treating early infant–caregiver relationship disturbances. In C. H. Zeanah, Jr., (Ed.), *Handbook of infant mental health* (pp. 414–426). New York: Guilford Press.

Murray, L. (1992). The impact of postnatal depression on infant development. *Journal of Child Psychology and Psychiatry, 33,* 543–561.

Murray, L., & Cooper, P. J. (1997). The impact of postpartum depression on child development. *Psychological Medicine, 27,* 253–260.

Murray, L., Fiori-Cowley, A., Hooper, R., & Cooper, P. J. (1996). The impact of postnatal depression and associated adversity on early mother–infant interactions and later infant outcome. *Child Development, 67,* 2512–2526.

Murray, L., Hipwell, A., Hooper, R., Stein, A., & Cooper, P. J. (1996). The cognitive development of five year old children of postnatally depressed mothers. *Journal of Child Psychology and Psychiatry, 37,* 927–935.

Murray, L., Kempton, C., Woolgar, M., & Hooper, R. (1993). Depressed mothers' speech to their infants and its relation to infant gender and cognitive development. *Journal of Child Psychology and Psychiatry, 34,* 1083–1101.

Richman, N., & Graham, P. (1971). A behavioural screening questionnaire for use with three-year-old children: Preliminary findings. *Journal of Child Psychology and Psychiatry, 12,* 5–33.

Seeley, S., Murray, L., & Cooper, P. J. (1996). The outcome for mothers and babies of health visitor intervention. *Health Visitor, 69,* 135–138.

Spitzer, R. L., Williams, J. B. W., Gibbon, M., & First, M. B. (1989). *Structured Clinical Interview for DSM-III-R—Patient edition (with psychotic screen).* New York: Biometrics Research Department, New York State Psychiatric Institute.

Stern, D. (1995). *The motherhood constellation.* New York: Basic Books.

9

The Treatment of Depressed Mothers and Their Infants

Tiffany Field
University of Miami School of Medicine

Mothers who remain depressed over their infants' first year of life have infants who show a profile of behavioral, physiological, and biochemical dysregulation. Thus, identifying postpartum depressed mothers who are likely to continue being depressed is critical for targeting those high-risk mother–infant dyads who need intervention. This chapter reviews data on dysregulation in infants of depressed mothers, on identifying mothers who remain depressed, and on some brief and some intensive interventions.

CONTRIBUTION OF INFANTS TO DISTURBED MOTHER–INFANT INTERACTIONS

Infants of depressed mothers may be affected prenatally (and/or genetically) and show problems as early as birth that may contribute to early interaction disturbances. Some investigators note that newborns born to mothers who were depressed during pregnancy were more fussy and less consolable than infants of nondepressed women (Whiffen & Gottlib, 1989; Zuckerman, Als, Bauchner, Parker, & Cabral, 1990). In a recent study at our laboratory, newborns were assessed on the Brazelton Neonatal Assessment Scale. The performance of 20 infants whose mothers were identified as depressed using the BDI (Beck Depression Inventory) and the DISC (Diagnostic Interview for Children) shortly after giving birth was compared to that of 20 infants of mothers from the same population who were not depressed (Abrams, Field, Scafidi, & Prodromidis, 1995). They had less developed motor tone, lower activity levels and more irritability, and less robustness and endurance during the examination. Infants of depressed mothers also performed more poorly on the orientation cluster; specifically, they did not localize the sound of a shaking rattle or track a moving bell as well as did newborns of nondepressed mothers. Their minimal responding to the inanimate versus the animate stimuli suggests that they may have higher sensory thresholds and require the more arousing animate stimuli for optimal responding. This may contribute to early interaction disturbances inasmuch as Brazelton orientation scores have been related to later interaction behaviors (Abrams et al., 1995).

Decreased motor tone and lower activity levels on the "depressed" cluster and lesser robustness in the neonates of depressed women are perhaps not surprising given that lower activity level, lethargy, and unavailability are the behaviors often reported for 3-month-old infants of depressed mothers. These infants also have elevated norepinephrine levels and indeterminate sleep patterns at the newborn stage (difficult-to-code patterns because they cannot be coded as deep sleep or active sleep) (Field, 1995) (see Table 9.1).

In a more recent study, similarly inferior performance was noted on the Brazelton scale by newborns, and their expressivity (facial expression responses to the Brazelton items) and imitative behavior was more limited on a neonatal imitation procedure (Lundy, Field, & Pickens, in press).

Further evidence for physiological dysregulation which may contribute to disturbed mother–infant interactions was found in our study on brain electrical activity in 3-month-old infants of depressed mothers (Field, Fox, Pickens, & Nawrocki, 1995). In this study, electroencephalograms (EEGs) were recorded from left and right frontal and parietal scalp regions in depressed and well mothers and their infants. In comparison to the control group, both depressed mothers and their infants displayed right frontal EEG asymmetry. The demonstration of right frontal asymmetry in these infants suggests that this pattern is present early in the first year of life among this high-risk group. In addition to the group average indicating this pattern, a greater number of depressed mothers and their

TABLE 9.1. Means for Newborn Variables

	Newborns of depressed mothers (*n* = 47)	Newborns of nondepressed mothers (*n* = 36)
Brazelton scores		
Orientation	4.8	5.6[*]
Inanimate auditory	5.5	6.9[**]
Inanimate auditory and visual	4.4	5.4[*]
Depression	3.3	2.3[*]
Robustness	5.0	5.8[*]
Indeterminate sleep	19.3	2.7[***]
Norepinephrine	141.2	58.4***

[*]$p < .05$; [**]$p < .01$; [***]$p < .001$.

infants displayed the right frontal EEG asymmetry pattern (see Figure 9.1). Thus, the depressed affect exhibited by the infants of depressed mothers is associated with a pattern of brain electrical activity similar to that found in inhibited infants and children and in some depressed adults. Further research is required to determine whether the EEG pattern is a marker of current or chronic mood state.

More recent data suggest that right frontal EEG asymmetry may be present even earlier from birth and may remain stable across at least the first 3 years of life. In a recent study, compared to well mothers' infants, infants of depressed mothers were found to have more right frontal EEG asymmetry as early as 1 month of age (Jones, Field, Fox, Lundy, & Davalos, 1997). This asymmetry was in turn negatively related to indeterminate sleep in the infants (right frontal activation was associated with more indeterminate sleep). This relation is problematic inasmuch as Sigman and Parmelee (1989) reported a negative correlation between indeterminate sleep in the newborn period and later childhood performance on IQ tests.

Data on the stability of right frontal EEG asymmetry come from a study in which we followed the development of 3-month-old infants of depressed mothers until they were 3 years of age (Jones et al., 1997). Right frontal EEG asymmetry was significantly stable across this period. Right frontal EEG asymmetry at 3 months was also predictive of inhibited behavior at 3 years, not unlike the data of Fox and colleagues suggesting a similar relation from 4 months to 14 months (Calkins, Fox, & Marshall, 1996).

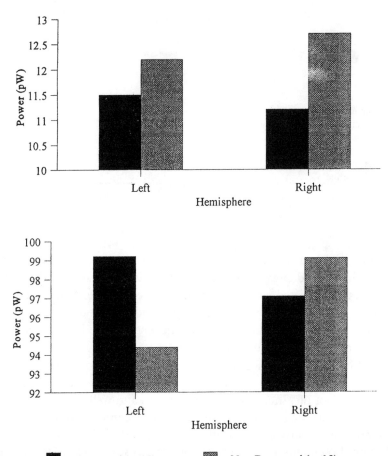

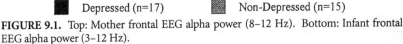

FIGURE 9.1. Top: Mother frontal EEG alpha power (8–12 Hz). Bottom: Infant frontal EEG alpha power (3–12 Hz).

Other evidence for physiological dysregulation in infants of depressed mothers has been noted as early as one week of age (Jones, et al., 1997). In that study newborns had not only right frontal EEG but also lower vagal tone and less mature sleep patterns. Lower vagal tone has also been reported for 3- to 6-month-old infants of depressed mothers (Field, Pickens, Fox, Nawrocki, & Gonzalez, 1995). In that study, we explored developmental changes in vagal tone. In addition, we rated mother–infant interactions on the Interaction Rating Scale, and administered the Infant Neurological Battery. Finally, we also explored the relations between vagal tone and the other infant measures. The developmental increase in vagal tone that occurred between 3 and 6 months for infants of nondepressed mothers did not occur for the infants of depressed mothers. Lower vagal tone at 6 months was also correlated with fewer vocalizations during interactions and less optimal neurological scores, suggesting a lesser degree of autonomic development and control by infants of depressed mothers.

Lower vagal tone has also been noted in infants of depressed mothers during their interactions with both their mothers and nondepressed strangers (Field et al., 1988). Vagal tone could be responsive to contextual factors such as stress and changes in attention during interactions. Contextual demands could be different for infants of depressed and nondepressed mothers. For example, depressed mothers are notably less expressive, and their infants may become more agitated in their attempts to elicit more responsivity. It is not clear whether the differences reflect a neuroregulation difference determined by the complexity of genetics and previous experience with the mother or whether the differences reflect different demands placed on the two groups in the interaction situation. The absence of a developmental increase in vagal tone in the infants of depressed mothers could relate to cumulative effects of maternal depression, including the continuing elevated norepinephrine levels noted in these infants. Another complex finding emerged in a study in which we recorded both facial expressions and vagal tone (Pickens & Field, 1993). In that study, interest and joy expressions were significantly correlated with vagal tone in infants of nondepressed mothers. However, for infants of depressed mothers, more negative behaviors, including gaze aversion and sad and angry expressions, were positively correlated with vagal tone.

The combination of less orienting behavior, more depressed behavior, more stress behaviors, more indeterminate sleep, right frontal EEG activation, lower vagal tone, and higher norepinephrine levels suggests a profile of dysregulation in the infant at a very early age. This profile, at least behaviorally, is likely to have some negative impact on early mother–infant interactions independent of the contribution of the mother's depressed behavior.

CONTRIBUTION OF THE MOTHERS' CONTINUING DEPRESSION

For many mothers who are depressed in the postpartum period, the depression subsides in the first few months of the infant's life (O'Hara,

Chapter 1, this volume). We have observed that mothers who were depressed during the first few months of their infants' life but were no longer depressed by 6 months had infants who also no longer behaved in a depressed-like fashion. Their development was normal at 1 year (Field, 1992). In contrast, mothers who remained depressed over the infants' first 6 months of life had infants who developed a "depressed" style of interacting and later at 1 year showed inferior Bayley Mental and Motor Scale performance (Bayley, 1969) and were at lower weight percentiles. Maternal depression persisted for 1 year for 75% of that sample, and the children eventually had externalizing or internalizing behavioral problems at the preschool stage (Field, Lang, et al., 1996).

Identifying those mothers who will remain depressed is extremely important because their infants, as already mentioned, begin to show growth and developmental delays at 1 year, suggesting they need early intervention. Behavioral predictors of chronic depression have been unreliable. However, physiological and biochemical markers may be more promising. In one of our data sets, for example, 51% of the variance in continuing depression (mothers still being depressed at 6 months) could be explained by variables collected at 3 months. These included the mother's right frontal EEG asymmetry, which explained 31% of the variance. The variables that explained the remaining 20% included low vagal tone and serotonin and elevated norepinephrine and cortisol levels. This profile may be promising for identifying mother–infant dyads who need intervention. Finding cost-effective interventions is then the next problem.

COST-EFFECTIVE INTERVENTIONS

The most commonly reported parenting problems for depressed mothers include their depressed mood state and their lesser sensitivity to their infants' emotional cues. The mothers' depressed affect (mood) is a problem because the infant does not receive feedback for his or her own behaviors, and the mothers' depressed behavior is also a model for the infant's developing depressed behavior. A parsimonious intervention would focus on these common problems.

Altering the mother's mood state may help change her behavior at least during interactions with her infant. Potential mood alteration techniques include music mood induction, visual imagery, aerobics, yoga, relaxation, and massage therapy. In one study we used relaxation and massage therapy techniques. Positive effects occurred for both intervention groups, although the effects were more dramatic for the massage therapy group subjects (Field, Grizzle, Scafidi, & Abrams, 1996) (see Table 9.2). Following a 30-minute massage, the mothers' anxiety levels and salivary cortisol levels (stress hormones) decreased. After a 4-week period of two massages per week, the mothers were significantly less depressed and their urinary cortisol levels were lower than the mothers who received relaxation, suggesting stable decreases in anxiety, depression, and stress.

Similar effects were noted for music mood induction. However, in this case we also recorded frontal and parietal EEG (Field, Grizzle, Scafidi,

TABLE 9.2. Means for Massage Therapy (*n* = 16) Group Mothers and for Relaxation Therapy (*n* = 16) Group Mothers

	Day 1		Day 10	
	Pre	Post	Pre	Post
State Anxiety Scale	35.67*	28.67	33.89*	28.28
	(34.73)*	(31.55)	(33.09)*	(30.73)
POMS Depression	19.44*	11.43	20.39*	9.06
	(18.37)	(19.40)	(18.56)	(17.12)
Behavior Observation Scale				
State	2.22	2.29	2.09	2.11
	(2.20)	(2.10)	(2.45)	(2.00)
Affect	1.72*	2.67	1.67*	2.83
	(2.55)	(2.45)	(2.64)	(2.55)
Activity	1.61	1.67	1.69	1.50
	(1.82)	(1.82)	(1.91)	(1.73)
Vocalization	1.44*	1.83	1.50*	1.94
	(1.82)	(1.64)	(2.09)	(1.86)
Anxiety	1.83*	1.06	1.94*	1.06
	(1.55)	(1.55)	(1.18)	(1.09)
Cooperation	2.56*	2.89	2.17*	2.89
	(2.82)	(2.55)	(2.55)	(2.64)
Fidgetiness	1.61*	1.11	1.61*	1.11
	(1.36)	(1.00)	(1.09)	(1.01)
Pulse	85.06*	77.76	87.88*	77.65
	(84.00)	(85.56)	(77.78)	(75.78)
Saliva cortisol	1.21*	.84	1.55*	1.16
	(1.55)	(1.65)	(1.87)	(1.80)
Urine cortisol	166.95*		120.08	
	(165.50)		(168.39)	

Note. Means for relaxation therapy group are given in parentheses. Asterisks indicate significant differences between adjacent means at *p* < .05.

& Abrams, 1996). Chronically depressed adults have right frontal EEG activation which remains even when their behavioral symptoms are in remission, suggesting that this pattern would be difficult to alter. However, after only 20 minutes of music (a selection of 5 rock music pieces) 10 out of the 12 depressed adolescents showed an attenuation of right frontal EEG activation, moving towards symmetry or towards left frontal EEG activation (see Figure 9.2). The two adolescents whose EEG pattern did not change claimed that they did not enjoy the rock music. When their favorite music (classical) was played, they too experienced a shift toward symmetry. Although it is not clear how long-lived these effects are, it was surprising that the right frontal EEG activation, thought to be a marker of chronic depression, could be altered by only 20 minutes of music.

In the next intervention we attempted to enhance the mothers' sensitivity to their infants' cues and to improve the infants' mood state. Depressed adolescent mothers giving their infants a massage were compared to depressed mothers who rocked their infants. Each intervention was administered for 15-minute periods on 12 days over a 6-week period (Field, Grizzle, Scafidi, & Abrams, 1996) (see Table 9.3). During the session, the massage therapy versus the rocked infants spent more time in active alert and active awake states, and they cried less. After the massage, they had lower salivary cortisol levels, suggesting lower stress levels. They also spent less time in an active awake state after the session, suggesting that massage may be more effective than rocking for inducing sleep. Ap-

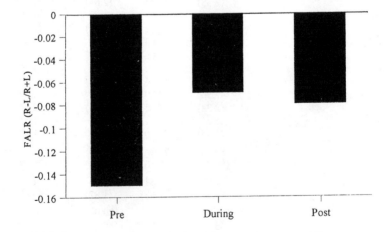

FIGURE 9.2. Mood music induction

TABLE 9.3. Means for Variables Measured at Beginning and End of Study Period for Massage Therapy and Rocking Group Infants

Variables	Massage therapy ($n = 20$)		Rocking ($n = 20$)		p
	Day 1	Day 12	Day 1	Day 12	
Weight (lb.)	14.7$_a$	16.3$_b$	14.9$_a$	15.4$_a$	.001
Formula intake	7.0$_a$	8.4$_a$	8.0$_a$	10.8$_a$	NS
Temperament					
Emotionality	13.7$_a$	12.2$_b$	13.6$_a$	13.0$_a$	.05
Activity	17.9$_a$	17.6$_a$	16.4$_a$	16.0$_a$	NS
Sociability	18.5$_a$	19.9$_b$	19.1$_b$	18.4$_a$	.05
Soothability	16.5$_a$	18.5$_b$	15.8$_a$	15.6$_a$	.05
Persistence	16.5$_a$	16.7$_a$	16.1$_a$	16.8$_a$	NS
Food adaptation	14.1$_a$	13.4$_a$	14.1$_a$	13.9$_a$	NS
Interaction rating	2.3$_a$	2.6$_b$	2.2$_a$	2.2$_a$	.05
Biochemical variables					
Norepinephrine	245.3$_a$	119.7$_b$	195.0$_a$	180.0$_a$	.05
Epinephrine	21.5$_a$	10.6$_b$	16.0$_a$	23.6$_a$	.05
Serotonin (5-HIAA)	944.9$_a$	1,427.9$_b$	1,001.5$_a$	1,132.4$_a$	.05
Cortisol (urine)	1,382.9$_a$	656.4$_b$	1,225.4$_a$	1,016.8$_a$	.05

Note. Different-letter subscripts (a's and b's) denote significant differences at $p < .05$ or less revealed by post hoc comparisons. For emotionality, norepinephrine, epinephrine, and cortisol, lower values are optimal. For sociability, soothability, interaction rating, and serotonin, higher values are optimal.

parently, rocked infants sleep during the rocking and wake up when it is over, and massaged infants are awake during the massage and sleep when it is over. After the 6-week follow-up period, the massage group as compared to the rocking group infants gained more weight and they improved on emotionality, sociability, and soothability temperament dimensions and face-to-face interaction ratings: They also showed decreased urinary stress hormones/catecholamines (norepinephrine, epinephrine, cortisol) and increased serotonin levels, suggesting less depression.

Interaction coaching is another technique for altering the mother's sensitivity to her infant's cues and for improving the mother–infant interaction. Maternal imitation is one of the most effective interaction coaching techniques (Field, 1977). The mother becomes less active and more sensitive to her infant's cues of being under- or overaroused when she uses this technique. The infant in turn becomes more attentive and responsive. We hypothesized that this technique would be very effective with depressed mothers who were intrusive. A more active, stimulating technique, "attention getting," in which mothers were coached to keep their infants' attention was expected to be more effective with withdrawn, depressed mothers. Depressed mothers were randomly assigned to one of these conditions, after investigators made independent ratings of the mother's style of interaction (i.e., intrusive or withdrawn). The data were consistent with our expectations. The imitation technique was more effective with overstimulating, intrusive mothers and the attention-getting technique was more effective with withdrawn mothers (Malphurs et al., 1996). For the mothers' touching behavior, for example, the intrusive mothers' touching decreased during the imitation session, and the withdrawn mothers' touching increased during the attention-getting game-playing session. The infants' facial expressions, in turn, were more frequent during the imitation session in the case of the intrusive mother–infant dyads, and facial expressions increased during game-playing in the case of the withdrawn mother–infant dyads.

Touching was also used as an intervention technique. Depressed mothers are noted to touch their infants less frequently. Their touch is also typically more negative, such as poking, punching, and pinching. To demonstrate the effectiveness of touching, we asked both depressed and nondepressed mothers to show a still face and remain quiet and inexpressive (Pelaez-Nogueras, Field, Cigales, Gonzalez, & Clasky, 1995). We then asked the mothers to massage their infants' legs as they retained the still-face position. Adding the touching led to increased infant smiling and decreased infant gaze aversion, particularly in the depressed mother–infant dyads.

We also attempted to modify the infants' interaction behavior by introducing the "depressed" infant to a nondepressed adult (Field et al., 1988). Unfortunately, the infant showed a generalized depressed mood state with nondepressed adults. Because this circumstance might relate to the nondepressed adult not being a mother herself, we introduced infants of depressed mothers to nondepressed mothers and observed the interactions of depressed mothers with nondepressed infants (Martinez et al., 1996). This intervention was also relatively ineffective because the infants made very little change, whether they were depressed infants interacting with nondepressed mothers or infants of nondepressed mothers interacting with depressed mothers. Even though the infants of nondepressed mothers appeared to be trying harder with the depressed mothers, the depressed mothers looked much the same whether they were with their own or another mother's infant. At least the depressed mothers did not negatively affect the infants of nondepressed mothers.

Introducing 3-month-old infants of depressed mothers to nondepressed teachers who were familiar (they were the infants' day-care teacher and primary caregiver), in contrast, improved the infants' interaction behaviors (Pelaez-Nogueras et al., 1995) (see Table 9.4). Compared to their behavior with their mothers, these infants showed more positive facial expressions and vocalizations when with their day-care teacher. Fathers can also buffer the negative effects, as improvement is noted when infants of depressed mothers interact with their fathers (Hossain, Field, Pickens, & Gonzalez, 1995) (see Table 9.5). The fathers showed more positive facial expressions and vocalizations than mothers did, and, in turn, the infants of depressed mothers showed more positive facial expressions and vocalizations when interacting with their fathers. These data suggest that nondepressed fathers and nondepressed infants' nursery teachers can compensate for the negative effects of depressed mothering.

TABLE 9.4. Mean Interaction Ratings of Infants ($n = 18$) with Depressed Mothers and Nondepressed Teachers

	Mother		Teacher		
	M	SD	M	SD	p
Infant interaction behaviors					
State	2.72	(0.57)	2.72	(0.75)	NS
Physical activity	2.50	(0.71)	2.83	(0.51)	NS
Head orientation	2.33	(0.59)	2.89	(0.47)	***
Gaze behavior	2.06	(0.54)	2.77	(0.42)	****
Facial expressions	2.39	(0.85)	2.94	(0.24)	*
Fussiness	2.06	(0.80)	2.72	(0.46)	***
Vocalizations	2.11	(0.83)	2.11	(0.83)	NS
Summary rating	2.31	(0.31)	2.72	(0.23)	****
Mother–teacher interaction behaviors					
State	2.28	(0.57)	2.94	(0.24)	****
Physical activity	2.06	(0.73)	2.89	(0.32)	****
Head orientation	2.61	(0.70)	3.00	(0.00)	*
Gaze behavior	2.78	(0.43)	3.00	(0.00)	*
Silence during infant gaze aversion	2.00	(0.00)	2.39	(0.61)	*
Facial expressions	2.17	(0.50)	3.00	(0.00)	****
Vocalizations	1.89	(0.47)	2.78	(0.42)	****
Infantalized behaviors	1.72	(0.67)	2.89	(0.32)	****
Contingent responsivity	2.22	(0.55)	3.00	(0.00)	****
Game playing	1.50	(0.62)	2.83	(0.51)	****
Summary rating	2.12	(0.31)	2.88	(0.12)	****

Note. Higher scores are optimal for all ratings.

*$p < .05$; **$p < .01$; ***$p < .005$; ****$p < .001$.

TABLE 9.5. Mean Interaction Ratings of Infants (n = 26) with Nondepressed Fathers and Depressed Mothers

	Father		Mother		
	M	SD	M	SD	p
Parent interaction behaviors					
State	2.5	(0.5)	2.1	(0.3)	.005
Physical activity	1.6	(0.5)	1.7	(0.7)	NS
Head orientation	2.9	(0.3)	2.9	(0.3)	NS
Gaze behavior	2.8	(0.4)	3.0	(0.0)	NS
Silence during infant gaze aversion	1.9	(0.8)	1.7	(0.8)	NS
Facial expressions	2.4	(0.7)	1.8	(0.4)	.01
Vocalizations	2.6	(0.9)	1.5	(0.5)	.001
Infantalized behaviors	2.0	(0.7)	1.8	(0.8)	NS
Contingent vocalizations	2.2	(0.4)	2.0	(0.9)	NS
Game playing	2.0	(0.9)	1.3	(0.6)	<.05
Summary score	2.3	(0.2)	1.9	(0.3)	<.005
Infant interaction behaviors					
State	2.8	(0.5)	1.8	(0.7)	<.001
Physical activity	2.3	(0.9)	2.5	(0.5)	NS
Head orientation	2.0	(0.7)	2.0	(0.6)	NS
Gaze behavior	2.7	(0.5)	2.1	(0.7)	<.05
Facial expressions	2.8	(0.6)	1.7	(0.5)	<.001
Fussiness	2.2	(0.9)	1.9	(0.7)	NS
Vocalizations	2.3	(0.8)	1.5	(0.5)	<.005
Summary score	2.4	(0.4)	1.9	(0.4)	<.005

Note. Gender-of-parent effect: $F(8,15) = 3.86, p < .01$; Wilks's lambda = .32.

MORE COMPREHENSIVE INTERVENTIONS

Comprehensive intervention programs for depressed mother–infant dyads are rare. One of the biggest problems in working with depressed mothers is finding them an educational/vocational experience that might attenuate their depression and finding their infants substitute caregiving so the mothers can pursue something for themselves and the infants will have less exposure to their mothers' depression. To help ameliorate these problems we arranged a 3-month social/educational/vocational rehabilitation program, as well as free day care in a model infant nursery in a local public vocational high school. Although we had not previously tried this kind of intervention with depressed mothers, we successfully used similar intensive interventions with nondepressed teenage mothers (Field, Widmayer, Greenberg, & Stoller, 1982). In addition, we provided music mood induction, relaxation therapy, massage therapy, and infant massage and interaction coaching. In this program the mothers attended vocational high school in the mornings and participated in social and vocational rehabilitation activities and aerobics in the afternoons; their infants received all-day model day care on a daily basis for 3 months. The mothers also spent approximately 1 hour per day in the infant nursery helping the teachers take care of their infants. The mothers and infants together were given interaction coaching.

In the first part of this study we developed a risk index for identifying those mothers who would remain depressed and would need intervention to prevent infant depression. Behavioral, psychophysiological, and biochemical assessments were made at the neonatal, 3-,and 6-month periods on a sample of depressed mothers, 20% of whom were expected to no longer be depressed by the 6-month assessment period. Using a regression model, the predictor variables from the neonatal and 3-month assessments were used to identify those mothers who would remain depressed at 6 months.

A sample of 160 depressed mothers and 100 nondepressed mothers and their infants were followed over the first 6 months to assess the infant's development and to identify potential markers from the first 3 months that predicted chronic depression in the mothers. The markers were then used to identify a second sample of chronically depressed mothers to receive an intervention.

In the longitudinal sample, a syndrome of dysregulation was noted in the infants, including lower Brazelton scores, more indeterminate sleep and elevated norepinephrine, epinephrine and dopamine at the neonatal period, right frontal EEG activation, lower vagal tone, and negative interactions at the 3- and 6-month periods. A group of variables contributed to 51% of the variance in the mothers' continuing depression, including right frontal EEG activation, lower vagal tone, and elevated norepinephrine, serotonin, and cortisol levels. In the second sample identified by these markers, depressed mothers and their infants received the 3-month intervention and were compared to depressed and nondepressed control groups.

Although the intervention mothers continued to have higher depression scores than did the nondepressed mothers, their interaction behavior became significantly more positive and their biochemical values and vagal tone normalized or approximated the values of the nondepressed control group (see Table 9.6). The infants in the intervention (day care) group also showed more positive interaction behavior, better growth, fewer pediatric complications, and normalized biochemical values, and by 1 year they had superior Bayley Mental and Motor scores. Thus, chronically depressed mothers could be identified and this relatively cost-effective intervention attenuated the typical delays noted in growth and development for this group.

CONCLUSION

In summary, the combination of less orienting behavior, more depressed behavior, more stress behaviors, more indeterminate sleep, right frontal activation, lower vagal tone, and higher norepinephrine levels suggests a profile of dysregulation in infants of depressed mothers at a very early age. This profile, at least behaviorally, is likely to have some negative impact on early mother–infant interactions independent of the contribution of the mother's depressed behavior. If the mother's depression persists for the infant's first 6 months of life, the infant shows growth and developmental delays at 1 year. Fortunately, those mothers who remained depressed could be identified for early intervention. Fifty-one percent of the variance in continuing depression could be explained by variables collected at 3 months, including mothers' right frontal EEG asymmetry, low vagal

TABLE 9.6. Six-Month Outcome Variables Following Intervention

	Groups			
Variables	Depressed control ($n = 40$)	Depressed intervention ($n = 40$)	Nondepressed intervention ($n = 40$)	p
Maternal interview				
Beck Depression Inventory	13.0_a	10.9_b	6.5_c	.05
DISC dysthymia (%)	22.7_a	14.3_b	0.0_c	.05
Background stress	20.5_a	21.3_a	22.3_a	NS
Interaction ratings				
Mother	2.0_a	2.3_b	2.5_b	.01
Infant	2.0_a	2.4_b	2.5_b	.05
Interactions (% time)				
Mother negative	14.8_a	6.8_b	10.3_b	.05
Mother neutral	43.2_a	27.2_b	33.9_b	.01
Mother positive	41.9_a	66.1_b	55.6_b	.005
Infant negative	5.9_a	3.9_b	3.0_b	.05
Infant neutral	69.6_a	64.9_a	62.5_a	NS
Infant positive	21.6_a	31.2_b	34.5_b	.05
Infant physical measures				
Vagal tone	2.9_a	4.7_b	3.8_b	.05
Weight	$8,048.9_a$	$9,211.0_b$	$11,982.7_c$	.05
Length	67.2_a	67.1_a	67.9_a	NS
Head circumference	42.4_a	42.1_a	43.7_a	NS
Neurological	69.7_a	69.8_a	68.3_a	NS
Pediatric complications	101.5_a	109.4_b	119.1_b	.05

Note. Different-letter subscripts (a's and b's) denote significant differences between means.

tone and serotonin, and elevated norepinephrine and cortisol levels. Brief interventions, including music and massage therapy techniques, were effective in altering the mothers' EEG asymmetry and cortisol levels, and providing the infants with massage therapy lowered their stress hormones and improved their face-to-face interaction ratings. A more comprehensive 3-month social/educational/vocational rehabilitation program for the mothers, as well as free day care in a model infant nursery for the infants, attenuated the growth and developmental delays typically noted for this group. Developmental follow-up studies are needed to determine whether these intervention effects persist, and prenatal intervention research is critical for attenuating the dysregulation noted in these infants as early as birth.

ACKNOWLEDGMENTS

We would like to thank the infants and parents who participated in these studies and the researchers who assisted with data collection. This research was supported by a National Institute of Mental Health Research Scientist Award (No. MH00331) and a National Institute of Mental Health Research Grant (No. MH46586) to Tiffany Field and a grant from Johnson & Johnson to the Touch Research Institute.

REFERENCES

Abrams, S. M., Field, T., Scafidi, F., & Prodromidis, M. (1995). Newborns of depressed mothers. *Infant Mental Health Journal, 16,* 231–237.

Bayley, N. (1969). *Bayley Scales of Infant Development.* New York: Psychological Corporation.

Calkins, S. D., Fox, N. A., & Marshall, T. R. (1996). Behavioral and physiological antecedents of inhibited and uninhibited behavior. *Child Development, 67,* 523–540.

Field, T. (1977). Effects of early separation, interactive deficits, and experimental manipulations on infant–mother face-to-face interaction. *Child Development, 48,* 763–771.

Field, T. (1992). Infants of depressed mothers. *Development and Psychopathology, 4,* 59–66.

Field, T. (1995). Infants of depressed mothers. *Infant Behavior and Development, 18,* 1–13.

Field, T., Fox, N., Pickens, J., Nawrocki, T., & Soutullo, D. (1995). Right front EEG activation in 3- to 6-month-old infants of "depressed" mothers. *Developmental Psychology, 31,* 358–363.

Field, T., Grizzle, N., Scafidi, F., & Abrams, S. (1996). Massage therapy for infants of depressed mothers. *Infant Behavior and Development, 19,* 107–112.

Field, T., Healy, B., Goldstein, S., Perry, S., Bendell, D., Schanberg, S., Zimmerman, E. A., & Kuhn, C. (1988). Infants of depressed mothers show "depressed" behavior even with non-depressed adults. *Child Development, 59,* 1569–1579.

Field, T., Martinez, A., Nawrocki, T., Pickens, J., Fox, N., & Schanberg, S. (in press). Music mood induction shifts in frontal EEG of depressed adolescents. *Adolescence.*

Field, T., Pickens, J., Fox, N., Nawrocki, T., & Gonzalez, J. (1995). Vagal tone in infants of depressed mothers. *Development and Psychobiology, 7,* 227–231.

Field, T., Lang, C., Martinez, A., Yando, R., Pickens, J., & Bendell, D. (1996). Preschool follow-up of children of dysphoric mothers. *Journal of Clinical Child Psychology, 25,* 275–279.

Field, T., Widmayer, S., Greenberg, R., & Stoller, S. (1982). Effects of parent training on teenage mothers and their infants. *Pediatrics, 69*(6), 703–707.

Hossain, Z., Field, T., Pickens, J., & Gonzalez, J. (1995). Infants of "depressed" mothers interact better with their nondepressed fathers. *Infant Mental Health Journal, 15,* 348–357.

Jones, N., Field, T., Fox, N., Lundy, B., & Davalos, M. (1997). EEG asymmetry in one-month old infants of depressed mothers. *Development and Psychopathology.*

Lundy, B., Field, T., & Pickens, J. (in press). Newborns of mothers with depressive symptoms are less expressive. *Infant Behavior and Development.*

Malphurs, J., Larrain, C., Field, T., Pickens, J., Pelaez- Nogueras, M., Yando, R., & Bendell, D. (1996). Altering withdrawn and intrusive interaction behaviors of depressed mothers. *Infant Mental Health Journal, 17,* 152–160.

Martinez, A., Malphurs, J., Field, T., Pickens, J., Yando, R., Bendell, D., DelValle, C., & Messinger, D. (1996). Depressed mothers' and their infants' interactions with non-depressed partners. *Infant Mental Health Journal, 17,* 74–80.

Pelaez-Nogueras, M., Field, T., Cigales, M., Gonzalez, A., & Clasky, S. (1995). Infants of depressed mothers show less "depressed" behavior with their nursery teachers. *Infant Mental Health Journal, 15,* 358–367.

Pickens, J., & Field, T. (1993). Facial expressivity in infants of "depressed" mothers. *Developmental Psychology, 29,* 986–988.

Sigman, M., & Parmelee, A. (1989, January). *Longitudinal predictors of cognitive development.* Paper presented at the meeting of the American Association for the Advancement of Science, San Francisco.

Whiffen, V. E., & Gottlib, I. M. (1989). Infants of postpartum depressed mothers: Temperament and cognitive status. *Journal of Abnormal Psychology, 98,* 274– 279.

Zuckerman, B., Als, H., Bauchner, H., Parker, S., & Cabral, H. (1990). Maternal depressive symptoms during pregnancy, and newborn irritability. *Developmental and Behavioral Pediatrics, 11,* 190–194.

10

~

Psychodynamic Perspectives on the Treatment of Postpartum Depression

Bertrand Cramer
University of Geneva

The search for specific etiological factors is a constant concern for clinicians trying to devise effective treatments. The therapeutic approach to postpartum depression would indeed be enhanced if specific factors (e.g., those related to the birth) could be implicated as causal or contributing agents.

However, the definition of such specific agents has not been—so far—very convincing. Indeed, the concept of postpartum depression as a specific clinical entity has been challenged, as has been the supposed higher incidence of depressive episodes in the postpartum period compared to other periods in a woman's life (Cooper, Murray, & Stein, 1991). There is little published work on specific psychotherapeutic treatment of postpartum depression (Trout, 1991; Brockington, 1992; Halberstadt-Freud, 1993; Gruen, 1993).

Yet, the term "postpartum depression" is still being used and the clinical impression remains that, indeed, there is such an entity as a depression linked to childbirth. Moreover, it is well accepted now that 1 out of 10 women will present a depressive pathology in the early postpartum period (Murray, 1989), and many more present more or less pronounced and durable dysphoria over many months following childbirth.

In the quandary about the specificity or lack of specificity of postpartum depression (and therefore of birth-related stressors) there is a variety of points of view, and some authors have suggested that there are different forms of postpartum depression. It appears that various stressors have different impact according to the socioeconomic status (SES) of women: In low SES women, nonspecific adverse events are most likely to predict postpartum depression; in middle-class populations, the cumulative effect of "nonspecific" life events seems less powerful and childbirth may be seen more clearly to act as a life event with pathogenic influences related to postpartum depression. In this spectrum of different forms of postpartum depression, some may be related to "difficulties, or vulnerability factors particular to child bearing and child rearing" (Murray, 1989, p. 24).

The hypothesis that some postpartum depressions are specifically birth-related events receives support from some studies (Hopkins, Campbell, & Marens, 1987), including a longitudinal study of postpartum and nonpostpartum affective episodes (Cooper & Murray, Chapter 8, this volume). It is also supported by treatment studies of this condition. Brockington and Cox-Roper (1988, p. 11), for example, argued that some of the postpartum depressions are not secondary to basic depressive tendencies but, rather, are primary disorders. They refer to patients "in whom the successful treatment of a profound disturbance of the mother–infant relationship has been followed by prompt recovery from prolonged and treatment resistant depression." The point that needs to be stressed in this quote is that the treatment addresses the *mother–infant relationship* and not the mother alone.

The more recent work by Murray and Cooper (1992; Cooper & Murray, Chapter 8, this volume) on the treatment effects on postpartum depression demonstrated that brief therapies with *mother and infant* improve both the maternal depression and aspects of the infant's developmental progress. It is most important in this research that treatment be addressed to the failing *relationship* between mother and infant and not to the mother alone; moreover, therapeutic results affect both the mother's mood *and* the infant's achievements. These changes suggest that both partners are involved in the clinical condition called postpartum depression which, therefore, could be labeled a "relationship disorder" (Sameroff & Emde, 1985).

My own work (Cramer, 1993) has tested the hypothesis that some postpartum depressions are to be considered a relationship disorder between mother and infant and received confirmatory evidence from two sources: longitudinal research on outcome of brief forms of mother–infant psychotherapies and clinical data. I first briefly review the research data, limiting the review to the study of treatment effects on child and mother when the mother shows depressive features.

MATERNAL DEPRESSION AND BRIEF MOTHER–INFANT PSYCHOTHERAPIES

I present some data of a study* that attempted to evaluate the effects of brief mother–infant psychotherapies (for an exhaustive description of the psychotherapeutic technique, see Cramer & Palacio-Espasa, 1993) on such outcome variables as infant symptoms, maternal representations, and mother–infant interactions. This research evaluated the capacity to predict our prognosis of the therapy as well as the differential effects of two forms of therapy: a psychodynamic psychotherapy and a "here-and-now"–oriented therapy known as interactional guidance (for a description of the research's design and instruments, see Robert-Tissot et al., 1996).

The population consisted of middle-class families with a young child (less than 30 months old) presenting symptoms such as sleep and eating difficulties, behavioral problems, fears, and so on. We excluded from the study children showing pervasive developmental disorders or severe emotional deprivation symptoms. We excluded mothers if they exhibited psychotic features, severe personality disorders, and—important for our topic—*major* depressive disorders.

We evaluated mother and child with various instruments that rated their interactions, emotions, symptoms, and maternal representations before therapy was conducted. We reevaluated them at the end of the therapy and again 6 and 12 months later.

Psychodynamic psychotherapy consisted of formulating a focal conflictual relationship between mother and child and interpreting it in relation to the mother's own past familial conflicts. Interactional guidance consisted of analyzing with the mother video recordings of her play with

*This research was funded by the Swiss National Research Fund No. 3-830.0.86.

the infant. The mother was supported when her interactions proved successful; she was generally encouraged to understand the mechanisms of interactions with her child.

The mean duration of these two treatments was between six and seven sessions. The most significant changes were obtained on symptoms: All functional symptoms (sleep, feeding) improved, separation difficulties diminished; behavioral disorders improved less. Some interactions were modified: Maternal sensitivity to infant's signals increased while intrusive control decreased. Infants became more cooperative, less compulsive-compliant, and showed more happiness. Changes in maternal representations were the least marked; the maternal representation that improved most, however, was the item "self-esteem," which we used as an important marker for the therapeutic effect on depressive mood.

When we tried to establish correlations between these therapy-induced changes and the level of depressive affect in mothers, we were surprised to find that a rather high level of depressive mood was found in our population. We used the Beck Depression Inventory questionnaire to evaluate the self-reports of depressive mood and found that the mothers fell into three groups:

- Thirty-three percent showed no depressive mood (score of 0–7 points).
- Forty-one percent showed mild depressive mood (8–15 points).
- Twenty-six percent showed medium to severe depressive mood (16–32 points).

The mean was 11 points, with a range from 0 to 32. It must be underlined that none of these mothers with high Beck scores presented psychotic depressive disorders; none of them had to be treated with high doses of medication or had been hospitalized.

We present here three items correlated with levels of depressive mood: an infant's symptom (sleep disturbance), an interactive measure (infant distress), and a measure of maternal self-esteem. We found that infants' symptoms (such as sleep disorders) and interactive features (such as infant distress during play episodes) correlated with levels of depressed mood before therapy and ceased to do so after therapy. Maternal self-esteem differed between the three groups before therapy and remained different after therapy, although all showed significant increase.

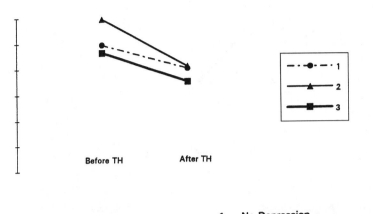

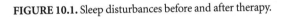

Before Therapy : p. 05
After Therapy : p. ns

1 = No Depression
2 = Mild Depression
3 = Medium to Severe Depression

FIGURE 10.1. Sleep disturbances before and after therapy.

Sleep Disturbances

Infants of depressed mothers in our study often exhibited sleep disorders. Other studies (Guedeney & Kreisler, 1988; Zuckerman, Stevenson, & Bailey, 1987; Murray, 1992) also reported this result. This finding is not specific, however, to maternal depression because sleep disorders occur frequently in a nonclinical population and also represent the most frequent symptom in the overall population of our outcome study. However, we found that sleep disorders diminished after therapy. After therapy, the correlation between the symptom and the level of maternal depressed mood was no longer significant.

It is interesting to note that infants of mothers with mild depressed mood received the highest score on sleep disturbances. This finding corroborates a study by Wrate, Rooney, Thomas, and Cox (1985), which reported a higher incidence of disturbed sleep in children of mildly depressed mothers as compared with those of severely depressed mothers.

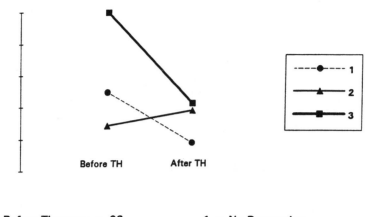

Before Therapy : p. 02   1 = No Depression
After Therapy   : p. ns   2 = Mild Depression
                           3 = Medium to Severe Depression

FIGURE 10.2. Infant distress during interaction before and after therapy.

Infant Distress

Infants of mothers with a medium to severely depressed mood scored much higher on distress during interactions than infants of mothers in the two other groups. After therapy, those differences no longer reached significant levels, with infants showing much lower levels of distress. The therapy seemed to decrease distress levels and influence the association between distress and depressive mood.

Maternal Self-Esteem

Mothers with postpartum depression show more doubts about their maternal competence, as has previously been reported (Gordon et al., 1989; Hopkins, Marcus, & Campbell, 1984; Wrate et al., 1985; Teti & Gelfand, Chapter 6, this volume). Our data indicated that before therapy, there was a significant association between self-esteem levels and the score on the Beck Depression Inventory. As expected, self-esteem was lower in the medium-to-severe depression group. Although therapy significantly raised the levels of self-esteem in the three groups, following treatment a significant relationship remained between self-esteem and depression, with lower self-esteem scores in the medium-to-severe depression group. The improvement in maternal self-esteem provided evidence for the positive effect of therapy on subjective maternal representations.

These data suggest that mother–infant psychotherapies modify in a positive way such symptoms as sleep disturbances and some areas of interactions (e.g., infant distress during interaction). Therapy brings about a decoupling of maternal depressed mood and infant sleep disturbances and distress, and maternal self-esteem is significantly increased. The therapy has not removed the depression completely but has altered it significantly so that it no longer correlates with symptoms and interactions (Luborsky, Crits-Christoph, Mintz, & Auerbach, 1988).

Notably, the greatest improvements were found in the mothers who were most depressed and were rated initially as presenting poor indications for improvement. This corroborates the "law of initial value" effect (or the "ceiling effect") (Luborsky et al., 1988), which proposes that more disturbed patients initially have a greater chance of demonstrating wide variations in improvement than do better adjusted patients.

This greater rate of improvement in mothers who received a "poor indication" score challenges the clinical notion that more depressed mothers necessarily require protracted treatment. It may indicate that the

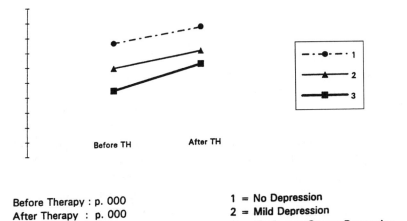

Before Therapy : p. 000
After Therapy : p. 000

1 = No Depression
2 = Mild Depression
3 = Medium to Severe Depression

FIGURE 10.3. Maternal self-esteem before and after therapy.

involvement of the child in conjoint mother–infant therapy has a particularly powerful effect on lifting maternal depressed mood. If this were indeed the case, it would strongly support our hypothesis that a conflictual mother–infant relationship is a determinant stressor contributing to postpartum depression.

These findings suggest that therapy simultaneously improves infant symptoms, characteristics of mother–infant interactions, and maternal subjective feelings. It is impossible to determine which of these comes first: Does the therapeutic effect act first on maternal mood and secondarily on infant symptoms? This theory would follow the model of change in maternal efficiency proposed by Teti and Gelfand (1991). However, it may be that it is a change in the mother's representations of the child that brings the initial therapeutic relief, with interactive strategies and maternal self-esteem secondarily improving.

These findings suggest that we have treated a group of mothers with depressed mood whose depression was intimately linked to the production and maintenance of infant and interactive symptoms, and whose improvement affects the whole mother–infant system. The apparently simultaneous impact of treatment on mother, infant, and mother–infant interactions supports the idea of interrelational pathology explaining at least some common pathologies of infants in the postpartum. What we want to add to this already fairly well known relational theory of infant disorders (Sameroff & Emde, 1985) is that some pathologies of mothers in the postpartum period and, in particular, some forms of postpartum depressions, can also be seen as a relationship disorder. In this approach, it is the relationship of the mother to the infant, and the burden of its care, that would be a major determinant of postpartum depression.

It is important to underline the role of this relational factor as an etiological agent for several reasons. First, it indicates that treatment of some postpartum depression needs to focus on the mother–infant relationship, as has been done in several approaches (Cooper & Murray, Chapter 8, this volume; Cramer, 1993), and not on the mother alone. Second, those postpartum depressions that may be selectively related to motherhood and child caring may turn out to have more adverse effects of infant development (Murray, 1992) than do other forms of postpartum depression linked, for example, to a primary depressive tendency or to strain in the marital relationship. Thus, the *form* of postpartum depression must be considered an important mediating factor in determining and predicting adverse child effects.

Other findings in the outcome study mentioned earlier gave a strong impetus to the clinical impression that child related factors determine some postpartum depressions. First, we were impressed to observe that one-quarter (26%) of mothers in our study showed medium-to-severe depressive mood. These women consulted our child guidance clinic for symptoms *in their infants,* not for their depression, and it was only through our evaluation that we found the high level of depressive mood. This suggested that concern over the infant is linked to depressive affect and that, indeed, these child-oriented anxieties may be an important correlate to postpartum depression.

The fact that the treatment was brief further strengthened the relational factor theory in postpartum depression. Our therapeutic interventions consisted of, on average, six to seven 1-hour sessions. The fact that such brief interventions could bring a marked improvement in maternal self-esteem and in other representations of the mother as an efficient maternal agent was baffling because standard treatment of depression is generally longer. Although we cannot claim that brief mother–infant psychotherapy *cured* maternal depression, we were impressed to see the rapid improvement in the maternal subjective state. Not only did self-esteem increase, but after treatment, the mothers represented themselves as having significantly improved in a number of dimensions: They saw themselves as calmer, easier, and more affectionate, trustful, and good looking. They also perceived the child as more trustful, easier, and more independent. This illustrates that rather wide changes in the mother's perception of herself and of her child can be achieved with this brief form of treatment. Moreover, some interactive parameters also changed significantly, which surprised us as interactions are usually quite resistant to change.

We were impressed to observe—when we evaluated the amplitude of improvement correlated with our initial prognosis—that the dyads with the most depressed mothers were those that showed the greatest improvement. This suggests we were dealing with a special form of depression, characterized by a strong reactive factor linked to caring for a young infant. Our treatment selectively focused on issues of mother–infant relationships and improvement was obtained when the attendant conflict was resolved.

Clinical Configuration

When we turn to the *content* of what the therapy of these mothers and infants revealed, we can best grasp the links between depression and the conflicts involved in dealing with a younger infant. The type of therapy referred to in the following development is psychodynamic. Although we did not find that psychodynamic therapy brought about greater improvement than another variety of noninterpretative therapy (interactional guidance), and although the specific ingredients bringing about change have not been, as yet, teased out, the psychodynamic framework is particularly useful in shedding light on the psychological processes at work in the subjective experience linked to various psychopathologies. Moreover, in cases of conflictual mother–infant relationships in the postpartum period, there is a particular expressiveness of mental contents that is not found at other times. This increased access to consciousness of contents that, usually, remain hidden enhances understanding of underlying process. This seems to be a specific feature of psychological functioning in the postpartum period, as other clinicians have noted (Bibring, Dwyer, Huntington, & Valenstein, 1961; Blos, 1985; Bydlowski, 1991) and is enhanced by the presence of the infant in the psychotherapy process. Fraiberg (1980) referred to this process of increased expressiveness, noting that the infant acts as a catalyst, enhancing representations and affects in mothers and mobilizing links with their own infantile experiences. Our clinical experience has taught us that what Winnicott (1969) called "primary maternal preoccupation" affects maternal psychological functioning in profound ways, with a peak in the first months after birth but with continuing influences over a longer period (up to 15 or 20 months) than has been generally recognized (Lyons-Ruth, Zoll, Connell, & Grunebaum, 1986).

Meaning Attributions and Projective Identifications

The most striking and ubiquitous feature of maternal functioning in this prolonged postpartum period is referred to as meaning attribution, which corresponds—in the psychodynamic literature—to the process of projective identification. New parents (and this is stronger in mothers than in fathers) inject meanings into all the attributes and attitudes of the infant. These meanings are shaped by the parents' own store of representations and feelings about basic issues (e.g., gender, aggression and affection, activity and passivity, dependency and separation, pleasure-seeking activities, feeding, sleeping, and motor activity).

These processes are called projective identifications (Sandler, 1987) because they are simultaneously based on identification (the mother "sees" her own attributes or tendencies in the baby, thus identifying the baby with herself) and projections (the mother externalizes on to the baby—by projection—that which really belongs to her own mental contents). Through this process, the mother creates familiarity with the newcomer who is her baby. She thus introduces the baby to her own interpretations of basic life issues. But in so doing she also lends to the child motivations and anxieties with which she has to cope within herself. She thus transmits to the infant intentions that may be problematic or conflictual for her. This process of meaning attribution is so powerful that it creates a sense of conviction that the infant, indeed, harbors these intentions that were—primarily—hers.

Secondarily, the mother reacts to the infant as if indeed he or she has intentions that have, in fact, their origins in the mother's store of unwanted motivations. She then defends herself against the anxiety provoked by the activation in the child of forbidden or dangerous tendencies by the formation of counterattitudes. It is at this juncture that the role of interactions becomes crucial. What was—so far—a forbidden mental content in the mother is now projected onto the child, and the mother attempts to curb these tendencies by initiating counteractions, expressed in the form taken by interactions. Some forms of infant anorexia provide a good example. In the first months, an infant might show head aversion when offered food. The mother insists, to the point of becoming intrusive, which leads to the common form of oppositional anorexia seen frequently in the second semester. When the dyad is seen in joint psychotherapy, the therapist uncovers a hidden scenario that determines the failure of feeding interactions. For various reasons, related to her conflicts over food and over the control of bodily needs, the mother unconsciously impedes the infant's free expression of appetite and subtly interferes with its alimentary initiative. This is done through interactive tactics that are unknown to the mother, and which can be best detected during frame-by-frame analysis of video recording of feeding interactions. The therapist can then objectify microepisodes of enacted forbidding by the mother of the infant's alimentary initiatives. Although the mother complains about the child's lack of appetite, the interactions reveal that she hinders the free expression of hunger needs in the child.

The impact of therapy occurs at three levels. First, the clinician must determine the nature of the symptom and confront the mother with her own conflict over eating, as it is transferred onto the child. The role of projective identification must be revealed, and the mother must see that she transfers onto the child unbridled tendencies such as, for example, to eat voraciously. Second, the therapist must try to detect examples of the enactment of maternal inhibitions of the child's eating initiative and of *his* or *her* signs of appetite. The therapist then establishes a link between these failed interactions and the corresponding mental conflict in the mother. The third level consists of establishing links between the *present* conflict between mother and child and corresponding *past* conflicts in the mother's own history.

Technical Factors

An exhaustive discussion of therapeutic technique in brief mother–infant psychotherapy is not the object of this chapter (for such a discussion, see Cramer & Palacio-Espasa, 1993). I present only two technical aspects here, briefly, as they have a bearing on the conditions for the feasibility of such therapies. Brief mother–infant therapies can bring meaningful improvement of symptoms, interactions, and maternal representations when two conditions are met; namely, the achievement of a therapeutic focus in the first sessions and the achievement of a positive working alliance.

Therapeutic Focus

In brief therapies, the early identification of a focus is an essential prerequisite (Strupp & Binder, 1984). The focus consists of a constellation made up of anxieties, modes of relationships, and defensive maneuvers typical for an individual. It is repetitive and compulsive, and although the patient is capable of describing this constellation, he or she is not aware of all its components. This central constellation has been studied in psychotherapy research. Its best known illustration is found under the term "core conflictual relationship theme" (CCRT) in the work of Luborsky and associates (Luborsky et al., 1988). In mother–infant therapies this focus consists of maternal conflicts enacted in the relationship with the child. It is revealed by the nature of the child's main symptom, by corresponding conflicts in the mother and projections onto the child, and attendant symptomatic interactions between the two. There are two principal reasons why there is a need to determine the details of this central configuration. First, the definition by therapist and mother of this focus early in the treatment is essential—as a working model—to achieve a dynamization of the therapeutic process, bringing about change in a brief period. In an ongoing study of the process of these therapies, we found that such a focus was determined within the *first* session in about 75% of the cases. When we evaluated the mother's understanding of and adhesion to this focus, we found that they reached the same level as the therapist during the third session (Cramer et al., 1994). Such a high level of achievement of patient–therapist consensus in early phases of treatment is unusual and seems to be a feature specific to mother–infant therapies. Second, it is the study of this focus that reveals the nature of conflicts, painful affects, and defenses that characterize the types of postpartum depression that can be dealt with in such a format.

Working Alliance

This concept refers to the active collaboration by the mother with the therapist's efforts. Mothers in fact demonstrate an active interest in understanding the problems and evince a minimum resistance to the therapist's probing and confrontations. Mothers develop this participation within an atmosphere of positive attachment to the therapist (Bordin, 1979). As with the determination of an early focus, most mothers adhere to treatment in a positive and collaborative way, and resistances were evaluated as generally low (Cramer et al., 1994).

These data on the early determination of the focus and on a working alliance confirm a clinical impression found among workers in the field of early interventions; that is, during the early phases of mother–infant attachment, there is an unusually high level of openness to insight and motivation for change. This is found in mothers with various forms of psychopathology and with varying levels of depression.

PSYCHOLOGICAL CONFIGURATIONS IN CASES OF POSTPARTUM DEPRESSIONS

Contents found when mothers are depressed tend to focus on a certain number of basic issues.

Guilt

In our outcome study, we found that before therapy, guilt was associated with the level of depression. The mothers with no depressed mood had low guilt scores; those with mild depressed mood had intermediate guilt scores, whereas those with medium to severe depressed mood had the highest guilt scores. Data were obtained with a questionnaire evaluating various feelings and representations in mothers. The maternal representation interview (Stern, Robert-Tissot, De Muralt, & Cramer, 1989) consists of open-ended questions completed in an evaluation by the mother of her feelings on a bipolar scale. We were not surprised to find particularly high levels of guilt in the most depressed group, as guilt about childrearing is typical in postpartum depressions (Campbell, Cohn, Flanagan, Popper, & Meyers, 1992). Of particular interest here is that the questionnaire addresses the topic of guilt in terms of feelings the mother has *about the child*. The content of guilt in these depressed mothers is primarily determined by a feeling of doing harm to the child, as we see in clinical reports from three mothers with postpartum depression.

Clinical Illustrations

Guilt is easily detected in the following three mothers, each of whom felt she had harmed her baby. Ms. F felt very concerned that she might have permanently damaged her child's development when she decided to go back to work, when Delia, her baby girl, was 5 months old. Ms. P explained that she developed fears of "causing his permanent misery" right after her son's birth. Ms. T was extremely concerned that she might crush her son if she were to impose any limits on him. She would feel like a torturer and berated herself that she caused his state of vulnerability and weakness (birthweight: 4½ pounds, or 2,090 grams).

At the level of interactions, the effects of such guilt are illustrated in characteristic ways. The mother cannot bear to frustrate the infant. She submits to all his demands, running to him several times at night whenever he emits a noise, bending backwards to fulfill all his wishes, and never imposing any discipline. Secondarily, this contributes to the creation of a tyrannical child, who rules his parents and drives them to exhaustion. Depressive feelings develop further, as the mother becomes increasingly angry at the child's selfish demands while not being able to express her resentment, which is experienced as potentially damaging to the child.

Corresponding infantile conflicts are revealed in her own past. Ms. F experienced intense rivalry with her sister and brother, whom she perceived as more successful than herself. This was reported (or transferred) onto her daughter who became, in turn, her rival. She left her daughter to go back to work, to become professionally successful in a belated attempt to compete with her siblings. Ms. P had always envied boys and would have preferred to be a man. She berated her son, who "forced" her to act as a woman and mother, just as she had hated her own father who treated her in a domineering way and who considered her "inferior" because she was a girl. Ms. T experienced her son as an inflexible ruler who imposed his will on her, just as, in her childhood, her paranoid mother imposed unyielding control over her.

These three mothers showed depressive symptoms since the birth of their own child, or in the early postpartum months and guilt was a major component of their depression. In many depressive disorders in the postpartum period, guilt over conscious wishes to harm or kill the baby becomes a major source of maternal suffering.

Low Self-Esteem and Incompetence

We saw earlier that the lowest scores of self-esteem were found in the mothers with the highest levels of depression. One component of self-esteem in the mother is her sense of self-efficacy or competence in dealing with the child. It seems that maternal self-efficacy correlates with maternal competence, perception of infant difficulties, and maternal depression. Maternal self-efficacy has been found to be extremely low among depressed mothers who perceive their infants as difficult (Teti & Gelfand, 1991). Maternal sense of efficacy is thus particularly important to evaluate as it mediates actual competence in parenting. This item is one of the most promising candidates when we try to determine the mediating effects of maternal depression on children, because a sense of poor self-efficacy in dealing with the child is frequently found in postpartum depressions.

Ms. F described herself as so anxiety-ridden that she could not deal coherently with her daughter's needs. She anxiously ran around after her, in constant anguish that she would do something wrong with her. Ms. P cried bitterly when she explained that she would have loved to give her son a better image of what a mother ought to be. She actually apologized to her 2-year-old son for not being more joyful and fun. Ms. T felt totally incompetent in dealing with her 16-month-old boy. He intimidated her so that she spent her time running around after him and trying to satisfy all his demands. She could never initiate an interaction, as she let him overrule her. This made her feel very weak.

At the *level of interactions*, this is illustrated by tentativeness of maternal attitudes and incoherence in educative strategies. Corresponding infantile conflicts are revealed in their own past. Thus, Ms. F had a gnawing sense of incompetence in her childhood, critically linked to a sense of inferiority in relation to her siblings and to a feeling that she never paid back her parents for the sacrifices they went through in order to procure her a good education. Ms. P's sense of incompetence was selectively linked to her conviction that she would have been a more valuable person had she been a man. Ms. T's sense of incompetence had its roots in a lack of achievement of autonomy, as she had submitted to her mother's rigid rule.

The sense of maternal incompetence was particularly painful for these women. One of the main effects of the psychotherapy on the mothers was to achieve an awareness of competent patterns in interactions with the child. What evolved generally was a new representation of the child seen then as more cooperative and more friendly. We interpreted the significant increase in self-esteem found at posttreatment evaluations as related to a lessening of projections of negative images on to the child and as revealing a renewed confidence in dealing with it.

The Infant as a Drain and Hindrance

Popular imagery represents new mothers as overwhelmed with joy after birth and extremely gratified by the care of the baby. Several sources have questioned the pertinence of this idealized version of mother–infant relationships. Pioneers in the feminist movement were among the first to critically evaluate the characteristics of devotion, altruism, and sacrifice which had been the cornerstones of mothering (Friedan, 1963; Rich, 1979; Mitchell, 1971). A longitudinal study by Cowan and Cowan (1992) on becoming parents revealed a consistent finding of disenchantment with marriage in young parents and that 20% to 30% of them reported enough symptoms to be at risk for clinical depression during their children's early years. The high rate of divorce among parents whose first child is less than 18 months old reveals the burden that the arrival of a child can place on the woman and on the parental couple.

Among the most important factors implicated in this "deflation" are the increased frustrations, responsibilities, and efforts the newborn imposes on the parents, foremost on the mother. Many mothers in our clinical study, especially in the more depressed group, complained that the infant drained them of energy and absorbed them so thoroughly that they no longer had space and time for the pursuit of their own achievements. Mothers experienced their infants as making them prisoners of the infants' needs and wishes. In feminist writings, the woman goes from one form of submission (to patriarchal order) to another form of submission (to the child). The woman then sees the infant as a hindrance in her quest for self-achievements, as a tyrannical ruler whose care forbids women to pursue personal quests. Women experience this feeling particularly strongly when they have had to interrupt their career to take care of the baby. Because most women nowadays have entered the work force (in France, more than 75% of women with young children work), this problem of competition between mothering and career achievement has created a built-in conflict with which our society confronts women. It is a source of ambivalence and conflict for many mothers.

Ms. F gives an excellent illustration of this antagonism between the two roles and functions (i.e., mothering and working). She explained that children absorb mothers so much that this can bring about a total annihilation of the woman's identity. This fear prompted Ms. F to go back to work: "I had to go back to work. When you just take care of children at home, you become useless. You lose yourself. You are *nobody.*" When her daughter was 5 months old, Ms. F went back to work half-time but then developed intense guilt at leaving her child, fearing that she would damage her daughter forever. The result was that Ms. F felt too guilty at work to concentrate adequately on her task and resentful toward her child who "absorbed" Ms. F when she took care of her. This conflict became insurmountable. Ms. F felt that she had become incompetent in both domains simultaneously and so resented her daughter. She soon became depressed, with a powerful sense of helplessness in her attempts to resolve this conflict.

Ms. P was quite adamant in claiming that having a child is like falling into a trap because of the tasks imposed by mothering. She berated her son for having imprisoned her, saying: "When he was born, I knew I had taken a 20-year sentence." She felt that giving birth had trapped her into the constraint of a maternal identity, with such attendant chores as feeding, cleaning, and changing the baby. To Ms. P, this entailed a devalued representation of "woman at home," while hindering the continued development of intellectual pursuits.

Ms. T was the most articulate in claiming that her child (a 16-month-old boy) totally ruled her. She was convinced she had to submit to all his demands, which excluded any possibility of finding alternative activities.

It was as if Ms. T had abandoned all personal will while becoming the slave of her child.

In *interactions*, these mothers are striking in their excessiveness in submitting to their child's demands to the point of total exhaustion. Simultaneously, they powerfully resent the child's rule and have to develop a series of defensive maneuvers to protect themselves against the awareness of a real hatred of their child. This conflict makes an important contribution to depression. The mothers feel compelled to exert a particularly vigilant overprotectiveness toward the child; at the same time, they resent having to act in such an altruistic way, sacrificing themselves for an infant they represent as totally selfish and domineering. This tension between simultaneous hatred of the child and selfless caring for him ends up producing a feeling of powerlessness and pent-up rage that contributes to depression.

These women's past *histories* reveal that the tyrannical baby represents either a hated sibling rival in their childhood or images of themselves as demanding babies who exhausted their own mothers. They project now onto their child representations of this demanding, selfish baby and identify with their own exploited mothers, which fosters an identity of the suffering, self-sacrificing mothers of popular imagery. This image is nowadays devalued compared with that of the "new" woman, engaged in professional and economic pursuits rather than exclusively maternal tasks. The inflation of this devalued representation of an exploited mother contributes to depressed mood.

Identity Problems

The social definition and representations of mothering have changed, contributing to a conflict between "old" and "modern" images of mothering, that is, between an identity centered on mothering essentially—as in former traditions—and a more composite identity where women want to root their functioning in extrafamilial activities as well. Women have particularly felt this change since the 1960s. Three main factors played a role in this transmutation: the introduction of contraceptives, which placed women in charge of their body and fertility; the massive entry of women in the working and economic field; and the change in traditional distribution of roles according to gender.

In terms of the subjective experience of women becoming mothers, these factors have had a profound but not yet quite acknowledged influence on popular representations of mothering. One of the consequences of this shift is that many women can no longer mold themselves in the maternal role handed down by their mothers. They need to take distance from a sometimes despised model of womanhood based essentially on domestic functions. This need contributes to an identity crisis that often emerges in the postpartum period. In terms of predisposing factors to depression, the lack of support from an easy identification with the woman's own mother's role contributes to a sense of weakness and loneliness. This failure of a solid, trusted mothering model is particularly strong in women who experienced intense conflicts with their mothers and who harbor strong criticisms and contempt for their maternal image. When they in turn become mothers, they suffer from the lack of a firm model; at the same time, they fear that they might turn out to resemble, against their better judgment, the mother they devalued.

Ms. T strongly rejected the image of her own mother who was overly controlling and strict. She wanted to be exactly the opposite with her son but broke down when she realized that in having to force-feed her boy, who presented a severe oppositional anorexia, she—too—was becoming an intrusive, domineering mother. She expressed in dramatic ways how much she needed to deidentify with her own mother, saying: "I don't have one common feature with my mother. It is as if this person had been imposed on me."

Ms. P experienced this challenge to her identity in a different way. She experienced mothering as an external constraint that forced her to submit to a standard feminine role, which she found debasing. Mothering forced her to accept her feminine condition which, so far, she had been able to deny. It was not only the identification with her mother that she thereby rejected but an overall identification with women. Depression set in when she realized that she was trapped, in spite of herself, in a feminine role because the birth of the child forced her to acknowledge her womanhood.

Ms. F wanted to be mother only "half-time" to protect herself against the dangers of being totally sucked in by domestic chores, as her own mother had been. She needed to continue her professional career so as not to remain an educationless housewife as her immigrant mother had been.

This conflict between two representations of personal identity is a debilitating factor that brings about doubts about the definition of the self and a sense of incompetence in mothering tasks. As such, it contributes to depressive feelings.

In addition to this identity conflict with her own mother, the new mother's sense of identity may also be threatened by her own identification with the baby (Pines, 1982). We can define some of the most crucial rearrangements of psychological structures of mothers giving birth as determined by these various challenges to what they experienced—until then—as a solid identity.

CONCLUSION

Nosology and Etiology

There are different forms of postpartum depressions. In some cases postpartum depression is just one episode among several depressive breakdowns in a woman showing a tendency for depression. In these depressions, birth does not seem to act as a specific factor. There is a similar lack of specificity of birth-related factor in situations with high levels of socioeconomic stressors. In SES high-risk groups, the birth of a baby seems to be just one additional factor in a situation in which depressive features show generally a high incidence (Lyons-Ruth et al., 1986, reported up to 64% of depression among such high-risk groups; Celia, Alves, Behs, Nudelman, & Saraiva, 1992, in Brazil, have reported that 100% of a high-risk group of young mothers living in *favellas* experience depressive symptoms). I have argued that there is a group of postpartum depressions in which the transition to parenthood and the burden of caring for a child act as a specific destabilizing life event with the attendant emergence of several psychological conflicts. It seems as if in different forms of postpartum depression, some etiological agents appear more on the forefront either because of attendant determinants (e.g., SES levels) or because of the methodology used in the research. Obvious, easy-to-objectify codeterminants (e.g., economic factors or clear marital strain) may appear to correlate highly with postpartum depression in large epidemiological studies, whereas more fine-grained, subjective data such as mother–infant psychological conflicts do not reach significant levels due to their elusive nature when rating scales or questionnaires only are being used. When studies based on psychotherapeutic treatments are used as the basic framework (Murray & Cooper, 1992; Cramer et al., 1990), issues related to mother–infant conflicts and maternal subjective experiences may appear with more force.

My studies focused on mothers showing disturbed relationships with a symptomatic infant and on cases in which I did not find *major* depressive disorders. This restricts the generalization of findings to *all* forms of postpartum depression. Thus, I do not present my findings as excluding other etiological factors, such as possible biological changes or socioeconomic and maternal stressors that are prominent in epidemiological studies.

Transition to Parenthood

Becoming a parent has long been considered a form of upheaval or crisis that most often fosters attachment to the newborn but may also lead to pathology. I presented data testing the hypothesis that in this transition, conflicts, feelings, and interactions link mother and child in various forms of symptoms best described as a relational pathology. Although this does not preclude the role of intrinsic preexisting pathologies in the mother and the baby, it brings into focus the respective contribution of mother and infant in the development of symptoms in the dyad during an extended postpartum period. Although relational pathology has been used mainly to define infant pathology, I find it useful to adhere to this concept to describe some forms of depressive breakdowns in mothers.

A mother has to deal with many psychological tasks in the postpartum period. She has to adapt to a real baby while she maintained a relation to the imagined baby during pregnancy. From being her mother's daughter, she has to develop an identity as mother of her own child. From creating a dyad with her husband, she has to adapt to a threesome.

The most crucial change is caused by the demands made on the mother by the newborn. The baby's demands are enormous compared with those involved in usual social intercourse. Babies foster a state of continuous preoccupation and forced altruism, which may be experienced as selfish tyranny, entrapping the mother to the point where she may feel totally drained. She may abandon all care for herself to the point of neglecting her own basic needs.

This constellation of psychological stressors brings all sorts of dormant aspirations and frustrations to the fore. Moreover, babies trigger a powerful process of projections in which they are imbued with all sorts of intentions. If negative intentions are predominant, the baby will be perceived as hostile, utterly selfish, and omnipotent. Those factors may bring about the types of relational conflicts illustrated here by the clinical vignettes. The mother then compensates for her disappointments and converts anger into an exaggerated solicitude, with the attendant feelings of guilt, anxiety, and low self-esteem. It is at this point that depressive developments occur.

Implications for Treatment

In the cases of postpartum depression in which this conflictual relationship has developed with the baby, it is the mother–infant relationship that needs to be treated. The presence of the baby is useful in several ways:

- It concentrates the mother's brooding and anxious concerns on the relationship to the baby.
- It allows for the expression—in the joint session—of symptomatic mother-baby interactions. These interactions can then be interpreted in terms of maternal conflicts.
- It allows for an illustration of the mother's distorted perception of the infant.

When maternal conflicts are clarified and the attendant failing interactions are understood, the baby is perceived differently (as I have demonstrated with the modification of representations of the infant after therapy): from frustrating he becomes gratifying; from a partner in failing interactions, he becomes a new source of maternal competence.

When this is the case, the baby him- or herself can be seen as a powerful therapeutic partner, correcting feelings of inefficacy and low self-esteem.

In cases of postpartum depression, this form of therapy was efficient in lifting depressive features and self-esteem when representations of the child became more positive (i.e., less contaminated by negative projections) and when attendant distorted interactions were modified.

Although brief forms of conjoint mother–infant psychotherapies are usually not indicated for the very severe forms of depression or when major economic and marital stressors predominate, it may be very helpful to deal with issues related to child care and to the conflicts of transition to parenthood in most cases of postpartum depression.

REFERENCES

Bibring, G., Dwyer, T. F., Huntington, D. S., & Valenstein, A. F. (1961). A study of psychological processes in pregnancy of the earliest mother–child relationship. *Psychoanalytic Study of the Child, 16,* 9–27.

Blos, P. J. (1985). Intergenerational separation–individuation. Treating the mother–infant pair. *Psychoanalytic Study of the Child, 40,* 41–56.

Bordin, E. S. (1979). The generalisability of the psychoanalytic concept of the working alliance. *Psychotherapy: Theory, Research and Practice, 16,* 252–260.

Brockington, I. F. (1992). Disorders specific to the puerperium. *International Journal of Mental Health, 21*(2), 41–52.

Brockington, I., & Cox-Roper, A. (1988). The nosology of puerperal mental illness. In R. Kumar & I. F. Brockington (Eds.), *Motherhood and mental illness* (Vol. 2, pp. 1–16). London: Butterworth.

Bydlowski, M. (1991). La transparence psychique de la grossesse. *Etudes Freudiennes, 32,* 135–142.

Campbell, S. B., Cohn, J. F., Flanagan, C., Popper, S., & Meyers, T. (1992). Course and correlates of postpartum depression during the transition to parenthood. *Development and Psychopathology, 4,* 29–47.

Celia, S., Alves, M. O., Behs, B., Nudelman, C., & Saraiva, J. (1992, May). *A strategy on primary prevention. Vida Centro-Humanistico. A community experience in bond formation.* Paper presented at the IACAPAP meeting, Budapest.

Cooper, P. J., Murray, L., & Stein, A. (1991). Postnatal depression. In J. Seva (Ed.), *European handbook of psychiatry* (pp. 1255–1262). Zaragosa, Spain: Anthropos.

Cowan, C. P., & Cowan P. A. (1992). *When partners become parents.* New York: Basic Books.

Cramer, B. (1993). Are postpartum depressions a mother–infant relationship disorder? *Infant Mental Health Journal, 14*(4), 283–297.

Cramer, B., & Palacio-Espasa, F. (1993). *La pratique des psychothérapies mères-bébés.* Paris: Presses Universitaires de France.

Cramer, B., Robert-Tissot, C., Rusconi Serpa, S., Pous, O., Favez, N., Palacio-Espasa, F., Bachman, J. P., Knauer, D., & Berney, C. (1994). *Processus et changements dans les psychothérapies mère–bébé: Foyer, alliance et interventions thérapeutiques.* Final report, FNRS no. 32-31323.91.

Cramer, B., Robert-Tissot, C., Stern, D. N., Serpa Rusconi, S., De Muralt, M., Besson, G., Palacio-Espasa, F., Bachmann, J. P., Knauer, D., Berney, C., & D'Arcis, U. (1990). Outcome evaluation in brief mother–infant psychotherapy: A preliminary report. *Infant Mental Health Journal, 11,* 278–300.

Fraiberg, S. (1980). *Clinical studies in infant mental health: The first year of life.* New York: Basic Books.

Friedan, B. (1963). *The feminine mystique.* New York: Norton.

Gordon, D., Burge, D., Hammer, C., Adrian, C., Jaenicke, C., & Hiroto, D. (1989). Observations of interactions of depressed women with their children. *American Journal of Psychiatry, 146,* 50–55.

Gruen, D. (1993). A group psychotherapy approach to postpartum depression. *International Journal of Group Psychotherapy, 43*(2), 191–203.

Guedeney, A., & Kreisler, L. (1988). Troubles sévères du sommeil dans les 18 premiers mois de la vie. In B. Cramer (Ed.), *Psychiatrie du bébé* (pp. 431–450). Paris: Eshel.

Halberstadt-Freud, H. C. (1993). Postpartum depression and symbiotic illusion. *Psychoanalytic Psychology, 10*(3), 407–423.

Hopkins, J., Campbell, S. B., & Marens, M. (1987). The role of infant related stressors in postpartum depression. *Journal of Abnormal Psychology, 96*(3), 237–241.

Hopkins, J., Marcus, M., & Campbell, S. B. (1984). Postpartum depression: A critical review. *Psychological Bulletin, 95*(3), 498–515.

Luborsky, L., Crits-Christoph, P., Mintz, I., & Auerbach, A. (1988). *Who will benefit from psychotherapy? Predicting therapeutic outcomes.* New York: Basic Books.

Lyons-Ruth, K., Zoll, D., Connell, D., & Grunebaum, H. V. (1986). The depressed mother and her one year old infant. In T. Field & E. Tronick (Eds.), *Maternal depression and child disturbance* (New Directions for Child Development, No. 34, pp. 31–46). San Francisco: Jossey-Bass.

Mitchell, J. (1971). *Women's estate.* New York: Random House.

Murray, L. (1989). Childbirth as a life event: The Cambridge study of postnatal depression and infant development. In J. Cox & E. S. Paykel (Eds.), *Life events and postpartum psychiatric disorders* (pp. 23–37). Southampton, England: Southampton University Press.

Murray, L. (1992). The impact of postnatal depression on infant development. *Journal of Child Psychology and Psychiatry, 33*(3), 543–561.

Murray, L., & Cooper, P. J. (1992). *The impact of postnatal depression on infant development. A naturalistic study.* Paper presented at the WAIPAD Fifth World Congress, Chicago.

Pines, D. (1982). The relevance of early psychic development to pregnancy and abortion. *International Journal of Psychoanalysis, 63,* 311–319.

Rich, A. (1979). *Of woman born.* New York: Norton.

Robert-Tissot, C., Cramer, B., Stern, D. N., Rusconi-Serpa, S., Bachmann, J. P., Palacio-Espasa, F., Knauer, D., De Muralt, M., Berney, C., & Mendiguren, G. (1996). Outcome evaluation in brief mother–infant psychotherapies: Report on 75 cases. *Infant Mental Health Journal, 17*(2), 97–114.

Sameroff, A., & Emde, R. (1985). *Relationship disturbances in early childhood: A developmental approach.* New York: Basic Books.

Sandler, J. (1987). *Projection, identification, projective identification.* London: Karnac Books.

Stern, D. N., Robert-Tissot, C., De Muralt, M., & Cramer, B. (1989). Le KIA-Profil: Un instrument de recherche clinique pour l'évaluation des états affectifs du jeune enfant. In S. Lebovici, P. Mazet, & J. P. Visier (Eds.), *L'évaluation des interactions précoces entre le bébé et ses partenaires* (pp. 131–149). Paris: Eshel.

Strupp, H. H., & Binder, J. L. (1984). *Psychotherapy in a new key.* New York: Basic Books.

Teti, D. M., & Gelfand, D. M. (1991). Behavioral competence among mothers of infants in the first year: The mediational role of maternal self-efficacy. *Child Development, 62*(5), 918–929.

Trout, M. (1991). Perinatal depression in four women reared by borderline mothers. *Pre and Peri Natal Psychology Journal, 5*(4), 297–325.

Winnicott, D. (1969). *De la pédiatrie à la psychanalyse.* Paris: Payot.

Wrate, R. M., Rooney, A. C., Thomas, P. F., & Cox, J. (1985). Postnatal depression and child development. A three year follow-up study. *British Journal of Psychiatry, 146,* 622–627.

Zuckerman, B., Stevenson, J., & Bailey, V. (1987). Sleep problems in early childhood: Continuities, predictive factors, and behavioral correlates. *Paediatrics, 80,* 664–671.

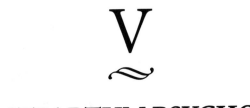

POSTPARTUM PSYCHOSIS

11

⁓

The Impact of Postpartum Affective Psychosis on the Child

Alison E. Hipwell
University of Cambridge

R. Channi Kumar
University of London

The past decade has seen growing recognition of possible adverse sequelae in infants of mothers suffering from nonpsychotic postnatal depressive disorder (see reviews by Rutter, 1990; Murray, 1992; Cummings & Davies, 1994). In contrast to this body of evidence, there have been few analogous investigations of the impact on infants of maternal affective psychotic illnesses. Although postpartum affective psychosis is 100 times rarer than nonpsychotic depression in the postnatal period (the latter has generally been found to occur after 10% of live births; see review by Kumar, 1994), its incidence is, nevertheless, markedly and significantly raised following childbirth (Kendell, Chalmers, & Platz, 1987). The fact that year after year about 1 in every 1,000 new mothers is afflicted with a severe and often unexpected episode of mental illness merits attention. Few systematic investigations have been made of the precise nature of the impact of maternal affective psychosis on the developing child and little is known about either immediate or longer-term effects. In terms of the mediation of any effects on the infant, the quality of caregiving among psychotic mothers has generally been described as disorganized, insensitive, and/or erratic (e.g., Gochman, 1985; Margison, 1990), but there are many possible indirect effects of such an illness that must also be taken into account.

Cases of infanticide provide the most extreme example of the adverse consequences of severe maternal mental illness for the young child. The law of England and Wales (Infanticide Act, 1938) explicitly recognizes that infants may have been fatally "at risk" because the mother's balance of mind was, at the time, disturbed "by reason of childbirth or lactation." The origins of this legislation can be traced back to cases of infant homicide occurring in the context of maternal postpartum affective psychosis (see Kumar & Marks, 1992). Fortunately, cases of infant homicide are relatively rare (Marks & Kumar, 1993) and in most instances occur in the context of depression or personality disorder (D'Orban, 1979; Marks & Kumar, 1995). There is no comparable information available about the prevalence of non-fatal cases of harm to infants through impulse or neglect, and the general questions that must be addressed are as follows: What are the consequences for infants' psychological, social, and physical development of the presence of maternal severe depression, or of a severe, acute, and florid affective psychosis, during the first few months of the child's life? Are there adverse sequelae that can be linked to particular features of maternal psychopathology (e.g., its nature, severity, timing and duration)?

Any evaluation of outcome in infants of psychotic mothers is likely to be confounded by a variety of such other factors as possible comorbid conditions in the mother, including mental impairment, personality disorder, and substance abuse, as well as her personal, family, marital, and social circumstances and, of course, the characteristics and health of the baby. In the case of postpartum affective psychosis, other important factors include the nature of the treatment that may have been provided and the circumstances of the mother's hospitalization, if any. Was her admission separate from, or jointly with, the infant? What was the quality of the milieu into which they were jointly admitted, or, if they were separated, who looked after the baby and how? What was the extent and nature of the contact between mother and baby during the illness?

Postpartum psychosis typically has an excellent short- to medium-term outcome, with most mothers being able to leave hospital after about 2 months (Kumar, Marks, Platz, & Yoshida, 1995) although it may take up to a year before they feel fully recovered (Hipwell, 1992). The illnesses therefore permit us to examine the consequences for infants of early and largely limited perturbations of the mother–infant relationship in terms of the nature of the mother's condition and its time course. The findings of research may help to improve the provision of clinical services and they may also, by looking for possible sequelae of the illness for the infant, shed some light on normal developmental processes. In the relevant research to date, small sample sizes and methodological disparity have limited the generalizability of findings. This review attempts to uncover the emerging picture of effects while highlighting questions about methodology that must be considered in any future research.

The topics reviewed are as follows: (1) nature of the exposure of the infant to psychotic symptoms in the mother, (2) timing of onset and duration of symptoms (i.e., the impact according to the developmental stage of the child), (3) nature of psychiatric treatment and management (i.e., the impact on the infant of continuous contact with or separation from mother, and substitute caregiving), (4) familial and social factors, (5) nature of the assessment of the child, and (6) characteristics of the child.

NATURE OF THE EXPOSURE OF THE INFANT TO PSYCHOTIC SYMPTOMS IN THE MOTHER

Studies of postnatally depressed mothers have highlighted the ways in which depression may influence their interactions with their infants, ranging from withdrawal and apathy, including reduced levels of reciprocity, consistency, dialogue, and proactive behavior, to overt hostility and intrusiveness (e.g., Cohn, Campbell, Matias, & Hopkins, 1990; Cohn, Matias, Tronick, Connell, & Lyons-Ruth, 1986; Field, 1987; Field, Healy, Goldstein, & Guthertz, 1990; Fleming, Ruble, Flett, & Shaul, 1988; Murray, 1992; Murray, Fiori-Cowley, Hooper, & Cooper, 1996; Pound, Cox, Puckering, & Mills, 1985). However, not every depressed mother behaves in such ways, and investigators increasingly recognize that a clinical diagnosis of major or minor (nonpsychotic) depression does not automatically warrant concern about parenting quality. Some recent studies have suggested that it is the interaction of depression with other factors, such as a history of poor parenting, marital friction, or more general characteristics of vulnerability, that may be more pertinent to difficulties in parenting than depression alone (e.g., Murray, 1992; Murray, Hipwell, Hooper, Stein, & Cooper, 1996; Stein et al., 1991; Kumar, in press).

There is reason to believe that a similarly diverse range of parenting behaviors may also exist among adults with a psychotic illness in the puerperium. In addition, it is possible that differences in the quality of parenting may reflect different categories or phases of maternal psychopathology. Thus, within individuals there may be extreme variability. For example, during an episode of bipolar illness, mothers may experience rapid and unpredictable mood swings, periods of severe depression, and/or periods of mania. Manic illness is characterized by such behaviors as overactivity, accelerated speech, distractibility, and grandiosity and such emotions as irritability and euphoria. The grandiose ideas may reach delusional intensity and can involve the infant such that the child is believed to have been born for a special purpose (e.g., to save the world) or to control the environment, influence the mother's thoughts, or change shape or appearance (Margison, 1990; Thiels & Kumar, 1987). The consequence for the infant of the mother's symptoms of a schizoaffective or bipolar manic depressive disorder is likely to be extreme variability in caregiving as a result of disturbed and unpredictable behavior, as well as sporadic emotional availability. An overactive and disinhibited mother may handle her infant excessively and roughly, and a depressed and agitated mother may not be able to leave her infant alone because she cannot complete routine caretaking tasks. Retardation and poor concentration in the mother may mean that substitute care of the infant is unavoidable. The mother may have delusions of guilt, fear about the infant's health, and regret about the possible harmful effects of her behavior on the infant. Overexaggerated beliefs of an inability to cope may affect management.

As well as having bizarre perceptions, a psychotic mother may also have distorted expectations of her infant's behavior. Margison (1982) has described the case of a mother who believed her infant was an angel and could therefore fly; disaster was averted by a diving catch by an alert nurse. Such incidents are, fortunately, extremely rare (see, e.g., Kumar et al., 1995), but as a result, information about possible risk factors is still scarce. For example, many mothers with delusions of nihilism, of possession, or of unusual powers vested in themselves or in the infant are intuitively believed to be a danger to their babies, especially if they are also subject to "command" hallucinations telling them to kill or to dispose of the baby, but systematic observations have not so far identified any reliable indicators of risk to infants (Kumar & Hipwell, 1996). Indeed, Margison (1986) has suggested that bizarre delusional ideas expressed concurrently with normal expressions of warmth toward the baby do not appear to seriously influence the subsequent mother–child relationship. In contrast, Thiels and Kumar (1987), who studied mothers and infants jointly admitted to a mother–baby unit (MBU), found that "Thinking disturbance" (an item on the Brief Psychiatric Rating Scale; Overall & Gorham, 1962), usually elevated in schizophrenics, was found to be most closely associated with disorganized infant care. These authors also reported that disturbances of maternal care activities were closely related to the severity of psychiatric illness, and recovery from the illness was associated with simultaneous improvements of maternal behavior.

Detailing the nature of the mother's symptoms, as opposed to simply reporting a psychiatric diagnosis, is also important because there is evidence that psychoses that arise in the postpartum period are clinically distinct from nonpuerperal psychoses. Thus, infants may be exposed to particular types of symptoms such as perplexity and disorganized speech if the mother has a postpartum manic episode, whereas such symptoms may not be characteristic of manic disorders occurring at any other time (Brockington, Winokur, & Dean, 1982). Similarly, psychotic depressive illnesses arising postnatally may be characterized by prominent symptoms such as agitation focused on the child, patchy disorientation (Dean & Kendell, 1981), confusion, sadness, and anxiety (Brockington et al., 1982) in comparison with nonpuerperal disorders with the same diagnoses. In spite of such suggested distinctions between postpartum and non-postpartum psychopathology, there is, as yet, no definitive evidence for a clinically distinct postpartum syndrome (Kumar, 1994). In a prospective study in Sweden, McNeil (1988) compared the lifetime episodes of psychotic illnesses of women who had had both pre- and postpartum occurrences with those who had had only prepartum illnesses; he reported that the former group of women had illnesses typically of greater severity and which led to longer hospital admissions (68% for more than 4 months; 23% for more than 1 year). The findings suggested that these two groups might have been suffering from two different forms of illness rather than simply reflecting a difference in the number of episodes of the same illness. Davies, McIvor, and Kumar (1995) drew a similar conclusion from their retrospective study of the case notes of 45 schizophrenic mothers jointly admitted with their infants to an MBU in the postpartum period. Therefore, there may be differences in causes and consequences of psychotic illnesses that occur only after childbirth in comparison with chronic or episodic illnesses that persist or happen to recur following delivery. Cooper and Murray (1995) have already provided evidence in favor of such a proposition in relation to postnatal depression.

With careful documentation of the nature of maternal disorders arising at this time and with efforts to reduce the heterogeneity of samples, it
is possible that we may be able to identify distinct difficulties in parenting
among mothers with a particular psychiatric diagnosis. In a study that
attempted to do this, Hipwell and Kumar (1996) gathered weekly ratings
by nurses of the quality of mother–infant interaction throughout the joint
admissions of 78 dyads to a psychiatric MBU. The diagnoses made independently by two psychiatrists were combined into three groups for
analysis: unipolar depression, bipolar disorder, and schizophrenia. Mothers diagnosed as schizophrenic were rated by the nurses as the most impaired during the week of admission, in the second week, and at the week
of discharge; they were followed by those with a bipolar disorder; finally,
mothers with unipolar depression were rated as the least impaired. These
group differences could not be explained by any variation in parity, maternal age, timing of admission, socioeconomic or marital status.

A large-scale study carried out in Sweden (McNeil, Näslund,
Persson-Blennow, & Kaij, 1985; Persson-Blennow, Näslund, McNeil,
Kaij, & Malmquist-Larsen, 1984; Persson-Blennow, Binett, & McNeil,
1988a, 1988b; Persson-Blennow, Näslund, McNeil, & Kaij, 1986) compared mothers with a history of psychosis (not differentiated in terms
of whether they relapsed in the puerperal period) with healthy controls. The investigators reported the results of a series of measures of
the quality of mother–infant interaction over the first 12 months
postpartum. There were more interactional difficulties across a range
of ages in the first year among the case-group dyads compared with
healthy controls (McNeil et al., 1985; Persson-Blennow et al., 1986,
1988a, 1988b). These difficulties were mainly due to maternal and not
to infant behaviors and were detected as early as day 3 postdelivery
(Persson-Blennow et al., 1984). From six sets of observations over the
first 12 months postpartum (3 days; 3 and 6 weeks; 3½, 6, and 12
months), the mothers with a history of psychosis (especially those
with lifetime diagnoses of Cycloid psychosis and Schizophrenia) repeatedly showed higher levels of tension, greater insensitivity and uncertainty regarding the infant's needs, less social contact and involvement with the infant, and less ability to create a positive emotional
climate during feeding. At two of the observation points, both of these
diagnostic groups of women showed a clear discrepancy between in-
tonation and content of speech, which was hypothesized to be similar

to the parental double-bind communication thought to be associated with the development of schizophrenia (Bateson, 1956). Unfortunately, no information was provided about the quality of interaction of dyads in which the mother had had a relapse in the puerperium compared with those who remained in remission. Thus, it is not possible to draw conclusions about the effects of exposure of the infant to current psychiatric symptoms in the mother. This issue is discussed further in the following section.

Although it would be helpful to isolate the independent effects of particular symptoms on the infant, there is evidence that the type of illness that the mother experiences is likely to be confounded with the timing of onset. Several studies have found that manic episodes of illness have an especially early onset (0–2 weeks postpartum), whereas depressive episodes of illness tend to arise at a later time (0–6 weeks postpartum) (Kendell, Rennie, Clarke, & Dean, 1981; Dean & Kendell, 1981; Meltzer & Kumar, 1985). Thus, not only will individual infants be exposed to particular clusters of psychiatric symptoms in the mother, but the timing of this exposure, and, therefore, the environmental correlates of onset, such as the need for clinical intervention, will also impinge upon the infant at differing developmental stages.

Summary

The studies reviewed in this section suggest that diagnostic labels in themselves may not be particularly informative about the actual environment experienced by the infant unless more detailed descriptions of symptom profiles are also provided. For example, the experience for the infant of a mother with a diagnosis of bipolar disorder with a recent manic episode but who is currently severely and persistently depressed may, during the depressed period, be indistinguishable from that for an infant of a mother with a unipolar depressive disorder. Furthermore, it has been suggested that the manifestations of postpartum psychoses may be somewhat different from psychoses arising at other times, and studies of infant outcome must therefore consider the precise nature of the concurrent symptoms to which the child has been exposed and comparisons made accordingly (see Kumar & Hipwell, 1994). In addition, a number of other critical issues must be tackled, such as the differential impact on the child of the mother's illness as a function of its timing and the extent to which the child is actually exposed to the symptoms and disturbed behavior.

TIMING OF ONSET AND DURATION OF SYMPTOMS: IMPACT ACCORDING TO THE DEVELOPMENTAL STAGE OF THE CHILD

It is now widely accepted that children are at increased risk of adult mental disturbance if their mothers have had a serious mental illness at some point in their lifetimes. Thus, in the case of severe maternal psychiatric illness arising in the postpartum period, we have the opportunity to examine the impact on the infant at a distinct, well-defined, and probably sensitive period in the developmental process, and to observe the possible longer-term effects of early maternal disturbance on child development. Although it is unlikely that early difficulties in the mother–infant relationship have a permanent impact on development for which there is no subsequent compensation (Murray, Hipwell, et al., 1996), it is likely that developmental shifts will temper or heighten the infant's vulnerability to the impact of severe disorders in maternal mental state across time. For example, toward the end of the first year, the infant begins to monitor more closely the affect expressed by adults. Radke-Yarrow (1987) described infants of this age as seeking more active emotional engagement with the mother when she becomes angry or distressed. Thus, it could be that affective disorders at this time have a particularly detrimental impact on the infant's emotional development. In fact, a number of studies of less severely disturbed samples have provided evidence that supports this notion. The results indicate that there is an association between a deterioration in the quality of the infant–mother attachment relationship between 12 and 18 months postpartum when the mother is "psychologically unavailable" during this time (Egeland & Sroufe, 1981; Schneider-Rosen, Braunwald, Carlson, & Cicchetti, 1985). Other investigators have suggested that it is the chronicity rather than the particular timing of episodes of the mother's illness that adversely affects infants (Sameroff et al., 1984; Gallant, 1982). However, the effect of chronicity has not been consistently reported in relation to psychotic episodes, and, frequently, the small sample sizes mean that statistical comparisons cannot be made.

There is a question whether the younger infant may be at risk even if the mother's episode of psychotic illness occurred prior to the child's birth. McNeil and Blennow (1988) reported a unique investigation that attempted to test whether serious maternal mental illness which persisted or recurred in the months following childbirth had a greater adverse effect on the child's development than a history of similar illness previously in a woman's life. The three groups compared were (1) mothers who had a history of psychosis but no episode in the 6 months postpartum (referred to as the non-Post Partum Psychosis [non-PPP] group), (2) mothers who had a history but also a postpartum episode of psychosis (PPP group), and (3) 104 healthy mothers who had never had an episode of psychiatric illness. During the first year the children's emotional development was documented using measures of attachment security and fear of strangers, temperamental measures were taken at 6, 12, and 24 months; at a follow-up at 6 years of age, further assessments were made of the children's mental health and development (McNeil & Kaij, 1987; McNeil, Persson-Blennow, Binett, Harty, & Karyd, 1988). Of the 25 women in the PPP group, 21 were described as being hospitalized during that time, and also the "vast majority" were separated from their infants "to some extent" (see relevant section of this chapter on the nature of psychiatric treatment and management for further discussion about mother–infant separations). No significant differences were reported in comparisons between the PPP and the non-PPP groups. However, in this study, there were also no differences between the PPP and the healthy control groups on *any* of the sets of child assessments. Although the investigators concluded that there were no important long-term negative effects for the child as a result of the timing of the mother's illness, or, in fact, as a result of severe maternal illness arising at any time in the woman's life, the numbers in the PPP group were relatively small (15, 12, and 17 for the three sets of data) and a number of trends were reported. Thus, in comparison with the offspring of mothers who had had a prior but no postpartum episode of illness (non-PPP), offspring of the PPP group tended to be more likely to be securely attached to their mothers at 1 year of age, less problematic temperamentally, and less likely to be mentally disturbed at 6 years. This trend is of interest because the PPP dyads were generally separated during the mother's illness whereas the children of the non-PPP group remained with their mothers throughout the postnatal period. As a result of the differences in the extent of separations, one would expect that, if anything, the infants in the non-PPP group would be somewhat *more* likely to show a fear of strangers and security in the attachment relationship and not the reverse (Bowlby, 1969/1984, 1973). However, as mentioned previously, some caution is required when considering these results because the group numbers were small and there were some difficulties with the measures of the mother–infant relationship employed, which is discussed further in the section on the nature of the assessment of the impact on the child.

Summary

It is not possible to reach general conclusions about effects of maternal illnesses on developing children because of differences between studies in both the ages of the infants at the time of exposure to maternal disturbance and their ages at the time of assessment. The longitudinal study conducted in Sweden provides some evidence that children do not experience any lasting adverse effects of a postpartum relapse of a psychiatric illness in the mother. However, neither the nature of the treatment received by the mothers nor the extent of the periods of separation from the infant during the illness was adequately described, and so the factors mediating child outcome cannot be determined. Little is known about the impact on the child in families in which the mother continues to experience chronic or subclinical symptoms or is intermittently and partially emotionally unavailable to the child because of episodic disturbances in her mental state. Furthermore, undesirable sequelae for the infants of severely mentally ill mothers may not always be immediate. Long-term prospective studies are essential if possible delayed effects are to be evaluated.

NATURE OF PSYCHIATRIC TREATMENT AND MANAGEMENT: IMPACT ON THE INFANT OF CONTINUOUS CONTACT WITH OR SEPARATION FROM THE MOTHER, AND EFFECTS OF SUBSTITUTE CAREGIVING

Hospital treatment is virtually inevitable for most mothers who experience severe mental illness in the postpartum period (Kendell et al., 1987); therefore, unless the dyad is jointly admitted to a specialist unit (see review by Kumar, 1992) during this period, there may actually be little contact between mother and infant. In the latter circumstances other factors are important. For example, the infant may experience an abrupt cessation of care by the primary caregiver and, in some cases also of breast feeding. When the pair is jointly admitted to hospital, clinicians attempt to help the mother to maintain some contact with her infant, although the reality is likely to be that variable periods of exposure to maternal disturbance will occur, as well as temporary separations. In such circumstances, the infant may be looked after by many caregivers.

On the one hand, it is likely that physical separation from the mother during all or part of an episode of illness will protect the infant from the potential risks of interaction with a severely mentally ill person. On the other hand, separating mother and infant throughout the episode of illness may, itself, have adverse effects on the way the relationship subsequently develops and may lead to additional feelings of guilt, inadequacy, and uncertainty in the mother. In normal samples characterized by repeated separations, increased rates of insecure infant–mother attachments have been systematically reported (Ainsworth, 1973; Blehar, 1974).

Infants who are admitted to hospital with their mothers may also experience benefits and costs of substitute caretaking: Admission may offer compensatory experiences and interrupt the potential course of disturbed mother–infant behaviors. Alternatively, care by continually changing shifts of nurses (even if efforts are made to employ a primary nurse care system) may be associated with problems that have been frequently highlighted by previous studies of multiple caretaking (e.g., Rutter, 1966; Provence & Lipton, 1962; Stevens, 1975). For example, caregivers may not have an adequate chance to learn the individual characteristics of the infant, nor may the infants have the chance to establish a dialogue with one (consistent) respondent. Such a situation is likely to have implications for the child's developing sense of "felt security" and self-efficacy. In spite of such concerns, there has been no convincing demonstration to date of any overriding disadvantages of joint mother–infant psychiatric admission and the variable substitute care that this inevitably entails (see Grunebaum, Weiss, Cohler, Hartman, & Gallant, 1975; Hipwell, 1992; Hipwell, Goossens, Melhuish, & Kumar, in press). For example, in a study of 11 mentally ill mothers who were admitted to hospital with their babies (between 3 days and 22 months old), Grunebaum et al. (1975) reported that, compared with 20 infants of "normal" mothers and 7 infants of mentally ill mothers not treated in hospital, the inpatients' offspring attained markedly higher developmental quotients than did the other groups, mainly as a result of higher scores on expressive language development. Despite the wide range of infant ages on admission and, therefore, differences in the developmental stages of the infants, the authors suggested that the infants' experience of multiple caretakers in the hospital proved to be beneficial at this time.

Hipwell (1992) followed up 25 mothers with severe affective disorders and their physically healthy infants who were jointly admitted to a specialist psychiatric unit within 10 weeks of childbirth. This sample was closely matched pairwise with healthy control dyads on five criteria: maternal age (within 2 years), parity, sex of the infant, social class, and ethnicity. The case-group mothers were given a range of psychiatric diagnoses but were grouped according to whether there was a manic component to the illness in the postpartum period so that the experiences for the infants could be closely compared. Developmental assessments and maternal interviews were carried out at 2, 6, and 12 months postpartum. Although few residual symptoms of maternal mental illness were detected at 1 year, the interactions of the case-group mothers with their infants at this time were described as being less sensitively involved and more likely to appear mechanical, controlling, and overstimulating than was the case for the healthy controls (Hipwell et al., in press). Fewer instances of reciprocal exchange and more conflict were also reported for the case group at this time. Although in the case group as a whole, there did not appear to be any adverse effect on the attachment relationship of severe maternal mental illness and joint hospitalization, there were differences in outcome according to diagnosis: A manic episode of illness in the postpartum period was associated with secure infant–mother attachment, whereas psychotic or nonpsychotic depression was associated with an insecure–avoidant pattern of infant behavior. This difference in the results within the case group was supported by the independent observations of concurrent patterns of mother–infant interaction; that is, those suffering from manic episodes showed more positive behavior in relaxed and reciprocal interactions with their children at 1 year than did those with depression. Mothers who had had a manic episode of illness in the postpartum period displayed more affectionate talk (i.e., more frequent vocalizations, encouragement, and praise), whereas their infants were observed to be more focused on, and persistent in, play. With regard to cognitive and physical development, no differences were found between the 1-year-old infants of previously mentally ill mothers and their controls. There was no association between the measures of child outcome and severity of the mother's illness, length of hospitalization, or time since recovery. In further research on cognitive outcome, a study conducted by Gamer, Gallant, and Grunebaum (1976) of 15 women admitted to hospital with psychosis between 1 and 11 months postpartum (and who, as a result, were separated from their infants for varying lengths of time) investigated infant performance on a test of object permanence (Piaget, 1954). Drawing links with the caregiving arrangements, the authors proposed that there were no unequivocal adverse effects on infant cognitive development at 1 year, of exposure to a psychotic mother and of variable separations from her.

The effects of discontinuities of child care associated with multiple caretaking and intermittent maternal care in the first months of life can be discerned to some extent in studies of the development of children brought up on a kibbutz. In this context, Oppenheim, Sagi, and Lamb (1988) and Sagi et al. (1985) suggested that the attachment relationship with the care provider in the kibbutz was influential as a precursor to later social and emotional development. Security in this relationship at 11 to 14 months predicted assertiveness and empathy 4 years later. However, extrapolation from such studies of the effects of multiple caregivers to psychiatric settings is obviously greatly limited by the differences in social and cultural circumstances, the impact of the mother's illness, the extent to which the parents have regular or irregular separations imposed upon them, and marked differences in the extent, training, and consistency of the substitute child caregivers.

It is apparent from the previously described research that the quality and consistency of alternative care must be examined as carefully as disruptions in mothers' caregiving behavior. Hipwell's (1992) study provides further evidence to suggest that the general absence of adverse outcome in the "jointly admitted" children of bipolar- and manic-disordered mothers may well have arisen because the infants' exposure to the maternal illness was limited rather than because there were genuinely no detrimental effects of the mothers' illnesses. Thus, although there were no differences in the lengths of hospital admission or illness between the mothers with different diagnoses, the inpatient depressed mothers in that study whose infants had relatively poor outcome appeared to be relieved of the care of their babies less often than mothers who had a manic/bipolar illness in the postpartum period. Infants of depressed mothers may thus have been exposed to more chronic maladaptive parenting and low-level affective symptoms that, although not being severe enough to warrant the provision of alternative child care, nevertheless had an adverse impact on the child (see Kochanska, 1991; Hipwell, 1992).

Any evaluation of the impact of maternal psychiatric disorder on infant outcome must therefore attempt to address the relative influence of treatment and management factors. Included within such factors are not only "together or apart" but also effects of drug treatments which obviously also vary according to the nature of the mother's illness. Antipsychotic or antidepressant medication may have different effects and side effects on the mother's behavior and feelings toward her infant and her ability to provide care, including breast feeding.

Summary

Differences in the type and extent of joint or separate inpatient care may be related to the nature of the mothers' current or previous illnesses (Hipwell et al., in press; McNeil, 1988). Unfortunately few studies have provided adequate details about the type of treatment and management of the mothers in the sample or of the extent of separations from the infant and the use and variation of substitute caregiving during the period of illness. The only evidence that is available on the costs and benefits to the child of joint admission suggests that there are no serious detrimental effects. Controlled comparisons are needed in which the alternative kind of care is equally carefully specified (e.g., with a foster family or within the extended family network, and with evaluation of the amount and quality of contact between mother and baby during the period of separation).

FAMILIAL AND SOCIAL FACTORS

Severe maternal mental illness and its management, such as joint mother–infant admission, may have other indirect consequences for the child in terms of the effect on the quality of familial relationships. It is highly likely that there will be a period of physical separation between the mother and her partner. In addition, either the father will be temporarily separated from the baby and may, as a result, experience difficulty in getting to know the newborn or, alternatively, he may find that he has become the primary caregiver during his partner's illness. Family members may feel anxiety about the infant's safety, blame the mother, or feel guilt about the occurrence of the illness. Little is known about the impact of these potential risk factors on the child.

There is evidence for assortative mating among couples in which one partner has a history of a severe breakdown in mental health. Alternatively, there may be a "contagion effect" whereby the partner becomes disturbed when the index spouse becomes ill. Thus, in studies of nonpsychotic depression, patients are frequently married to a depressed spouse (Merikangas, 1984). More recently, studies have also highlighted the relatively high rates of depressive symptoms in the postnatal period among partners and other relatives (Ballard, Davis, Cullen, Mohan, & Dean, 1994; Raskin, Richman, & Gaines, 1990; Areias, Kumar, Barros, & Figueiredo, 1996a, 1996b). Harvey and McGrath (1988) and Lovestone and Kumar (1993) focused on the mental health of the partners of women admitted to a psychiatric MBU and found high rates of depression among them. The latter study of 24 men also revealed that almost all the nine partners who had a lifetime diagnosis of psychiatric disorder experienced an episode of the disorder in the postpartum period that was more severe than previously, and, as the women recovered from their illnesses, so too did they.

In a case-note study of 40 married fathers with a bipolar affective disorder admitted to a research unit during a 9-year period, Davenport and Adland (1982) reported that 50% suffered a relapse within 1 year of their partner's delivery and more than half these "cases" became ill while their partners were pregnant. The investigators suggested that there may be a subgroup of male bipolar patients for whom fathering a child represents a sharply increased risk for prenatal or postpartum psychosis. Their results showed that this subgroup may be characterized by an earlier age of onset of affective illness and a history of childhood bereavement in comparison with fathers with a bipolar illness but no birth-related episodes. Regardless of the potential effects of these additional correlates, the findings indicate that the implications for the infant of having two mentally ill parents at this time must also be addressed. No such studies are known to have been carried out in the puerperium. However, reporting on a rather different sample (preschool-aged children of parents with bipolar affective disorder, of whom those with postpartum reactions were *excluded*), Radke-Yarrow, Nottleman, Martinez, Fox, and Belmont (1992) reported no *extra* adverse effect on the child if the father also experienced episodes of bipolar illness. These researchers suggest that among families in which there are two mentally ill parents, there may be well-established and effective social support systems that are set up when the child is very young. Such networks may play an important protective role for the child. The developmental stage of the children in this study, however, as well as the exclusion of women who experienced postpartum episodes, limits the degree to which the conclusions may be generalizable to postnatal populations.

In their study of women with a history of psychotic affective disorder after childbirth, Marks, Wieck, Seymour, Checkley, and Kumar (1992) found that the subsequent risk of postpartum relapse was correlated with low levels of emotional engagement by husbands with their wives during pregnancy (operationalized by rating both positive and negative levels of expressed emotion) (Vaughn & Leff, 1976; Vaughn, Snyder, Jones, Freeman, & Falloon, 1984). Further work is needed to establish whether such emotional reactions are indicative of enduring traits and whether they are also reflected in paternal attitudes and responses to the newborn infant.

Investigators are increasingly recognizing that parents behave towards their children differently according to the ordinal position of the child in the family (see review by Hoffman, 1991). Thus, further important consideration in assessing the impact of postnatal psychotic illness on the infant is the mother's prior experience of parenting. Thiels and Kumar (1987) suggested that the association between severity of mental illness and disturbances in mothering ability is weakened among multiparous women when prior experience of mothering may serve a protective function for the newborn. This evidence was derived from a study that examined the associations between aspects of psychopathology and disturbances of maternal behavior among a group of women suffering from severe puerperal psychoses who had been admitted to a specialized MBU. Because primiparity places a woman at increased risk of a psychotic breakdown in the postpartum period anyway (Kendell et al., 1987; Paffenbarger, 1964), such findings suggest that first-born infants are doubly at risk by being more likely to be exposed to a severely mentally ill mother as well as to more severe disturbance in care. Further research is needed to examine whether multiparity does indeed mitigate the effects of severe maternal disturbance on the infant's experience in the first months of life.

In samples of depressed parents, there is substantial evidence for the presence of marital conflict, and, in relation to postnatal depression, there is ongoing debate about whether it may be a cause or a correlate of the disorder (see Downey & Coyne, 1990; Cooper, Murray, Hooper, & West, 1996).

In contrast to the accumulating evidence of marital difficulties and psychiatric problems in the partners of women with postnatal psychosis, there is little evidence to suggest that psychotic disorders arising in the postpartum period are associated with general social adversity. Thus, in their unique prospective study of childbearing women with histories of affective disorder, Marks, Wieck, Checkley, and Kumar (1992) examined a number of social factors that could contribute to a recurrence of postpartum psychosis and found only the presence of a poor marital relationship to be significantly predictive. Other social factors such as marital status per se, number of children in the family, social class, the frequency of stressful life events, duration of marriage, and a lack of a confidant were not associated with either a psychotic or a nonpsychotic postpartum relapse. A similar lack of association between social disadvantage and onset of postpartum psychosis has been reported by Dowlatshahi and Paykel (1990) and Brockington, Martin, Brown, Goldberg, and Margison (1990). Both of these studies, using a retrospective design in which mothers who were hospitalized for psychotic illness in the postnatal period were interviewed following recovery, found no differences on measures of severe social stress and rates of independent life events between the inpatient group and healthy puerperal controls.

Among other studies that have examined the role of social factors, neither Seager (1960) nor Paffenbarger (1964) reported an increase in marital discord or domestic or social stress in mothers affected by postpartum psychosis compared with healthy controls. Similarly, McNeil (1988) found no association between a relapse of psychotic illness in the postpartum months and life stress, interpersonal difficulties, lack of support, problematic relationship with their own mothers, or negative attitude to the pregnancy compared with women who remained in remission in the period after childbirth when interviewed prospectively in pregnancy. Even more striking, McNeil reported *fewer* housing problems and pregnancy complaints, better preparation for the expected child, and a more positive attitude to the pregnancy among women who had a psychotic relapse after the birth (PPP group) compared with women who did not (non-PPP group). In addition, there was no particular pattern of difference revealed in comparisons between the PPP group and the healthy controls; that is, problems in current life situation and negative experience of pregnancy did not appear to be characteristics of a postpartum psychotic breakdown. It appears to be the case, therefore, that although there is an association between lower socioeconomic status, stressful life events, and the occurrence of nonpsychotic depression, this association does not appear to hold true for women experiencing postpartum psychotic illness (Brockington et al., 1982; Kumar, 1994; O'Hara & Zekoski, 1988; Paykel, Emms, Fletcher, & Rassaby, 1980; Watson, Elliott, Rugg, & Brough, 1984).

Summary

The extensive research on nonpsychotic postnatal depression has shown that factors associated with the disorder extending beyond the mother–infant pair, such as impaired familial functioning and social adversity, are likely to have an influence on the child's development. With regard to postpartum psychotic illness, although social adversity does not appear to be related to the disorder, qualities of the parents' own relationship, including the degree of emotional engagement between them and the presence of psychiatric disturbance in the partner, are likely to contribute to the wife's vulnerability to mental breakdown and its course and to have an impact on the couple's caregiving, attitudes, and relationship with the child, as well as a direct impact on the child's adjustment. Therefore, this is an important topic for future research.

NATURE OF THE ASSESSMENT OF THE IMPACT ON THE CHILD

Changes in nosological terminology in psychiatry as well as in diagnostic practices over the past decade have compromised comparisons between earlier and more recent studies (see Downey & Coyne, 1990). In addition, structured diagnostic interviews have generally replaced the self-report measures that were used in earlier studies. Although some studies appear to use the same procedures to assess mother–infant relationships, modifications have occasionally been made to their administration, and, as a result, their validity becomes questionable. D'Angelo (1986), for example, highlights the potential dangers of modifying the "strange situation" procedure (Ainsworth, Blehar, Waters, & Wall, 1978) for the assessment of infant–mother attachment with severely mentally ill groups of mothers and their offspring. Comparing the attachment classifications of infants of schizophrenic, depressed, and healthy control mothers, no association was revealed with maternal diagnosis when using the abbreviated three-episode procedure, whereas the converse was true for the standard seven-episode condition, with case group infants more likely than controls to evidence insecurity in their relationship with their mother. It was concluded that the abbreviated version of the strange situation could lead to overidentification of secure attachment among infants of mentally ill mothers.

In addition, most tests and rating scales have been developed and standardized in nonclinical samples; thus, their reliability and validity in psychiatric populations need to be established. For low-risk samples, much of the predictive power of early measures of infant functioning depends on an element of stability and continuity in family, social, and demographic characteristics. The patterns of infant behavior observed in the strange situation, for example, have been shown to be highly predictive of a range of later offspring outcome variables in stable family circumstances. Among families in which the mother is at risk of relapsing with a severe affective disorder, there may, by contrast, be little stability in the way the family functions, and thus this measure may not be useful other than in making comparisons between groups of dyads assessed concurrently.

The extreme nature of disturbances in severely mentally ill mothers' behavior also means that new instruments have to be developed so that comparisons within samples can be made (see Kumar & Hipwell, 1996). However, a measure that is designed to discriminate between the type and degree of severe maternal disturbance is likely to have little validity for a normal sample. Kumar and Hipwell (1996) described the psychometric properties of the Bethlem Mother–Infant Interaction Scale (BMIS) for a group of 78 jointly admitted mothers and infants and 55 healthy dyads. Inevitably, the range in the quality of mother–infant interactions was markedly less among the healthy sample and thus produced highly skewed data. A further potential problem that pertains to investigations of the behavior of mentally ill mothers and their infants is the issue of performance versus competence, and this also has a bearing on the context and format in which dyads are observed. Thus, overt displays of maternal hostility, which may occur more frequently among severely mentally ill mothers, are not generally observed in laboratory-based settings. For relatively limited periods mothers may be able to gather all their resources for short periods of observation of their caregiving behavior (Als, 1982).

Clinical assessments of a consecutive series of 20 schizophrenic women admitted with their infants into a specialized psychiatric unit (Kumar et al., 1995) showed that half of them were judged by staff as being unable to maintain consistent and safe care of their infants, with the consequence that alternative full-time caregivers had to be found for their infants. Among the more important factors evaluated were the mother's ability to understand, prioritize, and anticipate the infant's needs as far as possible independently to provide routine care, day and night, and to be able to engage in a sensitive and stimulating manner in play and dialogue with the baby. Incidents or episodes during which the baby might be "at risk" of harm were recorded in narrative form, such risk usually resulting from unintentional "neglect" because the mother's behavior was disorganized and only rarely because she was subject to impulses to harm the baby (e.g., because she believed it was "possessed" or because she was commanded to do so by voices). In extreme and severe cases of maternal illness it was relatively easy for observers to reach a consensus about lack of safety and inadequacy of parenting behavior. However, the real problem arises in less severely ill cases, when the mother's illness is not completely incapacitating or pervasive in its effects on her motivation and competence as a parent. There is a danger in such circumstances of being too demanding of the mother and setting too high standards simply because she is being assessed and also because, in relation to the infant's welfare, it is better to be safe than sorry (Ramsay & Kumar, 1996). The alternative approach is to attempt to define what is meant by "good enough" mothering in the particular case that is being assessed, which then opens the door to individual variations and prejudices, as well as raising questions about whether what is good enough for a 2-month-old will still be so for a 2-year-old.

Summary

The first priority must be the definition of criteria on which judgments about the mother's mental state and the child's adjustment are to be based. Assessments must then be made of the reliability, validity, and predictive power of measures when used with high-risk samples. Finally, as a way of standardizing the process of evaluation, observational and rating methods for assessing the mother–infant relationship and interactions must be systematically applied (see, e.g., Kumar & Hipwell, 1996).

CHARACTERISTICS OF THE CHILD

It must, of course, be remembered that there is a complex interaction between the mother and child that exists regardless of whether or not the mother is ill. When the mother suffers a psychotic episode in the postpartum period, the focus is generally on her as the deviant part of the dyad and little consideration is paid to the impact that the child may be having on her. However, the child may differ from the "norm" for a number of reasons (e.g., psychotropic medication during pregnancy or taken in as a result of breast feeding) and this may alter habituation and orienting responses as well as cuddliness and the frequency of smiling in the infant (Brazelton, 1969). To date, there is no clear evidence that there are more obstetric and perinatal complications among women who become severely mentally ill in the postpartum period than among healthy samples (McNeil & Blennow, 1988; Paffenbarger, 1982; Tetlow, 1955; Seager, 1960; Protheroe, 1961; Nott, 1982).

Using a sample of primiparous community-based women, Murray, Stanley, Hooper, King, and Fiori-Cowley (1996) reported that characteristics of the infants' behavior that were assessed in the immediate neonatal period predicted onset of postnatal nonpsychotic depression in the mother within 8 weeks of the delivery. However, because of the relatively low rate of severe psychiatric disorders that arise in the immediate postnatal period, no prospective studies have examined behavioral characteristics of the newborn that might have led to the onset of the mother's illness. Although there is no evidence to suggest that a temperamentally difficult infant can trigger the onset of maternal psychosis, it is possible that infant characteristics such as activity, irritability, and soothability or sociability could at least temper or heighten difficulties in the developing mother–child relationship. Brockington et al., (1982) reported increased rates of psychosis in biological relatives of women who developed postpartum psychosis, suggesting that genetic factors may be as important for the offspring's mental development as are short-term early disturbances in mothering behavior. It is clear that more detailed and systematic research is needed which focuses on the part played by the infant in the developing relationship with his or her psychotic mother and on characteristics of the child that are associated with measures of adverse or healthy developmental outcome.

CONCLUSION

Recently, attention has been turning increasingly to the urgent need for refinement of questions and design in research on the effects of severe postpartum maternal mental illness on the child. Although studies of postnatal nonpsychotic depression are beginning to identify the mechanisms by which aspects or different components of the mother's illness affect the infant and developing child, similar progress has not been made in the context of more severe disorders. The research that has been done has suffered from methodological inconsistencies and inadequacies, but the lack of progress is also a result of the complexity of the questions to be addressed.

Psychiatric conditions that occur, recur, or continue after childbirth must be considered in the context of their management as well as the family, marital, and social milieu if the impact on the child's adjustment is to be properly understood. There is also a need to assess intervening processes. For example, we cannot assume that a particular infant outcome such as performance on a cognitive assessment or the pattern of infant–mother attachment behavior has the same cause or course within a case group as it does in controls. A few studies have reported inconsistencies between antecedents and outcome measures for high-risk samples established among normal samples in stable family circumstances. Sameroff, Seifer, and Zax (1982) and Hipwell et al. (in press), for example, found little relationship between characteristics of mother–infant interaction in the early months postpartum among severely mentally ill mothers and their infants and the quality of the attachment relationship at 12 months. Although the experience of sporadic substitute care for these children may have been critical, along with other environmental factors, it is nevertheless plausible that the antecedents to attachment security or other developmental outcomes are different from those in healthy low-risk samples because of particular genetic factors that influence development.

The problem is that infants of severely mentally ill mothers may be adversely influenced by a number of factors which could contribute to a mother's vulnerability to become ill in the first place, to the particular course of the illness, or to difficulties in parenting. As far as the infant is concerned, such factors may include marital and family difficulties, a mentally ill father, genetic predispositions, and repeated separations due to the mother's hospitalizations. Surrogate care and multiple caretaking are also likely to be significant contributing factors in the course of children's development, but, at the moment, it is not clear what the relative impact is compared with exposure to maternal disturbance. The effects on the infant could be a result of these factors directly or a result an interaction with the mother's illness.

Differences between studies in their sample characteristics have limited the generalizability of the results that have been obtained so far. This problem may be lessened by providing more adequate descriptions of the groups studied and the nature of their clinical treatment, by selecting samples representative of the population from which they are drawn, and by closely matching them with appropriate controls. This latter problem is particularly difficult because of the inevitable co-occurrence of severe mental disturbance and the need for psychiatric care, which usually requires hospitalization. Thus, controlled comparisons are needed for severe maternal disturbance, institutionalization, and multiple caregiving and/or separation and substitute caregiving.

The studies described in this review have reported varying effects of severe maternal illness on the infant which may be specific to the nature of the particular samples investigated. Further examination of the positive characteristics and resources of mother, child, and family is needed. The literature indicates that there may be a variety of difficulties in parenting and effects on the developing child, but at present little is known about compensatory factors that come into play during and after the mother's illness, or about the ways in which the child's characteristics modify risk for future maladjustment.

REFERENCES

Ainsworth, M. D. S. (1973). The development of infant–mother attachment. In B. M. Caldwell & H. N. Ricciuti (Eds.), *Review of child development research* (Vol. 3, pp. 1–94). Chicago: University of Chicago Press.

Ainsworth, M. D. S., Blehar, M. C., Waters, E., & Wall, S. (1978). *Patterns of attachment.* Hillsdale, NJ: Erlbaum.

Als, H. (1982). The unfolding of behavioural organisation in the face of a biological violation. In E. Z. Tronick (Ed.), *Social interchange in infancy* (pp. 125–160). Baltimore: University Park Press.

Areias, M. E. G., Kumar, R., Barros, H., & Figueiredo, E. (1996a). Comparative incidence of depression in women and men, during pregnancy and after childbirth: Validation of the Edinburgh Postnatal Depression Scale in Portugese mothers. *British Journal of Psychiatry, 169,* 30–35.

Areias, M. E. G., Kumar, R., Barros, H., & Figueiredo, E. (1996b). Correlates of postnatal depression in mothers and fathers. *British Journal of Psychiatry, 169,* 36–41.

Ballard, C. G., Davis, R., Cullen, P. C., Mohan, R. N., & Dean, C. (1994). Prevalence of postnatally psychiatric morbidity in mothers and fathers. *British Journal of Psychiatry, 164,* 782–788.

Bateson, G. (1956). Toward a theory of schizophrenia. *Behavioural Science, 1,* 251–264.

Blehar, M. C. (1974). Anxious attachment and defensive reactions associated with day care. *Child Development, 46,* 683–692.

Bowlby, J. (1973). *Attachment and loss: Vol 2. Separation* New York: Basic Books.

Bowlby, J. (1984). *Attachment and loss: Vol 1. Attachment* (2nd ed.). New York: Basic Books. (Original work published 1969)

Brazelton, T. B. (1969). *The effect of prenatal drugs on the behaviour of the neonate.* Paper presented to the American Psychological Association, Miami Beach, FL.

Brockington, I. F., Martin, C., Brown, G. W., Goldberg, D., & Margison, F. (1990). Stress and puerperal psychosis. *British Journal of Psychiatry, 157,* 331–334.

Brockington, I. F., Winokur, G., & Dean, C. (1982). Puerperal Psychosis. In I. Brockington & R. Kumar (Eds.), *Motherhood and mental illness* (Vol. 1, pp. 37–69). London: John Wright.

Cohn, J. E., Campbell, S. B., Matias, R., & Hopkins, J. (1990). Face-to-face interactions of postpartum depressed and non-depressed mother–infant pairs at two months. *Developmental Psychology, 26,* 15–23.

Cohn, J. E., Matias, R., Tronick, E. Z., Connell, D., & Lyons-Ruth, D. (1986). Face-to-face interactions of depressed mothers and their infants. In E. Z. Tronick & T. Field (Eds.), *Maternal depression and infant disturbance* (New Directions for Child Development, No 34, pp. 31–45). San Francisco: Jossey-Bass.

Cooper, P. J., & Murray, L. (1995). Course and recurrence of postnatal depression. Evidence for the specificity of a diagnostic concept. *British Journal of Psychiatry, 166,* 191–195.

Cooper, P. J., Murray, L., Hooper, R., & West, A. (1996). The development and validation of a predictive index for postpartum depression. *Psychological Medicine, 26,* 627–634.

Cummings, E. M., & Davies, P. T. (1994). Maternal depression and child development. *Journal of Child Psychology and Psychiatry, 35,* 73–112.

D'Angelo, E. J. (1986). Security of attachment in infants with schizophrenic, depressed and unaffected mothers. *Journal of Genetic Psychology, 147,* 421–422.

Davenport, Y. B., & Adland, M. S. (1982). Postpartum psychoses in female and male bipolar manic–depressive patients. *American Journal of Orthopsychiatry, 52,* 288–297.

Davies A., McIvor, R. J., & Kumar, R. (1995). Impact of childbirth on a series of schizophrenic mothers: A comment on the possible influence of oestrogen on schizophrenia. *Schizophrenia Research, 16,* 25–31

Dean, C., & Kendell, R. E. (1981). The symptomatology of puerperal illness. *British Journal of Psychiatry, 139,* 128–133.

D'Orban, P. T. (1979). Women who kill their children. *British Journal of Psychiatry, 134,* 560–571.

Dowlatshahi, D., & Paykel, E. S. (1990). Life events and social stress in puerperal psychoses: Absence of effect. *Psychological Medicine, 20,* 655–662.

Downey, G., & Coyne, J. C. (1990). Children of depressed parents: An integrative review. *Psychological Bulletin, 108,* 50–76.

Egeland, B., & Sroufe, L. A. (1981). Attachment and early maltreatment. *Child Development, 52,* 44–52.

Field, T. M. (1987). Interaction and attachment in normal and atypical infants. *Journal of Consulting and Clinical Psychology, 55*(6), 853–859.

Field, T., Healy, B., Goldstein, S., & Guthertz, M. (1990). Behavior-state matching and synchrony in mother–infant interactions in non-depressed versus depressed dyads. *Developmental Psychology, 26,* 7–14.

Fleming, A., Ruble, D., Flett, G., & Shaul, D. (1988). Postpartum adjustment in first-time mothers: Relations between mood, maternal attitudes and mother–infant interactions. *Developmental Psychology, 24,* 71–81.

Gallant, D. H. (1982). Children of mentally ill mothers. In H. Grunebaum, J. Weiss, B. Cohler, C. Hartman, & D. H. Gallant (Eds.), *Mentally ill mothers and their children.* Chicago: Chicago University Press.

Gamer, E., Gallant, D. H., & Grunebaum, H. U. (1976). Children of psychotic mothers. *Archives of General Psychiatry, 33,* 311–317.

Gochman, E. R. (1985). Bi-polar mothering: Case description, mother–infant interaction, and theoretical implications. *Child Psychiatry and Human Development, 16*(2), 120–125.

Grunebaum, H. U., Weiss, J. L., Cohler, B. J., Hartman, C. R., & Gallant, D. H. (Eds.). (1975). *Mentally ill mothers and their children.* Chicago: University of Chicago.

Harvey, I., & McGrath, G. (1988). Psychiatric morbidity in spouses of women admitted to a mother and baby unit. *British Journal of Psychiatry, 152,* 506–510.

Hipwell, A. E. (1992). *Postpartum maternal mental illness and the psychological development of the infant.* Doctoral dissertation, University of London.

Hipwell, A. E., Goossens, F. A., Melhuish, E. C., & Kumar, R. (in press). Severe maternal psychopathology, "Joint" hospitalisation and infant–mother attachment. *Development and Psychopathology.*

Hipwell, A. E., & Kumar, R. (1996). Maternal psychopathology and prediction of outcome based on mother–infant interaction ratings (BMIS). *British Journal of Psychiatry, 169,* 655–661.

Hoffman, L. W. (1991). The influence of the family environment on personality: Accounting for sibling differences. *Psychological Bulletin, 110,* 187–203.

Kendell, R. E., Chalmers, J. C., & Platz, C. (1987). Epidemiology of puerperal psychoses. *British Journal of Psychiatry, 150,* 662–673.

Kendell, R. E., Rennie, D., Clarke, J. A., & Dean, C. (1981). The social and obstetric correlates of psychiatric admission in the puerperium. *Psychological Medicine, 11,* 341–350.

Kochanska, G. (1991). Patterns of inhibition to the unfamiliar in children of normal and affectively ill mothers. *Child Development, 62,* 250–263.

Kumar, R. (1992). Mentally ill mothers and their babies: What are the benefits and risks of joint hospital admission? In K. Hawton & P. Cowen (Eds.), *Practical problems in clinical psychiatry* (pp. 184–197). Oxford, England: Oxford University Press.

Kumar, R. (1996). Postnatal mental illness: A transcultural perspective. *Social Psychiatry and Psychiatric Epidemiology, 29,* 250–264.

Kumar, R. (in press). Severe disturbance of mothers' relationships with their newborn infants: Evidence for a disorder of mother–infant bonding. *British Journal of Psychiatry.*

Kumar, R., & Hipwell, A. E. (1994). Implications for the infant of maternal puerperal psychiatric disorders. In M. Rutter, E. Taylor, & L. Hersov (Eds.), *Child and adolescent psychiatry: Modern approaches* (pp. 759–775). Oxford, England: Blackwell Scientific.

Kumar, R., & Hipwell, A. E. (1996). Development of a clinical rating scale to assess mother–infant interaction in a psychiatric mother and baby unit. *British Journal of Psychiatry, 169*, 18–26.

Kumar, R., & Marks, M. (1992). Infanticide and the law in England and Wales. In J. A. Hamilton & P. N. Harberger (Eds.), *Postpartum psychiatric illness: A picture puzzle* (pp. 256–273). Philadelphia: University of Pennsylvania Press.

Kumar, R., Marks, M., Platz, C., & Yoshida, K. (1995). Clinical survey of a psychiatric mother and baby unit: Characteristics of 100 consecutive admissions. *Journal of Affective Disorders, 33*, 11–22.

Lovestone, S., & Kumar, R. (1993). Postnatal psychiatric illness: The impact on partners. *British Journal of Psychiatry, 163*, 210–216.

Margison, F. (1982). The pathology of the mother–child relationship. In I. Brockington & R. Kumar (Eds.), *Motherhood and mental illness* (Vol. 1, pp. 191–222). London: John Wright.

Margison, F. R. (1986). Assessment of mother–infant interaction and attachment—An overview. In J. L. Cox, R. Kumar, F. R. Margison, & L. J. Downey (Eds.), *Current approaches in puerperal mental illness* (pp. 29–33). Southampton, England: Duphar.

Margison, F. R. (1990). Infants of mentally ill mothers: The risk of injury and its control. *Journal of Reproductive and Infant Psychology, 8*(2), 137–146.

Marks, M., & Kumar, R. (1993). Infanticide in England and Wales. *Medicine Science and the Law, 33*, 329–339.

Marks, M., & Kumar, R. (1995). Parents who kill their infants. *British Journal of Midwifery, 3*, 249–253.

Marks, M. N., Wieck, A., Seymour, A., Checkley, S. A., & Kumar, R. (1992). Women whose mental illnesses recur after childbirth and partners' levels of expressed emotion during late pregnancy. *British Journal of Psychiatry, 161*, 211–216.

Marks, M. N., Wieck, A., Checkley, S. A., & Kumar, R. (1992). Contribution of psychological and social factors to psychotic and non-psychotic relapse after childbirth in women with previous histories of affective disorder. *Journal of Affective Disorders, 29*, 253–264.

McNeil, T. F. (1988). Women with nonorganic psychosis: Psychiatric and demographic characteristics of cases with versus without postpartum psychotic episodes. *Acta Psychiatrica Scandinavica, 78*, 603–609.

McNeil, T. F., & Blennow, G. (1988). A prospective study of postpartum psychoses in a high-risk group. 6. Relationship to birth complications and neonatal abnormality. *Acta Psychiatrica Scandinavica, 78*, 478–484.

McNeil, T. F., & Kaij, L. (1987). Swedish high-risk sample: Sample characteristics at age 6. *Schizophrenia Bulletin, 13,* 373–381.

McNeil, T. F., Näslund, B., Persson-Blennow, I., & Kaij, L. (1985). Offspring of women with nonorganic psychosis: Mother–infant interaction at three-and-a-half and six months of age. *Acta Psychiatrica Scandinavica, 71,* 551–558.

McNeil, T. F., Persson-Blennow, I., Binett, B., Harty, B., & Karyd, U.-B. (1988). A prospective study of postpartum psychoses in a high-risk group. 7. Relationship to later offspring characteristics. *Acta Psychiatrica Scandinavica, 78,* 613–617.

Meltzer, E. S., & Kumar, R. (1985). Puerperal mental illness, clinical features and classification: A study of 142 mother-and-baby admissions. *British Journal of Psychiatry, 147,* 647–654.

Merikangas, R. R. (1984). Divorce and assortative mating for depression. *American Journal of Psychiatry, 141,* 74–76.

Murray, L. (1992). The impact of postnatal depression on infant development. *Journal of Child Psychology and Psychiatry, 33,* 543–561.

Murray, L., Fiori-Cowley, A., Hooper, R., & Cooper, P. J. (1996). The impact of postnatal depression and associated adversity on early mother–infant interactions and later infant outcome. *Child Development, 67,* 2512–2526.

Murray, L., Hipwell, A. E., Hooper, R., Stein, A., & Cooper, P. J. (in press). The cognitive development of five year old children of postnatally depressed mothers. *Journal of Child Psychiatry and Psychology, 37,* 927–935.

Murray, L., Stanley, C., Hooper, R., King, F., & Fiori-Cowley, A. (1996). The role of infant factors in postnatal depression and mother–infant interactions. *Developmental Medicine and Child Neurology, 38,* 109–119.

Nott, P. N. (1982). Psychiatric illness following childbirth in Southampton: A case register study. *Psychological Medicine, 12,* 557–561.

O'Hara, M. W., & Zekoski, E. (1988). Postpartum depression: A comprehensive review. In R. Kumar & I. Brockington (Eds.), *Motherhood and mental illness* (Vol. 2, pp. 17–63). London: John Wright.

Oppenheim, D., Sagi, A., & Lamb, M. E. (1988). Infant–adult attachments on the kibbutz and their relation to socioemotional development 4 years later. *Developmental Psychology, 24,* 427–433.

Overall, J. E., & Gorham, D. R. (1962). The Brief Psychiatric Rating Scale. *Psychological Reports, 10,* 799–812.

Paffenbarger, R. S. (1964). Epidemiological aspects of parapartum mental illness. *British Journal of Preventative Social Medicine, 18,* 189–195.

Paffenbarger, R. S. (1982). Epidemiological aspects of mental illness Associated with childbearing. In I. Brockington & R. Kumar (Eds.), *Motherhood and mental illness* (Vol. 1, pp. 19–36). London: John Wright.

Paykel, E. S., Emms, E. M., Fletcher, J., & Rassaby, E. S. (1980). Life events and social support in puerperal depression. *British Journal of Psychiatry, 136,* 339–346.

Persson-Blennow, I., Näslund, B., McNeil, T. F., Kaij, L., & Malmquist-Larsson, A.

(1984). Offspring of women with nonorganic psychosis: Mother–infant interaction at three days of age. *Acta Psychiatrica Scandinavica, 70,* 149–159.

Persson-Blennow, I., Näslund, B., McNeil, T. F., & Kaij, L. (1986). Offspring of women with nonorganic psychosis: Mother–infant interaction at one year of age. *Acta Psychiatrica Scandinavica, 73,* 207–213.

Persson-Blennow, I., Binett, B., & McNeil, T. F. (1988a). Offspring of women with nonorganic psychosis: Antecedents of anxious attachment to the mother at one year of age. *Acta Psychiatrica Scandinavica, 78,* 66–71.

Persson-Blennow, I., Binett, B., & McNeil, T. F. (1988b). Offspring of women with nonorganic psychosis: Mother–infant interaction and fear of strangers during the first year of life. *Acta Psychiatrica Scandinavica, 78,* 379–383.

Piaget, J. (1954). *The construction of reality in the child.* New York: Basic Books.

Pound, A., Cox, A. D., Puckering, C., & Mills, M. (1985). The impact of maternal depression on young children. *Journal of Child Psychology and Psychiatry Monograph* (suppl. 4).

Protheroe, C. (1961). Puerperal psychoses: A long term study 1927–1961. *British Journal of Psychiatry, 11,* 9–30.

Provence, S., & Lipton, R. C. (1962). *Infants in institutions: A comparison of their development with family-reared infants during the first year of life.* New York: International Universities Press.

Radke-Yarrow, M. (1987). *Attachment in the context of psychopathology.* Paper presented at a conference on fruits of attachment theory: Findings and applications across the life cycle, London.

Radke-Yarrow, M., Nottelmann, E., Martinez, P., Fox, M., & Belmont, B. (1992). Young children of affectively ill parents: A longitudinal study of psychosocial development. *Journal of American Academy of Child and Adolescence Psychiatry, 31,* 68–77.

Ramsay, R., & Kumar, R. (1996). Ethical dilemmas in perinatal psychiatry. *Psychiatric Bulletin, 20,* 90–92.

Raskin, J. D., Richman, J. A., & Gaines, C. (1990). Patterns of depressive symptoms in expectant and new parents. *American Journal of Psychiatry, 147,* 658–660.

Rettersöl, N. (1968). Paranoid psychoses associated with impending or newly established fatherhood. *Acta Psychiatrica Scandinavica, 44,* 51–61.

Rutter, M. (1966). *Children of sick parents.* London: Oxford University Press.

Rutter, M. (1990). Commentary: Some focus and process considerations regarding the effects of parental depression on children. *Developmental Psychology, 26,* 60–67.

Sagi, A., Lamb, M. E., Lewkowicz, K., Shoham, R., Dvir, R., & Estes, D. (1985). Security of infant–mother, –father, and –metapelet attachments among kibbutz-reared Israeli children. In I. Bretherton & E. Waters (Eds.), Growing points of attachment theory and research. *Monographs of the Society for Research in Child Development, 50*(1–2, Serial No. 209).

Sameroff, A. J., Seifer, R., & Zax, M. (1982). Early development of children at risk for emotional disorder. *Monographs of the Society for Research in Child Development, 50*(Serial No. 199).

Sameroff, A. J., Barocas, R., & Seifer, R. (1984). The early development of children born to mentally ill women. In N. Watt, E. J. Anthony, L. Wynne, & J. Rolf (Eds.), *Children at risk for schizophrenia.* New York: Cambridge University Press.

Schneider-Rosen, K., Braunwald, K. G., Carlson, V., & Cicchetti, D. (1985). Current perspectives in attachment theory: Illustration from the study of maltreated infants. In I. Bretherton & E. Waters (Eds.), Growing points of attachment theory and research. *Monographs of the Society for Research in Child Development, 50*(1–2, Serial No. 209).

Seager, C. P. (1960). A controlled study of post-partum mental illness. *Journal of Mental Science, 106,* 214–230.

Stein, A., Gath, D. H., Bucher, J., Bond, A., Day, A., & Cooper, P. J. (1991). The relationship between postnatal depression and mother–child interaction. *British Journal of Psychiatry, 158,* 46–52.

Stevens, A. (1975). *Attachment and polymatric rearing.* Unpublished master's thesis, University of Oxford.

Tetlow, C. (1955). Psychoses of childbearing. *Journal of Mental Science, 101,* 629–639.

Thiels, C., & Kumar, R. (1987). Severe puerperal mental illness and disturbances of maternal behaviour. *Journal of Psychosomatic Obstetrics and Gynecology, 7,* 27–38.

Vaughn, C. E., & Leff, J. P. (1976). The influence of family and social factors on the course of psychiatric illness. *British Journal of Psychiatry, 129,* 125–137.

Vaughn, C. E., Snyder, K. S., Jones, S., Freeman, W. B., & Falloon, I. R. (1984). Family factors in schizophrenic relapse: Replication in California of British research on expressed emotion. *Archives of General Psychiatry, 41,* 1169–1177.

Watson, J. P., Elliott, S. A., Rugg, A. J., & Brough, D. I. (1984). Psychiatric disorder in pregnancy and the first postnatal year. *British Journal of Psychiatry, 144,* 453–462.

Afterword

~

Maternal Depression and Infant Development: Cause and Consequence; Sensitivity and Specificity

Michael Rutter
Institute of Psychiatry, London

It has been known for a long time that parental mental disorder, including maternal depression, is associated with a substantially increased risk of various forms of adverse outcomes in children (see Cummings & Davies, 1994; Downey & Coyne, 1990; Rutter, 1966, 1989a). Some of this increase in risk is likely to be mediated genetically (see McGuffin, Owen, O'Donovan, Thapar, & Gottesman, 1994; Plomin, DeFries, McClearn, & Rutter, 1997), but it has been shown that parental mental disorder is also associated with impairments in parenting (see Rutter, 1990a; Weissman & Paykel, 1974) and with an increase in family discord, disruption, and disorganization (Rutter, 1989a; Rutter, Maughan, Meyer, et al., in press). The finding that parental mental disorder is associated with an increased risk for a broad range of psychopathology in children, and not just that mirroring the parental disorder (see Rutter, Maughan, Meyer, et al., in press), together with evidence that *within* families with a mentally-ill parent, family discord and hostility are associated with disorder in the child, strongly suggests that an important part of the risk is environmentally mediated.

Although so much is well known and generally accepted, the research described earlier in this book has increased our understanding in several very important, and sometimes dramatic, ways. To begin with, it has explicitly recognized that maternal depression is a risk *indicator*, and not necessarily a risk mechanism. That is, the consistency of the association between maternal depression and disorder in the child across a wide range of studies suggests that it reflects some form of causal process, but nevertheless the research challenge to determine the nature of the risk mechanisms involved remains. As the editors point out in the preface to the volume, the focus is on the effects of postpartum depression on mother–infant interactions, but it is not assumed that these necessarily constitute the key mediating variables.

A second strength of this book is that the authors directly take on board the need to examine two-way effects (see Bell, 1968; Bell & Chapman, 1986; Rutter, Champion, Quinton, Maughan, & Pickles, 1995; Rutter, Dunn, et al., in press). Parents undoubtedly influence children, but children have equally important effects on their parents (as well as on other people who interact with them). When researchers first began to appreciate this possibility, they emphasized the determination of the relative importance of each direction of effect. Research findings then went on to demonstrate the importance of cycles of interaction by which child characteristics shaped parental behavior, which, in turn, influenced the course of child behavior (see, e.g., Martin, Maccoby, & Jacklin, 1981; Patterson, 1982, with respect to oppositional behavior). The studies described here carry on that tradition in their emphasis on the ongoing dynamics of dyadic parent–child interactions.

A third key feature of the research described in this book is the explicit recognition of the need to consider the social context of the parent–child interaction. Nearly 20 years ago, Bronfenbrenner (1979) underlined this need when he outlined the ways in which individual behavior is shaped by social interactions and the ways in which social systems function in a nested fashion. Parent–child dyads are shaped by the family context in which they arise and family interactions, in turn, are influenced by the extended kin network and by the social nexus provided by peer groups and the community. It is a decided strength of this volume that the research with which it deals spans low- to high-risk samples, and the socially privileged to the socially deprived.

A fourth strength stems from the diversity of outcomes and range of mediating and moderating mechanisms considered. Thus, the infant outcomes extend from cognitive impairment to insecure attachment to behavioral deviance. Similarly, the processes range from cognitive patterns to emotional states to effects on brain development. Throughout the chapters, there is an explicit developmental focus both in terms of consideration of possible sensitive period effects and of the need to consider the ways in which immediate effects may lead to long-term sequelae or, alternatively, dissipate with time or alter with changing life circumstances.

In this afterword, it seems appropriate to consider a few of these overarching issues in terms of their conceptual and empirical research implications, rather than seek to comment on any one program of research in detail. Three, perhaps, are of the greatest fundamental importance: (1) the testing of hypotheses on causal mechanisms, (2) the interplay between soma and psyche, and (3) sensitive-period effects.

TESTING CAUSAL HYPOTHESES

Most of the literature of psychosocial risks has rested content with the identification of risk indicators. The chapters in this book have been refreshing in their rejection of this unhelpful and unambitious complacency and in their explicit attempts to tackle the difficult question of just which mechanisms mediate the risk effects, while considering the range of important moderating variables (i.e., those that increase or decrease the risk consequences, given the operation of a specified risk factor—see Baron & Kenny, 1986; Rutter, 1990b).

Child Effects

The first issue is whether any association between a maternal variable and a child variable reflects an effect of the former on the latter, or vice versa. Murray and Cooper (Chapter 5, this volume) tackled the question using the time-honored and powerful research strategy of examining within-individual change (Farrington, 1988) through the availability of longitudinal data (Rutter, 1994). Their finding that neonatal characteristics (poor motor functioning and irritability) substantially increased the risk of postpartum depression is provocative and important (Murray, Stanley, Hooper, King, & Fiori-Cowley, 1996). The effect was substantial (albeit based on relatively small numbers): a fourfold increase in risk for the combination of these two neonatal characteristics as compared with the risk when both were absent. The size of the effect appears puzzling in view of the transience of these infancy characteristics, and the mechanisms remain obscure in view of the relative lack of infant effects on mother–child interaction. There are implications, of course, for both the ongoing interplay between parent and child and for the nature of postnatal depression. As O'Hara's review (Chapter 1, this volume) clearly shows, postnatal depression has a great deal in common with depressive disorders arising at other times, but also a few distinctive features. We need to ask whether there was anything distinctive (in terms of correlates or course) about the postnatal depressions associated with neonatal irritability and poor motor control. How could there be such a marked effect on maternal depression without an effect on mother–child interaction? The possibility of some third-variable effect (such as a genetic liability in both mother and infant) needs to be considered, although it has to be said that there is no indication that this does in fact constitute the explanation.

The chapter by Hipwell and Kumar (Chapter 11, this volume) is notable for its highlighting of the important differences between the circumstances of postnatal depression and the much less common postnatal psychoses, which pose somewhat different issues of child care. Nevertheless, as they bring out very well in their review of their own and others' research findings, there is an equally pressing need to consider the processes of mother–infant interaction with respect to their effects on both partners in the dyad. The issues are important in terms of their implications for the treatment of these severe, but usually acute, maternal disorders. Also, the situation provides an invaluable "natural experiment" in which investigation of the effects of a severe perturbation in the mother's state can be used to study both dyadic interaction and the infant's psychological development.

An alternative strategy for examining child effects is provided by the various different forms of experimental manipulation. Thus, for example, gender effects have been examined in the past by the "baby X" tactic of studying adult responses to babies who are dressed ambiguously with respect to gender, and are randomly given male and female names (Smith & Lloyd, 1978; Condry & Ross, 1985). Anderson, Lytton, and Romney (1986) used a variant of this approach in their study of the effects of conduct disturbance through an examination of trios of dyads involving children with and without conduct disturbance interacting with their own and with someone else's mother. Brunk and Henggeler (1984) employed child actors to examine the effects of different styles of child behavior on patterns of response by adult strangers. Yarrow and Klein (1980) used the natural experiment of children's movement between foster families to examine the effects of child characteristics on caregiving patterns and responses. Field (Chapter 9, this volume) adopted a comparable strategy in her comparison of caregiver–child interaction with biological mothers and professional caregivers for infants whose mothers were depressed. No very straightforward conclusion is possible. Bates (1989) found only quite small inconsistent effects in relation to variations in infant characteristics within the normal range, but quite marked effects have been found for more extreme child features, as illustrated by the references cited (see Rutter, Dunn, et al., in press).

Third-Variable Effects

All social scientists are trained in the ever-present need to consider the possibility that a statistical correlation, or association between A and B, represents the operation of some third variable C, rather than any kind of causal mechanism between A and B. Thus, for example, the apparent environmental effects of maternal depression on children's psychological development, supposedly mediated via distortions of parenting interactions, could instead reflect either genetic mediation or the consequences of some variable (such as social disadvantage) antecedent and predisposing to the maternal depression. The standard approach in cross-sectional studies is to employ some form of multivariate statistical analysis to determine if the effects "hold up" after controlling for the influences of possible confounding variables. The approach is considerably strengthened if longitudinal data are available and, especially, if additional tests (such as a dose–response relationship and reversal effects) are employed (see Rutter, 1994). However, much greater research leverage on the causal hypothesis is provided by the use of experimental designs, either as they occur naturally or as contrived in the laboratory or clinical context.

Contrived Experiments

The power of experimental design has been recognized almost as long as science has existed. If through systematic planned manipulation across a range of different circumstances, a change in variable A always causes variable B to move, it is a reasonable assumption that a causal effect is involved. Treatment studies provide the most obvious and straightforward contrived experiment in the field of behavioral and development sciences. Unfortunately, few treatment studies have, in fact, been informative on mechanisms (Rutter, 1982). The problems have been that so many forms of treatment are designed to be broad ranging in their effects, that so many effects are nonspecific, and that very few investigations have sought to relate changes in the hypothesized mediating mechanisms (within the treated group) to changes in the outcome variable. Cooper and Murray's study (Chapter 8, this volume) was both innovative and informative in its comparison of different forms of treatment explicitly designed to influence a different target (Cooper, Murray, Hooper, & West, 1996). Interestingly, and perhaps surprisingly, all forms of treatment (whether focused on the depression or the mother–child interaction) were equally effective in relieving maternal depression but equally ineffective (relatively speaking) in influencing either mother–child interaction or infant behavior. The implication would seem to be that maternal depression cannot constitute the main risk mechanism; rather, its effects would seem to be indirect. On the other hand, the finding that the continuation of maternal depression (irrespective of treatment) *was* associated with infant outcomes suggests that the depression was not just an epiphenomenon. Rather, it is likely that it played some important role, albeit an indirect one, in the causal nexus. The importance of the chronicity of maternal depression in Campbell and Cohn's research (Chapter 7, this volume) points to the same conclusion.

Cramer (Chapter 10, this volume) also used the strategy of therapeutic intervention to investigate causal processes. He reports that a psychodynamic approach, in which mother–child conflict was related to the mother's past familial conflicts and interactional guidance, focusing on "here-and-now" aspects of mother–child interplay, did not differ in their effects. His findings, both quantitative and clinical, highlight the ways in which maternal depression is intertwined with potentially problematic aspects of mother–infant interaction. However, so far the findings do not separate the alternative explanation of the causal mechanisms. It would be informative, for example, to compare the effects (both on maternal depression and on mother–child interaction) of antidepressant medication on its own and psychological treatments focussing on the dyadic interaction on their own.

Natural Experiments

In addition to the leverage provided by deliberate manipulation of variables, natural experiments that pull apart variables that ordinarily go together serve the same purpose. Attention to the timing of maternal depression provides one approach. Thus, Stein et al. (1991) examined patterns of parent–child interaction in dyads where the mother had been depressed or mentally ill but was no longer so. Their finding that the patterns still differed from controls suggested that the effects probably derived from some continuing features of the mother and not from the depressive episode as such.

An alternative approach that does not seem to have been employed would be to focus on the outcomes for children of mothers who become depressed only after the supposed period of risk. For example, Hay (Chapter 4, this volume) proposes that the ill effects on children's cognitive development arise only when the maternal depression occurs during the children's first year of life. If so, the cognitive levels of older children (i.e., those already older than a year at the time of the maternal depression) should be systematically higher, and no different from control groups. Curiously, despite Plomin and Daniels's (1987) highlighting of the child specificity (i.e., nonshared nature) of most environmental effects, extraordinarily little research use has been made of sib–sib comparisons within the *same* families. Much greater use needs to be made of this research strategy. If child-specific effects are hypothesized (as is the case with the sensitive-period postulate), there is an obligation to make the necessary comparisons among different children in the same family.

An alternative approach would be to examine the effects of maternal depression on infant cognition in the absence of ongoing interaction—as is the case with depression in the biological mothers when children have been adopted or fostered. This is not a feasible approach when the postulated effects are subtle and minor but it would be practicable with respect to the quite substantial cognitive impairment associated with maternal depression in the studies reported by Hay (Chapter 4, this volume).

Yet another design is provided by situations in which the rate of mental depression is raised as a result of factors that play little or no role in the population as a whole. Families with twins provide the obvious possibility here (Rutter & Redshaw, 1991). The question, then, is whether within a twin sample, maternal depression is associated with cognitive impairment in the children and whether this effect accounts for any cognitive difference between twins and singletons.

Maternal depression is more likely to arise in the context of social deprivation and disadvantage. Accordingly, it is possible that the risks to the children statistically associated with maternal depression may arise from the accompanying social adversity rather than from the depression per se. If so, what is needed is a comparison across samples that differ in their social circumstances. This need was explicitly recognized by the investigators reporting their research in this book. The findings are helpful, but not conclusive, in their suggestion (which is not entirely consistent) that the greatest effects are seen in socially disadvantaged groups. Again, the implication is that depression forms part of the causal process but does not represent the main risk mechanism.

In that connection, we need to consider the role of replication and nonreplication in testing causal hypotheses. Consistency in findings across a wide range of samples and of social and physical circumstances is a useful guide to the likelihood of a true causal effect (Rutter, 1994). It constitutes a more general case of the specific experimental principle. That is, if the causal effect of *A* on *B* is real, it should be found even if all manner of associated variables (*C, D, E*, etc.) are varied. Conversely, nonreplication is equally powerful (Rutter, 1974). That is, if the apparent effect of *A* is in actuality due to *C*, the outcome *B* should *not* be increased in situations where *A* occurs in the absence of *C* (see Rutter, 1971, and Fergusson, Horwood, & Lynskey, 1992, for an application of this approach with respect to parent–child separation and family discord).

Of course, in practice, fine judgment is required in deciding what represents replication. Thus, as Hay (Chapter 4, this volume) points out, the apparent effects of maternal depression on infant cognition have been found across several rather different studies. But, as Hay also notes, sometimes the effects apply only to perceptual–motor skills and sometimes also to verbal skills, sometimes to boys only and sometimes to both sexes, sometimes they persist to age 5 and sometimes they do not. This could be interpreted as nonreplication. Of course, when dealing with relatively small samples, substantial variation arising by chance alone must be expected. Further research is needed to resolve the matter, but again, as emphasized by Hay, such research needs to be guided by theory in order to test competing hypotheses.

Finally, with respect to third-variable effects, it is necessary to draw attention to the importance of genetic designs for examining the proximal processes involved in nature–nurture interplay (Rutter et al., in press-a). There is a genetic contribution to virtually all human behavior in both parents and infants (including parenting features and family patterns) and it is possible that part of the risks may be genetically mediated (Plomin et al., 1997). Although it is most unlikely that this accounts for the bulk of the effects, usually the best way to test for environmental mediation is to use genetic strategies (such as twin and adoptee designs) that can pull apart nature and nurture (see Rutter et al., 1990).

Moderating Variables

All the studies reported in this book note the considerable variation in effects. Whatever the level of maternal depression, some children show impairment and some do not. That is a universal finding across a wide range of acute and chronic psychosocial risk experiences (Rutter, 1981, 1995a). At one time this led to a concept of "invulnerable" children but it is now apparent that that is a most misleading way of putting things (Rutter, 1995b). Some supposed "invulnerability" constitutes measurement error or a failure to assess an adequate range of outcomes. When the lack of ill effects is real, it is neither categorical nor absolute. That is, children vary in their degree of vulnerability and that feature applies to particular types of risks and circumstances and not to the whole of life. Moreover, the relative vulnerability may be a consequence of protective features in the environment, or of synergistic child–environment interactions (see Rutter, 1990b), rather than of some intrinsic characteristic of the child as an individual. Nevertheless, children vary greatly in their response to what seem to be the same set of experiences.

The qualifier "seem to be" is necessary because of the extensive evidence that so many environmental effects are relatively child-specific (Plomin & Daniels, 1987; Rutter, Dunn, et al., in press). Even when there is a risk factor that could impinge on the entire family (such as maternal depression, family discord, or social disadvantage), the extent to which it *actually* impinges varies among children. Some children are drawn into the risk situation and some remain relatively detached from it, some are scapegoated, some are used maladaptively as a source of comfort, some get drawn into vicious cycles of negative interaction, and some respond in ways that serve to break the cycle or initiate more positive modes of interchange (Rutter, 1987). In order to understand this variation, it is necessary to identify both the mediating and the moderating mechanisms; the latter cannot be studied adequately unless the former are known. The chapters by the Papoušeks (Chapter 2, this volume) and by Tronick and Weinberg (Chapter 3, this volume) set the scene by means of their reviews of what is known about early parent–infant interactions generally, and the theme is further explored in later chapters in relation to the specific effects of maternal depression.

Three different, although interrelated, sets of mechanisms need to be considered. First, there are those involved on the route from maternal depression to impaired caregiving or a maladaptive style of mother–infant interaction. Teti and Gelfand (Chapter 6, this volume) draw attention to the likely importance of cognitive features in relation to both the mother's self-concept and self-efficacy and the perception of the infant. Given the importance of aberrant social cognitions in depressive disorders (Teasdale & Barnard, 1993), that emphasis seems appropriate. Nevertheless, the focus on the direct effects of depression seems too narrow. Attachment theorists have long argued for the importance of a person's *own* experience of caregiving as an influence on the pattern of parental care they provide for their children (Belsky & Cassidy, 1994; Carlson & Sroufe, 1995; Rutter, 1995c; Cassidy & Shaver, in press). Although the empirical evidence to support this argument is limited, there are findings showing substantial connections (Fonagy, Steele, & Steele, 1991). The possibility that the effects of maternal depression on parenting will be influenced by the cognitive–affective set, and by the style of social interaction that the mother brings to the situation as a consequence of her own earlier experiences, certainly warrants much fuller exploration than it has received up to now (Rutter & O'Connor, in press). Also, however, it is likely that the interactional patterns associated with maternal depression will be influenced by the mother's social context, social supports, and other stresses/difficulties at the time (Rutter, 1989b). Parenting is not an isolated skill or habit; rather it constitutes an outcome of a diverse range of influences on the person's social behavior (Rutter & Rutter, 1993).

The second set of mechanisms concerns the immediate impact on the child. The question in this case is which of the varied altered features of mother–child interaction actually matter in terms of leading to adverse effects on the child. Those are the issues that constitute the focus of most of the chapters in this volume and it is clear that a rich array of good leads have been provided. Equally, it has to be accepted that there is still some way to go before it can be said that the key risk mechanisms for the various maladaptive outcomes have been determined and delineated.

Given the limited understanding of mediating mechanisms, it is not surprising that knowledge of moderator effects is even more limited. Protective mechanisms have mainly been studied in relation to older children (Rutter, 1990b, 1995b) and few data are available on effects in infancy. Extremes of temperamental variations may be influential (Rothbart & Bates, in press) but their importance in relation to maternal depression is largely unknown. As Hay (Chapter 4, this volume) discusses, there is some indication that boys may be more susceptible in some respects, but the limited evidence that is available suggests that the gender difference may not be particularly powerful or pervasive (Rutter, 1990a). The issue of age effects, that is, the suggestion that children of a certain age range are more vulnerable, is considered later in this chapter.

The third set of mechanisms concerns the link between the immediate adverse impact on the child and the eventual development and duration of psychopathology or developmental impairment. Surprisingly, psychosocial researchers have paid little attention to the effects of environmental stress or adversity on the organism. Yet, it has to be a key issue. Unless these are understood, it will remain difficult to devise rational plans for prevention or treatment. With respect to the links between the experience of child abuse and the development of disruptive behavior, the findings from the longitudinal study undertaken by Dodge and his colleagues (Dodge, Bates, & Pettit, 1990; Dodge, Pettit, Bates, & Valente, 1995) suggest that social cognitive processes may play a role. Earlier animal studies have also indicated that stress experiences can induce changes in the structure and function of the neuroendocrine system that may shape later responses to new stressors (Hennessey & Levine, 1979). Among the wider list of alternative mediators (see Rutter, 1989c) several chapters in this book draw attention to possible effects on neural functioning and brain development. These need to be considered in relation to the broader issue of what is known about the interplay between soma and psyche.

SOMA–PSYCHE INTERPLAY

Several chapters in this volume postulate somatic mediation of some of the effects of maternal depression on infants. Thus, Field (Chapter 9, this volume) uses her EEG data to argue that they suggest physiological dysregulation in both the depressed woman and their infants. She draws attention, however, to the corrective effects on the EEG of relaxation, massage, and positive mood induction. Presumably, therefore, the EEG findings represent a somatic concomitant of the psychological dysfunction rather than an underlying, persistent biological abnormality. Hay (Chapter 4, this volume) seems to go further in suggesting that early social experiences lead to permanent neural changes and that the offspring of depressed mothers already show a compromised integrity of the neuroregulatory system. Tronick and Weinberg (Chapter 3, this volume), too, point to animal research showing that caregiving variations affect the infant brain. Murray and Cooper (Chapter 5, this volume) similarly argue that there is accumulating evidence that experiential factors influence the course of infant brain development.

There is a danger of this sounding like unwarranted biological determinism, and it is important to make several distinctions. First, all mental activities are bound to involve some neural change. Regardless of whether or not the change can be demonstrated, it is bound to occur because the workings of the mind have to be based on the functioning of the brain. But in fact, it has been possible to demonstrate brain changes as a result of mental functioning. That constitutes the basis of functional brain imaging, and PET scan studies have been able to show which part of the brain has increased metabolic activity during particular mental processes (e.g. Paulesu, Frith, & Frackowiak, 1993; Fletcher et al., 1995). These metabolic changes are temporary and parallel in time the performance of the mental tasks. However, if there are lasting mental changes, it may be presumed that there must also be lasting brain changes. How else could the former be mediated? Again, research findings have confirmed the supposition. Thus, Horn (1990, 1993) demonstrated in animal studies the neural alterations that accompanied the learning process involved in imprinting.

It should not be assumed from these findings that either the psyche or the soma are primary; rather they represent different facets of the same process. Moreover, because that is so, two-way effects are likely to be found. That is, if changes are induced in the soma, there may well be psychological consequences. Conversely, changes in the psyche will have somatic concomitants. This has been shown in both human and animal studies with respect to neuroendocrine effects. Just as an induced rise in testosterone increases dominance, an induced alteration in dominance affects testosterone levels (Rose, Holaday, & Bernstein, 1971). For example, winners of fiercely fought tennis or chess matches show a rise in sex hormone level while losers show a fall (Mazur & Lamb, 1980; Mazur, Booth, & Dabbs, 1992). There are comparable two-way effects between mood changes and social cognitions. Thus, if depression is alleviated through the use of antidepressive medication, depressive cognitions improve; conversely, if cognitive treatment alleviates depressive cognitions, beneficial mood changes tend to follow (Hollon, Shelton, & Loosen, 1991). Neither form of treatment is more basic than the other, and therefore neither is inherently preferable. Superior efficacy should be established empirically and not presupposed on theoretical grounds.

Just as neither the soma nor the psyche has necessary primacy over the other, so also it cannot be assumed that somatic changes will be lasting. Some are and some are not. Moreover, even when some of the somatic changes are enduring, it does not necessarily follow that the associated functional impairment will be equally persistent. Thus, infants with well-documented cerebral palsy due to brain damage may show no detectable neurological signs when older (see Rutter, Chadwick, & Schachar, 1983; Nelson & Ellenberg, 1982). Animal studies have shown that severe, chronic malnutrition affects brain growth, but other studies suggest that restoration of normal nutrition and a normal pattern of upbringing in severely malnourished, psychologically deprived children results in a remarkable degree of cognitive catch-up, as well as restoration of normal physical growth (Lien, Meyer, & Winick, 1977; Winick, Meyer, & Harris, 1975; Rutter & the English and Romanian Adoptees [E. R. A.] Study Team, 1997). These findings do not necessarily mean that there are no somatic or psychological scars or sequelae, but they do negate the assumption that the effects of brain damage inevitably involve permanent functional consequences. The issue needs to be reframed in terms of a question of the circumstances under which changes either are, or are not, lasting. These are most conveniently considered under the topic of sensitive periods.

SENSITIVE PERIODS

As Hay (Chapter 4, this volume) discusses, the concept of sensitive periods has had its ups and downs over time. It had its heyday in the early years of studies of imprinting in birds when the evidence seemed to suggest that the time window of enhanced susceptibility to particular experiences was narrow, fixed, and biologically determined, and that the psychological sequelae were permanent. Subsequent research forced a rethinking of these assumptions as it became evident that all aspects of these claims had been overstated (Bateson, 1966, 1990). For a while, this was followed by a tendency to downplay sensitive periods almost to the point of extinction. In recent years, the pendulum has begun to swing the other way, and there is now something of a revival of sensitive period notions. With respect to the effects of postnatal depression on children's psychological functioning, several distinctions need to be drawn.

To begin with, there is the general issue of whether or not empirical evidence exists of age effects on children's responses to different experiences. Clearly, there is such evidence. However, it is necessary to appreciate that age indexes changing experiences as well as biological maturation (Rutter, 1989d). That is, older children differ from younger ones in the experiences they have had as well as in their greater degree of biological maturity. Also, age effects on environmental susceptibility may come about through several somewhat different mechanisms.

First, infants obviously differ from older children and adults in their cognitive processing skills, and thus their responses to experiences will differ. It is well established that infants' long-term memories of discrete events are different from those of adults (Rutter, Maughan, Pickles, & Simonoff, in press). The precise reasons why that is so are not fully understood but probably the differences stem more from the processes of recall rather than the initial encoding of memories. Either way, the end result is that people tend not to remember specific experiences encountered during the first 2 or 3 years of life. The implications of this relative infantile amnesia are poorly documented, but Kagan (1982) has suggested that the lack of mature cognitive transduction of early experiences means that the impact of such events is likely to be less enduring than that of similar experiences occuring when children are older.

Another age effect that seems to be largely a function of psychological maturity, is the relative lack of susceptibility to the stress of hospital admission before the age of 6 months or so and again after age 5 or thereabouts (Rutter, 1979, 1995a). Although the precise mechanisms have not been well delineated, it seems that these infants' relative immunity to ill effects derives from the fact that babies have yet to develop selective attachments and therefore do not have specific attachment relationships that could be broken. Also, because they are cognitively less able to anticipate the future, they are less likely to be apprehensive about all that a hospital stay might involve. School-age children, like post-infancy preschoolers, are vulnerable in both respects but are less susceptible to ill effects probably because of their growing ability to appreciate that relationships can be maintained during a separation and their greater ability to understand why they have been admitted to the hospital.

A second, rather different form of age effect concerns the possible role of physical traumata in disrupting or altering maturational brain processes. It is well established that major unilateral lesions of the dominant cerebral hemisphere in later childhood or adult life tend to result in severely impaired language functioning, aphasia, and accompanying verbal/cognitive deficits (McFie, 1975; Newcombe, 1969). By contrast, the effects of unilateral brain damage are not seen in babies (see, e.g., Vargha-

Khadem, Isaacs, van der Werf, Robb, & Wilson, 1992). It is not that early lesions are without effects; indeed, especially when they are accompanied by epilepsy, they may be particularly likely to lead to a substantial impairment in overall IQ. Brain immaturity makes a difference in the *patterns* of sequelae, rather than in overall susceptibility (Rutter, 1993).

A third way in which developmental immaturity may be important concerns the possibility of developmental programming, and it is this route that has been proposed for the supposed lasting effects of postnatal depression on infant cognition, and other aspects of psychological functioning. The phenomenon is certainly real. Thus, it is well established that patterned visual input in early life is crucial for the development of brain systems mediating vision (Blakemore, 1991; Held, 1993). Animal research has also suggested that perinatal sex hormones affect the pattern of brain development, with some functional implications, and there is some indication that something comparable may also apply in humans (Gorski, 1984; Swaab, 1991). Lucas, Morley, Cole, Lister, and Leeson-Payne (1992; Lucas, 1994; Morley & Lucas, 1994) have shown, through randomized controlled trials in preterm babies, that babies fed on breast milk (either by tube or breast feeding) had a higher IQ than those fed on formula. In explanation, he proposed a form of developmental programming. Other research has shown that diet in infancy influences both metabolic functioning and sensitivities to diets in adulthood (see Bock & Whelan, 1991). It may be concluded that the development of bodily systems, including the brain, is indeed influenced by a wide range of environmental inputs. Sometimes the effect applies generally and sometimes only to vulnerable subgroups. For example, Lucas et al. (1990) found that there was no overall effect on the risk of allergies of feeding preterm infants on cows' milk formulas, but early exposure to cows' milk did increase the risk in those with a family history of atopy.

Could something comparable apply with respect to the impact of postnatal depression, as suggested by Hay (Chapter 4, this volume)? Possibly, but some skepticism is warranted. To begin with, there is still some uncertainty about the robustness of age-specific effects on infant cognition. Sib–sib comparisons across large longitudinal samples (which are needed to examine an adequate range of possible confounders) are required. But if confirmed, could such relatively mild variations in infants' experiences make an appreciable impact on brain development? The well-demonstrated examples of effects on brain development all concern quite gross restrictions of specific experiences (such as patterned visual input) on specific brain systems. It is not by any means self-evident that the same will apply to mild, partial constraints on social experiences. Much of human development is set up to function adequately across quite a wide range of environments. Thus, although holding and looking are apparently crucial aspects of attachment behavior, limbless and vision-impaired infants nevertheless develop selective attachments (Rutter, 1981). Although it is possible that marked variations in mother–infant interaction have implications for normal brain development, these have yet to be demonstrated.

CONCLUSION

The research described in this volume has cast light on both the nature of postnatal depression and its effects on infants. These issues are of considerable practical importance both because of the frequency of postpartum depression and because the effects on infants seem to impinge on a wide range of psychological functions in the individual child as well as on crucial patterns of family interaction. Most importantly, the concepts and findings discussed by the authors have potential implications for a much broader range of issues, both theoretical and practical, with respect to early psychological development. The high quality research described in this book, especially that undertaken by the editors, has clearly shown how difficult developmental questions can be tackled rigorously while still retaining a sensitivity to the subtleties of parent–child interaction and to the nuances of individual psychological development.

REFERENCES

Anderson, K. E., Lytton, H., & Romney, D. M. (1986). Mothers' interactions with normal and conduct-disordered boys: Who affects whom? *Developmental Psychology, 22*, 604–609.

Baron, R. M., & Kenny, D. A. (1986). The moderator–mediator variable distinction in social psychological research: Conceptual, strategic, and statistical considerations. *Journal of Personality and Social Psychology, 51*, 1173–1182.

Bates, J. E. (1989). Applications of temperament concepts. In G. A. Kohnstamm, J. E. Bates, & M. K. Rothbart (Eds.), *Temperament in childhood* (pp. 321–355). Chichester: Wiley.

Bateson, P. (1966). The characteristics and context of imprinting. *Biological Reviews, 41*, 177–211.

Bateson, P. (1990). Is imprinting such a special case? *Philosophical Transactions of the Royal Society of London, 329,* 125-131.

Bell, R. Q. (1968). A reinterpretation of the direction of effects in studies of socialization. *Psychological Review, 75,* 81-95.

Bell, R. Q., & Chapman, M. (1986). Child effects in studies using experimental or brief longitudinal approaches to socialization. *Developmental Psychology, 22,* 595-603.

Belsky, J., & Cassidy, J. A. (1994). Attachment: Theory and evidence. In M. Rutter & D. Hay (Eds.), *Development through life: A handbook for clinicians* (pp. 373-402). Oxford: Blackwell Scientific.

Blakemore, C. (1991). Sensitive and vulnerable periods in the development of the visual system. In G. R. Bock & J. Whelan (Eds.), *The childhood environment and adult disease* (Ciba Foundation Symposium No. 156, pp. 129-146). Chichester, England: Wiley.

Bock, G. R., & Whelan, J. (Eds.). (1991). *The childhood environment and adult disease.* (Ciba Foundation Symposium No. 156). Chichester, England: Wiley.

Bronfenbrenner, U. (1979). *The ecology of human development, experiments by nature and design.* Cambridge, MA: Harvard University Press.

Brunk, M. A., & Henggeler, S. W. (1984). Child influences on adult controls: An experimental investigation. *Developmental Psychology, 20,* 1074-1081.

Carlson, E. A., & Sroufe, L. A. (1995). Contribution of attachment theory to developmental psychopathology. In D. Cicchetti & D. J. Cohen (Eds.), *Developmental psychopathology: Vol. 1. Theory and methods* (pp. 581-617). New York: Wiley.

Cassidy, P., & Shaver, J. (Eds.). (in press). *Handbook of attachment theory and research.* New York: Guilford Press.

Condry, J. C., & Ross, D. F. (1985). Sex and aggression: The influence of gender label on the perception of aggression in children. *Child Development, 56,* 225-233.

Cooper, P. J., Murray, L., Hooper, R., & West, A. (1996). The development and validation of a predictive index for postpartum depression. *Psychological Medicine, 26,* 627-634.

Cummings, E. M., & Davies, P. T. (1994). Maternal depression and child development. *Journal of Child Psychology and Psychiatry, 35,* 73-112.

Dodge, K. A., Bates, J. E., & Pettit, G. S. (1990). Mechanisms in the cycle of violence. *Science, 250,* 1678

Dodge, K. A., Pettit, G. S., Bates, J. E., & Valente, E. (1995). Social information-processing patterns partially mediate the effects of early physical abuse on later conduct problems. *Journal of Abnormal Psychology, 104,* 632-643.

Downey, G., & Coyne, J. C. (1990). Children of depressed parents: An integrative review. *Psychological Bulletin, 108,* 50-76.

Farrington, D. P. (1988). Studying changes within individuals: The causes of offending. In M. Rutter (Ed.), *Studies of psychosocial risk: The power of longitudinal data* (pp. 158-183). Cambridge, England: Cambridge University Press.

Fergusson, D. M., Horwood, L. J., & Lynskey, M. T. (1992). Family change, parental discord and early offending. *Journal of Child Psychology and Psychiatry, 33,* 1059–1075.

Fletcher, P., Happé, F., Frith, U., Baker, S., Dolan, R., Frackowiak, R., & Frith, C. (1995). Other minds in the brain: A functional imaging study of "theory of mind" in story comprehension. *Cognition, 57,* 109–128.

Fonagy, P., Steele, H., & Steele, M. (1991). Maternal representations of attachment during pregnancy predict the organization of infant–mother attachment at one year of age. *Child Development, 62,* 891–905.

Gorski, R. A. (1984). Critical role for the medial preoptic area in the sexual differentiation of the brain. In C. J. de Vries, J. P. C. de Bruin, H. B. M. Uylings, & M. A. Corner (Eds.), *Sex differences in the brain* (Progress in brain research 61, pp. 129–146). Amsterdam: Elsevier.

Held, R. (1993). Binocular vision: Behavioral and neuronal development. In M. H. Johnson (Ed.), *Brain development and cognition: A reader* (pp. 152–166). Oxford: Blackwell.

Hennessey, J. W., & Levine, S. (1979). Stress, arousal, and the pituitary-adrenal system: A psychoendocrine hypothesis. In J. M. Sprague & A. N. Epstein (Eds.), *Progress in psychobiology and physiological psychology* (pp. 133–178). New York: Academic Press.

Hollon, S. D., Shelton, R. C., & Loosen, P. T. (1991). Cognitive therapy and pharmacotherapy for depression. *Journal of Consulting and Clinical Psychology, 59,* 88–99.

Horn, G. (1990). Neural bases of recognition memory investigated through an analysis of imprinting. *Philosophical Transactions of the Royal Society, 329,* 133–142.

Horn, G. (1993). Brain mechanisms of memory and predisposition: Interactive studies of cerebral function and behavior. In M. H. Johnson (Ed.), *Brain development and cognition: A reader* (pp. 481–509). Oxford, England: Blackwell.

Kagan, J. (1982). *The nature of the child.* New York: Basic Books.

Lien, N. M., Meyer, K. K., & Winick, M. (1977). Early malnutrition and 'late' adoption: A study of their effects on development of Korean orphans adopted into American families. *American Journal of Clinical Nutrition, 30,* 1734–1739.

Lucas, A. (1994). Role of nutritional programming in determining adult morbidity. *Archives of Disease in Childhood, 71,* 288–290.

Lucas, A., Brooke, O. G., Morley, R., Cole, T. J., & Bamford, M. F. (1990). Early diet of preterm infants and development of allergic or atopic disease: Randomised prospective study. *British Medical Journal, 300,* 837–840.

Lucas, A., Morley, R., Cole, T. J., Lister, G., & Leeson-Payne, C. (1992). Breast milk and subsequent intelligence quotient in children born preterm. *Lancet, 339,* 261–264.

Martin, J. A., Maccoby, E. E., & Jacklin, C. N. (1981). Mothers' responsiveness to interactive bidding and nonbidding in boys and girls. *Child Development, 52,* 1064–1067.

Mazur, A., Booth, A., & Dabbs, J. M. (1992). Testosterone and chess competition. *Social Psychology Quarterly, 55,* 70–77.

Mazur, A., & Lamb, T. A. (1980). Testosterone, status, and mood in human males. *Hormones and Behavior, 14,* 236–246.

McFie, J. (1975). *Assessment of organic impairment.* London: Academic Press.

McGuffin, P., Owen, M. J., O'Donovan, M. C., Thapar, A., & Gottesman, I. I. (1994). *Seminars in psychiatric genetics.* London: Royal College of Psychiatrists.

Morley, R., & Lucas, A. (1994). Influence of early diet on outcome in preterm infants. *Acta Paediatrica (Suppl. 405),* 123–126.

Murray, L., Stanley, C., Hooper, R., King, F., & Fiori-Cowley, A. (1996). The role of infant factors in postnatal depression and mother–infant interactions. *Developmental Medicine and Child Neurology, 38,* 109–119.

Nelson, K. B., & Ellenberg, J. H. (1982). Children who "outgrew" cerebral palsy. *Pediatrics, 69,* 529–536.

Newcombe, F. (1969). *Missile wounds of the brain: A study of psychological deficits.* New York: Oxford University Press.

Patterson, G. R. (1982). *Coercive family processes.* Eugene, OR: Castalia.

Paulesu, E., Frith, C. D., & Frackowiak, R. S. (1993). The neural correlates of the verbal component of working memory. *Nature, 362,* 342–345.

Plomin, R., & Daniels, D. (1987). Why are children in the same family so different from one another? *Behavioral and Brain Sciences, 10,* 1–15.

Plomin, R., DeFries, J. C., McClearn, G., & Rutter, M. (1997). *Behavioral genetics.* New York: W. H. Freeman.

Rose, R. M., Holaday, J. W., & Bernstein, I. S. (1971). Plasma testosterone, dominance risk and aggressive behaviour in male rhesus monkeys. *Nature, 231,* 366–368.

Rothbart, M. K., & Bates, J. E. (in press). Temperament. In N. Eisenberg (Ed.), *Handbook of child psychology: Vol. 3. Social, emotional and personality development* (5th ed.). New York: Wiley.

Rutter, M. (1966). *Children of sick parents.* Oxford, England: Oxford University Press.

Rutter, M. (1971). Parent–child separation: Psychological effects on the children. *Journal of Child Psychology and Psychiatry, 12,* 233–260.

Rutter, M. (1974). Epidemiological strategies and psychiatric concepts in research on the vulnerable child. In E. Anthony & C. Koupernik (Eds.), *The child in his family: Children at psychiatric risk* (Vol. 3, pp. 167–179). New York: Wiley.

Rutter, M. (1979). Separation experiences: A new look at an old topic. *Journal of Pediatrics, 95,* 147–154.

Rutter, M. (1981). *Maternal deprivation reassessed* (2nd ed.). Harmondsworth, England: Penguin.

Rutter, M. (1982). Psychological therapies: Issues and prospects. *Psychological Medicine, 12,* 723–740.

Rutter, M. (1987). Psychosocial resilience and protective mechanisms. *American Journal of Orthopsychiatry, 57,* 316–331.

Rutter, M. (1989a). Psychiatric disorder in parents as a risk factor for children. In D. Shaffer, I. Philips, & N. B. Enzer (Eds.), with M. M. Silverman & V. Anthony (Assoc. Eds.), *Prevention of mental disorders, alcohol and other drug use in children and adolescents* (OSAP Prevention Monograph 2, pp. 157–

189). Rockville, MD: Office for Substance Abuse Prevention, U.S. Department of Health and Human Services.

Rutter, M. (1989b). Intergenerational continuities and discontinuities in serious parenting difficulties. In D. Cicchetti & V. Carlson (Eds.), *Child maltreatment* (pp. 317–348). New York: Cambridge University Press.

Rutter, M. (1989c). Pathways from childhood to adult life. *Journal of Child Psychology and Psychiatry, 30,* 23–51.

Rutter, M. (1989d). Age as an ambiguous variable in developmental research: Some methodological considerations from developmental psychopathology. *International Journal of Behavioral Development, 12,* 1–34.

Rutter, M. (1990a). Commentary: Some focus and process considerations regarding effects of parental depression on children. *Developmental Psychology, 26,* 60–67.

Rutter, M. (1990b). Psychosocial resilience and protective mechanisms. In J. Rolf, A. Masten, D. Cicchetti, K. Neuchterlein & S. Weintraub (Eds.), *Risk and protective factors in the development of psychopathology* (pp. 181–214). New York: Cambridge University Press.

Rutter, M. (1993). An overview of developmental neuropsychiatry [Special Issue]. *Education and Child Psychology, 10,* 4–11.

Rutter, M. (1994). Beyond longitudinal data: Causes, consequences, changes and continuity. *Journal of Consulting and Clinical Psychology, 62,* 928–940.

Rutter, M. (1995a). Maternal deprivation. In M. H. Bornstein (Ed.), *Handbook of parenting: Vol. 4. Applied and practical parenting* (pp. 3–31). Mahwah, NJ: Erlbaum.

Rutter, M. (1995b). Psychological adversity: Risk, resilience and recovery. *South African Journal of Child and Adolescent Psychiatry, 7,* 75–88.

Rutter, M. (1995c). Clinical implications of attachment concepts: Retrospect and prospect. *Journal of Child Psychology and Psychiatry, 36,* 549–571.

Rutter, M. & the English & Romanian Adoptees (E.R.A.) Study Team (1997). *Developmental catch-up, and deficit, following adoption after severe global early privation.* Manuscript submitted for publication.

Rutter, M., Bolton, P., Harrington, R., Le Couteur, A., Macdonald, H., & Simonoff, E. (1990). Genetic factors in child psychiatric disorders. I. A review of research strategies. *Journal of Child Psychology and Psychiatry, 31,* 3–37.

Rutter, M., Chadwick, O., & Schachar, R. (1983). Hyperactivity and minimal brain dysfunction: Epidemiological perspectives on questions of cause and classification. In R. E. Tarter (Ed.), *The child at psychiatric risk* (pp. 80–107). New York/Oxford, England: Oxford University Press.

Rutter, M., Champion, L., Quinton, D., Maughan, B., & Pickles, A. (1995). Understanding individual differences in environmental risk exposure. In P. Moen, G. H. Elder, Jr., & K. Lüscher (Eds.), *Examining lives in context: Perspectives on the ecology of human development* (pp. 61–93). Washington, DC: American Psychological Association.

Rutter, M., Dunn, J., Plomin, R., Simonoff, E., Pickles, A., Maughan, B., Ormel, J., Meyer, J., & Eaves, L. (in press). Integrating nature and nurture: Implications of person–environment correlations and interactions for developmental psychopathology [Special Issue]. *Development and Psychopathology.*

Rutter, M., Maughan, B., Meyer, J., Pickles, A., Silberg, J., Simonoff, E., & Taylor, E. (in press). Heterogeneity of antisocial behavior: Causes, continuities, and consequences. In D. W. Osgood (Ed.), *Nebraska Symposium on Motivation: Vol. 44. Motivation and delinquency.* Lincoln: University of Nebraska Press.

Rutter, M., Maughan, B., Pickles, A., & Simonoff, E. (in press). Retrospective recall recalled. In R. B. Cairns & P. C. Rodkin (Eds.), *The individual in developmental research: Essays in honor of Marian Radke-Yarrow.* Thousand Oaks, CA: Sage.

Rutter, M., & O'Connor, T. (in press). Implications of attachment theory for child care policies. In P. Cassidy & J. Shaver (Eds.), *Handbook of attachment theory and research.* New York: Guilford Press.

Rutter, M., & Redshaw, J. (1991). Annotation: Growing up as a twin: Twin–singleton differences in psychological development. *Journal of Child Psychology and Psychiatry, 32,* 885–895.

Rutter, M., & Rutter, M. (1993). *Developing minds: Challenge and continuity across the lifespan.* New York: Basic Books.

Smith, C., & Lloyd, B. (1978). Maternal behavior and the perceived sex of infant: Revisited. *Child Development, 49,* 1263–1266.

Stein, A., Gath, D. H., Bucher, J., Bond, A., Day, A., & Cooper, P. J. (1991). The relationship between postnatal depression and mother–child interaction. *British Journal of Psychiatry, 158,* 46–52.

Swaab, D. F. (1991). Relation between maturation of neurotransmitter systems in the human brain and psychosocial disorders. In M. Rutter & P. Casaer (Eds.), *Biological risk factors for psychosocial disorders* (pp. 50–66). Cambridge, England: Cambridge University Press.

Teasdale, J. D., & Barnard, P. J. (1993). *Affect cognition and change: Re-modelling depressive thought.* Hove, England: Lawrence Erlbaum.

Vargha-Khadem, F., Isaacs, E., van der Werf, S., Robb, S., & Wilson, J. (1992). Development of intelligence and memory in children with hemiplegic cerebral palsy: The deleterious consequences of early seizures. *Brain, 115,* 315–329.

Weissman, M. M., & Paykel, E. S. (1974). *The depressed woman: A study of social relationships.* Chicago: University of Chicago Press.

Winick, M., Meyer, K. K., & Harris, R. C. (1975). Malnutrition and environmental enrichment by early adoption: Development of adopted Korean children suffering greatly in early nutritional status is examined. *Science, 190,* 1173–1175.

Yarrow, L. J., & Klein, R. P. (1980). Environmental discontinuity associated with transition from foster to adoptive homes. *International Journal of Behavioral Development, 3,* 311–322.

Index